THE RELEASE OF
CATECHOLAMINES FROM
ADRENERGIC NEURONS

THE RELEASE OF CATECHOLAMINES FROM ADRENERGIC NEURONS

Edited by:

DAVID M. PATON

Professor and Head
Department of Pharmacology and Clinical Pharmacology
School of Medicine
University of Auckland, Auckland, New Zealand

Formerly Professor of Pharmacology and Assistant Dean
Faculty of Medicine, University of Alberta, Edmonton, Alberta, Canada

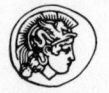

PERGAMON PRESS

OXFORD . NEW YORK . TORONTO . SYDNEY . PARIS . FRANKFURT

U.K.	Pergamon Press Ltd., Headington Hill Hall, Oxford OX3 0BW, England
U.S.A.	Pergamon Press Inc., Maxwell House, Fairview Park, Elmsford, New York 10523, U.S.A.
CANADA	Pergamon of Canada Ltd., 75 The East Mall, Toronto, Ontario, Canada
AUSTRALIA	Pergamon Press (Aust.) Pty. Ltd., P.O. Box 544, Potts Point, N.S.W. 2011, Australia
FRANCE	Pergamon Press SARL, 24 rue des Ecoles, 75240 Paris, Cedex 05, France
FEDERAL REPUBLIC OF GERMANY	Pergamon Press GmbH, 6242 Kronberg-Taunus, Pferdstrasse 1, Federal Republic of Germany

First edition 1979

British Library Cataloguing in Publication Data

The release of catecholamines from adrenergic neurons.
1. Adrenergic mechanisms 2. Catecholamines
I. Paton, David Murray
612'.89   QP365.5   78-40926
ISBN 0 08 021536 X hard case
ISBN 0 08 023755 X flexicover

In order to make this volume available as economically and as rapidly as possible the author's typescript has been reproduced in its original form. This method unfortunately has its typographical limitations but it is hoped that they in no way distract the reader.

Printed in Great Britain by
William Clowes & Sons Limited
London, Beccles and Colchester

To my wife
BETH
and our children
HEATHER AND FIONA

Generous financial assistance
for the publication of this volume
was provided by:

THE FACULTY OF MEDICINE, UNIVERSITY OF
ALBERTA, EDMONTON, ALBERTA, CANADA

CIBA-GEIGY CANADA LIMITED, DORVAL,
QUEBEC, CANADA

MERCK FROSST LABORATORIES, DORVAL, QUEBEC,
CANADA

CONTENTS

LIST OF CONTRIBUTORS

M.P. Blaustein
Department of Physiology and Biophysics
Washington University School of Medicine
St. Louis, Missouri, U.S.A.

A.S. Clanachan
Department of Pharmacology
University of Alberta
Edmonton, Alberta, Canada

M. Fillenz
Department of Physiology
University of Oxford
Oxford, England

M. Göthert
Pharmakologisches Institut
Universität Hamburg
Hamburg, Federal Republic of Germany

W. Haefely
Department of Experimental Medicine
Hoffman-LaRoche Co. Ltd.
Basel, Switzerland

G. Häusler
Department of Experimental Medicine
Hoffman-LaRoche Co. Ltd.
Basel, Switzerland

G. Henderson
Department of Pharmacology and Experimental Therapeutics
Loyola University Stritch School of Medicine
Maywood, Illinois, U.S.A.

J. Hughes
Department of Biochemistry
Imperial College of Science and Technology
London, England

I.J. Kopin
Laboratory of Clinical Science
National Institute of Mental Health
Bethesda, Maryland, U.S.A.

H.W. Kosterlitz
Unit for Research on Addictive Drugs
Marischall College
University of Aberdeen
Aberdeen, Scotland

S.Z. Langer
Department of Biology
Synthelábo
Paris, France

K. Löffelholz
Pharmakologisches Institut
Universität Mainz
Mainz, Federal Republic of Germany

J.C. McGrath
Department of Pharmacology
University of Glasgow
Glasgow, Scotland

E. Muscholl
Pharmakologisches Institut
Universität Mainz
Mainz, Federal Republic of Germany

D.M. Paton
Department of Pharmacology and Clinical Pharmacology
University of Auckland School of Medicine
Auckland, New Zealand

A.D. Smith
Department of Pharmacology
University of Oxford
Oxford, England

K. Starke
Pharmakologisches Institut
Universität Freiburg
Freiburg, Federal Republic of Germany

L. Stjärne
Department of Physiology
Karolinska Institute
Stockholm, Sweden

U. Trendelenburg
Pharmakologisches Institut
Universität Würzburg
Würzburg, Federal Republic of Germany

D.J. Triggle
Department of Biochemical Pharmacology
State University of New York at Buffalo
Buffalo, New York, U.S.A.

PREFACE

Thirty years have elapsed since von Euler demonstrated that noradrenaline is the principal catecholamine present in peripheral
adrenergic nerves. Since that time there has been a steadily
increasing interest in the biochemistry, physiology and pharmacology of adrenergic transmission. This was further increased
by the demonstration of noradrenergic and dopaminergic neurons
within the central nervous system.

Much work has been devoted to determining how catecholamines are
released from such neurons. An important advance was the demonstration that release was inhibited by noradrenaline acting on
presynaptic α-adrenoceptors, and by other agonists acting on presynaptic receptors. A number of drugs and procedures also modify
the release of catecholamines or themselves initiate release. The
aim of this volume is to provide a comprehensive and critical review of these advances in our understanding of the release of
catecholamines from adrenergic neurons. Each section is not simply a review of the author's own work, but rather represents an
attempt to present a balanced review of the relevant literature.

The volume is intended primarily for investigators studying the
release of catecholamines and other neurotransmitters but is also
intended for senior students and others wishing to obtain current
information on the release of catecholamines. The volume does
not deal with release of catecholamines from the adrenal medulla.

I should like to thank all the contributors to this volume for
their cooperation in completing their chapters and for their suggestions about the volume. These were greatly appreciated. I
wish also to thank those authors and publishers who have generous-
ly allowed us to reprint material from their publications.

Financial assistance for the publication of this volume was gener-
ously provided by Dr. D.F. Cameron, Dean, Faculty of Medicine,
University of Alberta; Ciba-Geigy Canada Ltd., Dorval, Quebec and
Merck Frosst Laboratories, Dorval, Quebec.

My former secretary at the University of Alberta, Mrs. Laurel
McLachlin, provided invaluable assistance as she proofread and
edited all the contributions, and typed many of the chapters in
camera-ready form. The volume would not have been completed without her assistance which was loyally provided at a time when there
was a serious illness in her immediate family. I also appreciate
very much the assistance received from the other members of the
secretarial staff at the University of Alberta and from
Dr. Thornton of Pergamon Press.

Finally, I should like to acknowledge the support and encourage-
ment I have received from my wife throughout the completion of
this volume, the final period of which coincided with our move
from Edmonton to Auckland.

Auckland, April 1978   David M. Paton

BIOCHEMICAL STUDIES OF THE MECHANISM OF RELEASE

A. D. Smith

Biochemical studies can contribute to our understanding of the fundamental mechanisms in the release of neurotransmitters at two levels of analysis: at the subcellular level and at the molecular level. Progress in studies at the molecular level depends, however, upon identifying the subcellular mechanisms involved in secretion and so it is hardly surprising that this is the first problem which attracted the interest of biochemists. Indeed, our knowledge of the molecular events in the release of noradrenaline from nerves is still fragmentary. In this chapter I shall give a short historical account of how biochemical methods have been applied to answer the question: how does noradrenaline pass from the store in synaptic vesicles to the extracellular space when the nerve is stimulated electrically or when release is evoked by drugs?

I   HISTORICAL INTRODUCTION

Biochemical studies on adrenergic nerves would have been far more difficult if pioneering work had not first been done on the adrenal medulla. This is true of studies on the biosynthesis (Blaschko, 1973), storage (Smith, 1972) and release of catecholamines. The biochemical approach to studies on the mechanism of release involves the following steps:

1. identification of the subcellular site of storage of the catecholamine;

2. determination of the characteristic chemical composition of the storage organelle and the distribution of these constituents between the membrane and soluble content;

3. examination of the perfusion fluid leaving an organ for the presence of soluble constituents of the storage organelle;

4. demonstration that release of noradrenaline and soluble constituents of the organelle can occur without release of substances from the cytosol of the cell.

Application of this approach to the adrenal medulla has led to the conclusion that, when secretion is evoked by acetylcholine (or analogous drugs), the release of catecholamines occurs quantitatively by exocytosis (detailed reviews are given by Smith & Winkler, 1972; Viveros, 1975). The most powerful argument for secretion by exocytosis from the chromaffin cell was the demonstration that high molecular weight proteins (chromogranins and

dopamine-β-hydroxylase) stored in the chromaffin granules were
secreted together with catecholamines, whereas proteins present
in the cytosol (tyrosine hydroxylase, lactate dehydrogenase) were
not released, neither were lipid constituents of the chromaffin
granule membrane.

When these findings on the chromaffin cell were reported, most
cell biologists were happy to accept them because they had studied
a similar mechanism of secretion in exocrine glands. However,
when I suggested that an analogous mechanism of secretion might
occur from sympathetic nerves, the idea was dismissed, in a discussion at a symposium in Leuven in 1967, by several distinguished
cytologists on the grounds that nerves were different because
neurotransmitters were only of low molecular weight and were known
to be synthesized in nerve terminals. It was also argued that
protein secretion by neurons was unlikely because the nerve terminal contained no ribosomes and so could not synthesize protein.
Such arguments could only be answered by experimental evidence;
accordingly my colleagues in Gent and I decided to see if we could
demonstrate the secretion of specific proteins by sympathetic
neurons. Our plan was based upon the fact that adrenal chromaffin
cells originate from the neural crest and so there was a good
chance first, that the fundamental mechanisms of release of catecholamines might be the same in sympathetic nerve and chromaffin
cell and, second, that the specific protein (chromogranin) of
chromaffin granules might also occur in the synaptic vesicles of
the nerves. The discovery by Kapeller and Mayor (1966) that
dense-cored vesicles accumulate in axons on the proximal side of
a ligation of a sympathetic nerve trunk seemed to provide a way
for protein synthesized in the cell body to be transported in
secretory vesicles to the nerve ending. We planned to prepare
antiserum to chromogranin A from bovine adrenal chromaffin granules, to use this antiserum to test for the presence of chromogranin in the noradrenergic vesicles of bovine splenic nerve and,
if the latter proved to be the case, to test for the release of
chromogranin into the perfusate upon stimulation of the ox splenic
nerve.

An unexpected discovery by Viveros, Arqueros and Kirshner (1968)
allowed us to make a short-cut in the plan: these authors found
that, contrary to previous views, not all the dopamine-β-hydroxylase activity of ox adrenal chromaffin granules was bound to the
membrane; as much as half of the enzyme of the particles was water-
soluble and, furthermore, this soluble enzyme was secreted upon
stimulation of the perfused gland. Dopamine-β-hydroxylase had
just been shown to be present in a particulate fraction (containing the noradrenergic vesicles) of ox splenic nerve (Stjärne, Roth
& Lishajko, 1967) and so we immediately started experiments to see
if the enzyme was secreted upon stimulation of the splenic nerve.
The dog spleen was chosen for the initial studies, because of the
expertise already available in Gent. It was indeed found that
dopamine-β-hydroxylase was secreted upon nerve stimulation and
that the release, like that of noradrenaline, was dependent upon
the presence of calcium ions in the perfusion fluid.

A communication describing the results of these experiments and proposing that the secretion of noradrenaline occurred by exocytosis was submitted to *Nature* in the autumn of 1968, but was not accepted for publication on the grounds "It is either too long or too specialised..." The referee's report stated "These findings merely add biochemical evidence for a release mechanism that has already been established [sic] by electrophysiological studies."

The results were eventually reported to the International Congress on Pharmacology in Basel in June 1969 (DePotter, Moerman, De Schaepdryver & Smith, 1969) and, together with subsequent quantitative studies on chromogranin release from calf splenic nerve, to the Physiological Society in July 1969 (De Potter, De Schaepdryver, Moerman & Smith, 1969). At the same meeting of the Physiological Society, Geffen, Livett and Rush (1969) reported that chromogranin and dopamine-β-hydroxylase accumulated on the proximal side of a ligature on the sheep splenic nerve and also presented qualitative immunochemical evidence of the release of these proteins upon stimulation of the sheep splenic nerve. The following year Gewirtz and Kopin (1970) reported that dopamine-β-hydroxylase was also released upon stimulation of the splenic nerve of the cat. These early studies on perfused organs led to the demonstration of dopamine-β-hydroxylase activity in the blood plasma of rat and man (Weinshilboum & Axelrod, 1971) and to evidence that the concentration of this enzyme may, in certain circumstances, reflect activity of the sympathetic nervous system (see chapter by Kopin).

II   CONSTITUENTS OF NORADRENERGIC VESICLES

The first step in the biochemical approach to the study of transmitter secretion should be the identification of the subcellular site of storage of the transmitter. Noradrenaline is found in several fractions of homogenates of sympathetic nerve trunks or innervated organs: some is always present in the supernatant fraction and the remainder occurs in particles. Fractionation of the particulate fraction by centrifugation has shown that at least two types of particle can store noradrenaline (Smith, 1972; Lagercrantz, 1976) and that these particles correspond to the large and small dense-cored vesicles identified by electron microscopy (see chapter by Fillenz). A further storage site has been postulated by cytochemical studies: exogenous 5-hydroxydopamine can be taken up into the tubular smooth endoplasmic reticulum of sympathetic neurons (Holtzman, 1971; Tranzer, 1972). The problem with the latter cytochemical studies is that they only show the localisation of 5-hydroxydopamine and not that of endogenous noradrenaline. If it turns out that some noradrenaline normally is present within the cisternae of endoplasmic reticulum, then it is likely that this noradrenaline would be released into the supernatant upon homogenization of the tissue; hence biochemical evidence of this store will never be convincing, for it can also be argued that most of the noradrenaline recovered in the cytoplasm is released from the storage vesicles, together with soluble vesicle proteins, as a result of damage during homogenization (De Potter, Smith & De Schaepdryver, 1970).

Biochemical analysis of the distribution of possible constituents
of the noradrenergic vesicles between the various subcellular
fractions is the most reliable way of identifying such constituents (Smith, 1972) although, now that highly purified fractions
of large dense cored vesicles can be obtained, it is also possible
to carry out a direct analysis of the vesicles (Lagercrantz, 1976).
The constituents positively identified are given in Table 1.

TABLE 1

Constituents of noradrenergic vesicles (references are to reviews,
where possible).

Large vesicles

    Noradrenaline   Smith (1972)
                                           Lagercrantz (1976)
    Adenosine 5'-triphosphate   (large vesicle reviews)

    Dopamine-β-hydroxylase (soluble and membrane)

    Chromogranin A

    Other chromogranins

Small vesicles

    Noradrenaline   Smith (1972)
                                           De Potter & Chubb (1977)
    Dopamine-β-hydroxylase

    Adenosine 5'-triphosphate (?)   Fried *et al*. (1978)

The importance of quantitative analysis of the constituents of
noradrenergic vesicles is shown by the discovery that the large
dense-cored vesicles of the splenic nerve become richer in noradrenaline, with respect to their content of dopamine-β-hydroxy-
lase and adenosine 5'-triphosphate (ATP), the more distal the seg-
ment of the nerve trunk that is analysed (De Potter, 1971;
Lagercrantz, 1976). This difference between 'proximal' and
'distal' vesicles is also reflected in an increase in equilibrium
density of the vesicles (De Potter, 1971; De Potter & Chubb, 1977)
and almost certainly means that the actual content of noradrenaline per vesicle is greater in the 'distal' vesicles. Because
it is not possible to isolate vesicles from a terminal network of
the neuron, without including some vesicles from preterminal axons,
there is little hope that biochemical methods can tell us the
ratios of the amounts of noradrenaline, ATP and vesicle proteins
within those noradrenergic vesicles that occur in terminal varicosities. This is most unfortunate, because these data are necessary if a quantitative statement is to be made concerning what

proportion of the noradrenaline released from the nerves is secreted by exocytosis (see Smith & Winkler, 1972; Smith, 1973 for
more detailed discussion).

A further complication is that, as shown in Table 1, there is
very little known for certain about the composition of the small
dense-cored vesicles, which comprise a large (often the predominant) part of the store for noradrenaline in terminal varicosities
(see chapter by Fillenz). Until a specific soluble constituent
of the small noradrenergic vesicles is identified, it will not be
possible to use the biochemical approach to look for evidence of
exocytosis from these vesicles.

   III   RELEASE OF CONSTITUENTS OF NORADRENERGIC VESICLES
         UPON NERVE STIMULATION

Proteins. In our studies on the release of dopamine-β-hydroxylase and chromagranin A, we chose the spleen as the most suitable
sympathetically innervated organ because of its 'open' type of
circulation; thus, macromolecules released from nerve endings on
blood vessels could pass directly into the venules. Since both
the proteins were relatively large (effective hydrodynamic radii
of the order of 12 nm) we thought that in any other organ the release would be difficult to demonstrate as the proteins would pass
into the lymphatic vessels. However, other workers have now shown
that it is possible to demonstrate release of dopamine-β-hydroxylase from the vas deferens into an organ bath and from the isolated perfused heart (Table 2). Furthermore, the enzyme has also

TABLE 2

Tissues from which release of protein constituents of noradrenergic vesicles has been demonstrated *in vitro* upon nerve stimulation

Tissue	Protein	Reference
Spleen		
calf	chromogranin A	Smith *et al.* (1970)
	dopamine-β-hydroxylase	Smith *et al.* (1970)
dog	dopamine-β-hydroxylase	Smith *et al.* (1970)
cat	dopamine-β-hydroxylase	Gewirtz & Kopin (1970)
Vas deferens		
guinea-pig	dopamine-β-hydroxylase	
Heart		
guinea-pig		
rabbit	dopamine-β-hydroxylase	Langley & Gardier (1977)

been detected in lymph (Åberg, Hansson, Wetterberg, Ross & Fröden, 1974; Ngai, Dairman, Marchelle & Spector, 1974) and in cerebro-spinal fluid (Goldstein & Cubeddu, 1976), where its concentration increased after cold stress in rabbits (De Potter, Pham-Huu Chanh, De Smet & De Schaepdryver, 1976).

There have been very few studies on the other vesicle proteins, largely because they have, so far, no recognisable enzymic activity and so have to be analysed immunochemically. It is note-worthy that although release of a protein cross-reacting with antiserum to chromogranin A has been shown to occur from calf and sheep splenic nerves, there are several other soluble chromogran-ins in the large noradrenergic vesicles (Bartlett, Lagercrantz & Smith, 1976) and it is likely that these would also be released at nerve terminals.

Most workers conclude that, if they can demonstrate release of a specific vesicle protein from a perfused organ upon nerve stimu-lation, the protein is actually secreted from the nerve terminals. In the early studies we felt it was necessary to exclude other possible sites of origin for the proteins, as shown in Table 3. This table also lists other criteria which should, ideally, be applied in any study where the release of protein from an organ is being studied. The more of these criteria that can be satis-fied, the more certain will be the conclusion that the protein released is derived from the terminals of the nerve that is stimu-lated. It is particularly important to exclude that the proteins are not released as a result of damage to the neurons in an iso-lated organ: this is best done by analysis of the perfusate for a protein (e.g., tyrosine hydroxylase or dopa decarboxylase) that occurs in the cytosol of the terminals. Of course, the sensiti-vity of the assay for cytosol proteins must be such that these could be detected in the perfusate if they leaked out of damaged nerves stoichiometrically with the vesicle proteins.

Adenine nucleotides. Although early attempts were made to demon-strate the release of adenine derivatives upon stimulation of the splenic nerve (Stjärne, Hedqvist & Lagercrantz, 1970) it is now clear that not only is this approach complicated by the presence of such nucleotides in non-nervous tissue, they are also present in purinergic nerves (Burnstock, 1972) and, furthermore, the act-ual amount of ATP in the large noradrenergic vesicles is very low (Lagercrantz, 1976). The molar ratio of noradrenaline to ATP in large noradrenergic vesicles of splenic nerve terminals is of the order of 50, which is very different from the value of about 5 in adrenal chromaffin granules (Winkler, 1976).

Finally, there is still no convincing evidence that the small nor-adrenergic vesicles contain ATP, since all the studies so far published have not excluded contamination of the vesicle fraction by fragments of the innervated muscular tissue (Fried, Lagercrantz & Hökfelt, 1978). Thus, caution is required in any discussion about the possible release of ATP from sympathetic nerves (Burnstock, 1976; Chubb, 1977; Smith, 1977).

TABLE 3

Criteria required to establish that protein is secreted from sympathetic nerve terminals

1. Exclude release from

   (a) chromaffin cells   dog and calf spleens   Smith *et al.* (1970)
   (b) blood pooled in tissue   dog and calf spleens   Smith *et al.* (1970)
   (c) unidentified sites sen-   dog and calf spleens   Smith *et al.* (1970)
       sitive to noradrenaline

2. Demonstrate that release

   (a) is proportional to that   calf spleen   Smith *et al.* (1970)
       of noradrenaline   guinea-pig vas deferens   Weinshilboum *et al.* (1971)

   (b) is calcium-dependent   cat spleen   Cubeddu *et al.* (1974a)
                                                  dog and calf spleen   Smith *et al.* (1970)
                                                  guinea-pig vas deferens   Johnson *et al.* (1971)

   (c) is blocked by drugs that   no report?
       inhibit noradrenaline re-
       lease (e.g., guanethidine)

   (d) occurs in the absence of re-   calf spleen   Smith *et al.* (1970)
       lease of proteins in cytosol

3. Characterise released proteins   calf spleen   Smith *et al.* (1970)
   to show identity with those in   rabbit cerebrospinal   De Potter *et al.* (1976)
   isolated vesicles   fluid

Biochemical studies

7

IV   IMPLICATIONS OF THE BIOCHEMICAL STUDIES

Release by exocytosis. The original biochemical studies were designed to test the hypothesis that release of noradrenaline from
sympathetic nerves occurs by exocytosis. The most rigorous biochemical test of this hypothesis, as applied in studies on the
adrenal medulla (Schneider, Smith & Winkler, 1967), requires the
demonstration:

1.   that the amount of vesicle protein released bears the same
      stoichiometric relationship to the amount of noradrenaline
      released as occurs in the vesicles isolated by centrifugation;

2.   that none of the membrane-bound constituents of the vesicle
      are released;

3.   that the vesicle protein is released without any release of
      proteins from the cytosol.

Although the stoichiometry is not firmly established, for the
reasons outlined in the section on the composition of noradrenergic vesicles, I have argued (Smith & Winkler, 1972; Smith, 1973)
that most of the noradrenaline released from the splenic nerve
probably is secreted by exocytosis. These arguments were put
forward before evidence that one of the vesicle proteins (dopamine-
β-hydroxylase) might also be present in another compartment of the
neuron (Brimijoin, 1974; 1976; see also chapter by Fillenz) and
before the report that the proportion of 'soluble' dopamine-β-hydroxylase in the large noradrenergic vesicles of splenic nerve
might be greater than previously estimated (Kirksey, Klein,
Baggett & Gasparis, 1978). It would, however, be a mistake to
think that because calculation of the stoichiometry of release is
now even more uncertain, the uncertainty applied to the occurrence
of exocytosis. Secretion of high molecular weight proteins
(dopamine-β-hydroxylase and chromogranin A) undoubtedly occurs
from sympathetic nerves and the most likely way in which this can
take place in the absence of release of cytosol proteins is by
exocytosis. Thus, since the proteins within the large noradrenergic vesicles are secreted by exocytosis upon electrical stimulation of the nerve, all other soluble constituents of these vesicles (including noradrenaline) must also be released in this way.

Functions of non-transmitter substances. Since we can only speculate about the extraneuronal actions (if any) of the vesicle proteins following their release, the reader is referred to the ex-
cellent discussion by Chubb (1977).

Drugs that act on noradrenergic terminals. The measurement of
dopamine-β-hydroxylase activity in the perfusate from an organ is
in many ways a more direct measure of the release of noradrenaline
from the terminals than the measurement of the amount of transmitter itself. This is because noradrenaline can suffer several
fates (metabolism by two enzymes, uptake into nerves or into
other cells) following its release. Of course, we have to assume,
for the time being, that the dopamine-β-hydroxylase released into
the perfusate is a constant proportion of that secreted from the

neuron. In spite of the risks of making such an assumption,
measurements of the concentration of the enzyme in perfusates
have already provided important evidence concerning the mode of
action of drugs. Increased release of dopamine-β-hydroxylase per
impulse occurs in the presence of α-adrenergic antagonists
(De Potter, Chubb, Put & De Schaepdryver, 1971) which argues for
a normal feedback inhibition by released noradrenaline acting via
presynaptic α-receptors (see chapter by Langer). Prostaglandins
inhibit the evoked release of dopamine-β-hydroxylase from the vas
deferens (Johnson, Thoa, Weinshilboum, Axelrod & Kipin, 1971).
Tyramine evokes the release of noradrenaline, but not of the
enzyme (Chubb, De Potter & De Schaepdryver, 1972) confirming that
this drug does not initiate secretion by exocytosis. Papaverine
increases the evoked release of dopamine-β-hydroxylase from the
spleen, indicating an increased efficiency of exocytosis (Cubeddu,
Barnes & Weiner, 1974b). Atropine increases, and acetylcholine
decreases, the output of dopamine-β-hydroxylase from the isolated
perfused heart during sympathetic nerve stimulation (Langley &
Gardier , 1977). Of particular interest is that pretreatment of
cats with reserpine, leading to almost total loss of noradrenaline
from the spleen, hardly affected the amount of dopamine-β-hydroxylase released upon stimulation of the splenic nerve (Cubeddu &
Weiner, 1975). It is to be hoped that other pharmacologists will
realise the value of measuring dopamine-β-hydroxylase activity in
extracellular fluids when they are trying to elucidate the mode
of action of drugs on noradrenergic transmission.

Extracellular vesicle proteins as a measure of sympathetic nervous activity. The hope that the level of dopamine-β-hydroxylase
in blood plasma, lymph and cerebrospinal fluid might indicate the
activity of noradrenergic nerves has only partly been fulfilled.
Technical problems in the assay of the enzyme, especially in cerebrospinal fluid (but see De Potter et al., 1976) have been one of
the difficulties. Another difficulty has been that individual
humans vary greatly in their 'resting' blood level of the enzyme;
this intriguing finding might lead to a better understanding of
genetic or environmental factors which influence the sympathetic
nervous system. The most promising application of such measurements so far have been in longitudinal studies on individual
patients, although it is important to realise that the rise in
concentration of the enzyme following a stimulus occurs after a
few minutes, in contrast to the nearly instantaneous rise in noradrenaline concentration (Mathias, Smith, Frankel & Spalding,
1976). Another complicating factor that has been discovered is
that although during chronic stress in man the level of dopamine-
β-hydroxylase in the plasma may rise in the acute stage, it falls
markedly soon afterwards to levels well below normal; in contrast,
the stress-induced rise in the concentration of catecholamines
persists after the acute period (Hörtnagl, Stadler-Wolffersgrün,
Brücke, Hammerle & Hackl, 1978). This can best be explained by a
depletion of the stores of releasable dopamine-β-hydroxylase in
sympathetic nerve endings; while noradrenaline can be made in the
endings, the enzyme can only be made in the cell body and has to
be transported to the endings. A fuller discussion of the studies
on human blood plasma is given in the chapter by Kopin.

Origin of synaptic vesicles. In the report of the finding of the
release of vesicle proteins to the Neuroscience Research Program
meeting in November 1969, it was suggested that the empty membrane
of the large noradrenergic vesicle might divide into two or more
fragments following its retrieval from the plasma membrane, and
that these fragments might turn into small noradrenergic vesicles,
which are so characteristic of terminal varicosities (Smith, 1970;
see also Smith *et al.*, 1970). This hypothesis was based on the
ultrastructural studies of Diner (1967) on the adrenal medulla
and it was subsequently put forward as a general hypothesis for
the origin of synaptic vesicles in all neurons (Smith, 1971; but
see also Holtzman, 1977). Quantitative studies (De Potter &
Chubb, 1977) on the distribution of noradrenaline and dopamine-β-
hydroxylase in the dog spleen following stimulation of the splenic
nerve has strongly supported the hypothesis: it was found that
small noradrenergic vesicles containing dopamine-β-hydroxylase are
only formed when the splenic nerve is stimulated in the presence
of calcium ions and that the membrane-bound dopamine-β-hydroxylase
lost from the large noradrenergic vesicles is almost quantitatively recovered in the small noradrenergic vesicles.

The latter studies give a further example of the value of applying
quantitative biochemical methods to the study of the subcellular
events involved in the release of neurotransmitters. The combination of such an approach with an understanding of the ultrastructure of the neuron is bringing us closer to a detailed picture of
the dynamic events in the nerve terminal which follow the arrival
of the action potential from the cell body. The diagram in Fig. 1
represents an attempt to summarise our present views about such
events in the terminal varicosity of a typical sympathetic neuron.

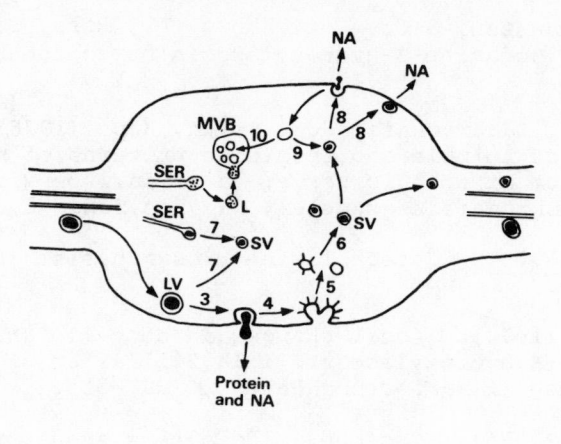

Fig. 1. Origin and fate of noradrenergic vesicles in a terminal
         varicosity of a sympathetic nerve (Smith, 1973).

The large vesicles are assembled from their constituents in the
cell body and arrive in the varicosity following fast transport
along the axon (events 1 and 2; not shown).

3: large vesicles secrete proteins and noradrenaline (NA) by
    exocytosis;

4: membrane of large vesicle is converted into small coated pits;

5: coated pits bud from plasma membrane to give coated vesicles
    which become electron-lucent small vesicles;

6: electron-lucent small vesicles take up or synthesize NA and
    become small noradrenergic vesicles;

7: alternative possible modes of formation of small vesicles -
    either by budding from smooth endoplasmic reticulum (SER) or
    by fission of intact large vesicle;

8: small vesicles release their content either by exocytosis or
    by forming a tight junction with plasma membrane;

9: empty small vesicles are recharged with NA;

10: empty small vesicles are ultimately digested in multivesicular
    bodies.

Abbreviations

L   primary lysosome
LV   large noradrenergic vesicle
MVB multivesicular body
NA   noradrenaline
SER smooth endoplasmic reticulum
SV   small noradrenergic vesicle

REFERENCES

Åberg, H.E., Hansson, H.E., Wetterberg, L., Ross, S,B, & Fröden,
    O. (1974). Dopamine-β-hydroxylase in human lymph. *Life Sci.*
    14, 65-71.

Bartlett, S.F., Lagercrantz, H. & Smith, A.D. (1976). Gel elect-
    rophoresis of soluble and insoluble proteins of noradrenergic
    vesicles from ox splenic nerve: a comparison with proteins
    of adrenal chromaffin granules. *Neuroscience* 1, 339-344.

Blaschko, H. (1973). Catecholamine biosynthesis. *Br. Med Bull.*
    29, 105-109.

Brimijoin, S. (1974). Local changes in subcellular distribution
    of dopamine-β-hydroxylase (EC 1.14.2.1) after blockade of
    axonal transport. *J. Neurochem.* 22, 347-353.

Brimijoin, S. (1976). Cycloheximide alters axonal transport and
    subcellular distribution of dopamine-β-hydroxylase activity.
    J. Neurochem. 26, 35-40.

Burnstock, G. (1972). Purinergic nerves. *Pharmacol. Rev.* 24,
    509-581.

Burnstock, G. (1976). Do some nerves release more than one
    transmitter? *Neuroscience* 1, 239-248.

Chubb, I.W. (1977). The release of non-transmitter substances.
    In: *Synapses* (eds.) G.A. Cottrell & P.N.R. Usherwood, Blackie,
    Glasgow, pp. 264-290.

Chubb, I.W., De Potter, W.P. & De Schaepdryver, A.F. (1972).
    Tyramine does not release noradrenaline from splenic nerve by
    exocytosis. *Naunyn Schmiedeberg's Arch. Pharmacol.* 274, 281-
    286.

Cubeddu, L.X., Barnes, E.M., Langer, S.Z. & Weiner, N. (1974a).
    Release of norepinephrine and dopamine-β-hydroxylase by nerve
    stimulation. 1. Role of neuronal and extraneuronal uptake
    and of *alpha* presynaptic receptors. *J. Pharmacol. Exp. Ther.*
    190, 431-450.

Cubeddu, L.X., Barnes, E. & Weiner, N. (1974b). Release of nor-
    epinephrine and dopamine-β-hydroxylase by nerve stimulation.
    2. Effects of papaverine. *J. Pharmacol. Exp. Ther.* 191, 444-
    457.

Cubeddu, L.X. & Weiner, N. (1975). Nerve stimulation-mediated
    overflow of norepinephrine and dopamine-β-hydroxylase. 3.
    Effects of norepinephrine depletion on the *alpha* presynaptic
    regulation of release. *J. Pharmacol. Exp. Ther.* 192, 1-14.

De Potter, W.P. (1971). Noradrenaline storage particles in splen-
    ic nerve. *Phil. Trans. R. Soc. Lond. B.* 261, 313-317.

De Potter, W.P., Moerman, E.J., De Schaepdryver, A.F. & Smith, A.D. (1969a). Release of noradrenaline and dopamine-β-hydroxy-lase upon splenic nerve stimulation. *Proc. 4th Int. Congr. Pharmacol*. Abst. P146, Basel:Schwabe & Co.

De Potter, W.P., De Schaepdryver, A.F., Moerman, E.J. & Smith, A.D. (1969b). Evidence for the release of vesicle-proteins together with noradrenaline upon stimulation of the splenic nerve. *J. Physiol. (Lond.)* 204, 102P-104P.

De Potter, W.P., Smith, A.D. & De Schaepdryver, A.F. (1970). Subcellular fractionation of splenic nerve: ATP, chromogranin A and dopamine β-hydroxylase in noradrenergic vesicles. *Tissue & Cell* 2, 529-546.

De Potter, W.P., Chubb, I.W., Put, A. & De Schaepdryver, A.F. (1971). Facilitation of the release of noradrenaline and dopamine-β-hydroxylase at low stimulation frequencies by α-blocking agents. *Arch. Int. Pharmacodyn. Ther.* 193, 191-197.

De Potter, W.P., Pham-Huu Chan, C., De Smet, F. & De Schaepdryver, A.F. (1976). The presence of dopamine-β-hydroxylase in the cerebrospinal fluid of rabbits and its increased concentration after stimulation of peripheral nerves and cold stress. *Neuroscience* 1, 523-529.

De Potter, W.P. & Chubb, I.W. (1977). Biochemical observations on the formation of small noradrenergic vesicles in the splenic nerve of the dog. *Neuroscience* 2, 167-174.

Diner, O. (1967). L'expulsion des granules de la médullosurrenale chez le hamster. *C.r.Lebd. Seanc. Acad. Sci., Paris D* 265, 616-619.

Fried, G., Lagercrantz, H. & Hökfelt, T. (1978). Improved isolation of small noradrenergic vesicles from rat seminal ducts following castration. A density gradient centrifugation and morphological study. *Neuroscience* 3 (in press).

Geffen, L.B., Livett, B.G. & Rush, R.A. (1969). Immunological localization of chromogranins in sheep sympathetic neurones, and their release by nerve impulses. *J. Physiol. (Lond.)* 204, 58P-59P.

Gewirtz, G.P. & Kopin, I.J. (1970). Release of dopamine-β-hydroxylase with norepinephrine during cat splenic nerve stimulation. *Nature (Lond.)* 227, 406-407.

Goldstein, D.J. & Cubeddu, L.X. (1976). Dopamine-β-hydroxylase activity in human cerebrospinal fluid. *J. Neurochem.* 26, 193-195.

Holtzman, E. (1971). Cytochemical studies of protein transport in the nervous system. *Phil. Trans. Roy. Soc. B. Lond.* 261, 407-421.

Holtzman, E. (1977). The origin and fate of secretory packages, especially synaptic vesicles. *Neuroscience* 2, 327-355.

Hörtnagl , H., Stadler-Wolffersgrün, R., Brücke, Th., Hammerle, A. & Hackl, J.M. (1978). Changes of dopamine-β-hydroxylase activity in human plasma during prolonged overactivity of the sympathetic nervous system in various diseases. *Naunyn-Schmiedeberg's Arch. Pharmacol.* (in press).

Johnson, D.G., Thoa, N.B., Weinshilboum, R., Axelrod, J. & Kopin, I.J. (1971). Enhanced release of dopamine-β-hydroxylase from sympathetic nerves by calcium and phenoxybenzamine and its reversal by prostaglandins. *Proc. Nat. Acad. Sci. (USA)* 68, 2227-2230.

Kapeller, K. & Mayor, D. (1966). Ultrastructural changes proximal to a constriction in sympathetic axons during the first 24 hours after operation. *J. Anat.* 100, 439-441.

Kirksey, D.F., Klein, R.L., Baggett, J.McC. & Gasparis, M.S. (1978). Evidence that most of the dopamine β-hydroxylase is not membrane bound in purified large dense cored noradrenergic vesicles. *Neuroscience* 3, 71-81.

Lagercrantz, H. (1976). On the composition and function of the large dense-cored vesicles of sympathetic nerves. *Neuroscience* 1, 81-92.

Langley, A.E. & Gardier, R.W. (1977). Effect of atropine and acetylcholine on nerve stimulated output of noradrenaline and dopamine beta-hydroxylase from isolated rabbit and guinea pig hearts. *Naunyn-Schmiedeberg's Arch. Pharmacol.* 297, 251-256.

Mathias, C.J., Smith, A.D., Frankel, H.L. & Spalding, J.M.K. (1976). Dopamine β-hydroxylase release during hypertension from sympathetic nervous overactivity in man. *Cardiovasc. Res.* 10, 176-181.

Ngai, S.H., Dairman, W., Marchelle, M. & Spector, S. (1974). Dopamine-β-hydroxylase in dog lymph - effect of sympathetic activation. *Life Sci.* 14, 2431-2439.

Schneider, F.H., Smith, A.D. & Winkler, H. (1967). Secretion from the adrenal medulla: biochemical evidence for exocytosis. *Br. J. Pharmacol.* 31, 94-104.

Smith, A.D. (1970). Proteins of vesicles from sympathetic axons: chemistry, immunoreactivity, and release upon stimulation. *Neurosci. Res. Prog. Bull.* 8, 377-382.

Smith, A.D. (1971). Some implications of the neuron as a secreting cell. *Phil. Trans. Roy. Soc. Lond. B.* 261, 423-437.

Smith, A.D. (1972). Subcellular localisation of noradrenaline in sympathetic neurons. *Pharmacol. Rev.* 24, 435-457.

Smith, A.D. (1973). Mechanisms involved in the release of noradrenaline from sympathetic nerves. *Br. Med. Bull.* 29,
123-129.

Smith, A.D. (1977). Dale's principle today: adrenergic tissues.
In: *Neuron Concept Today* (eds.) J. Szentagothai, J. Hamori &
E.S. Vizi, Akademiai Kiado, Budapest, pp. 49-61.

Smith, A.D., De Potter, W.P., Moerman, E.J. & De Schaepdryver,
A.F. (1970). Release of dopamine β-hydroxylase and chromogranin A upon stimulation of the splenic nerve. *Tissue & Cell*
2, 547-568.

Smith, A.D. & Winkler, H. (1972). Fundamental mechanisms in the
release of catecholamines. *Handb. Exp. Pharmacol.* 33, 538-617.

Stjärne, L., Hedqvist, P. & Lagercrantz, H. (1970). Catecholamines and adenine nucleotide material in effluent from stimulated adrenal medulla and spleen. *Biochem. Pharmacol.* 19,
1147-1158.

Stjärne, L., Roth, R.H. & Lishajko, F. (1967). Noradrenaline
formation from dopamine in isolated subcellular particles
from bovine splenic nerve. *Biochem. Pharmacol.* 16, 1729-1739.

Tranzer, J.P. (1972). A new amine storing compartment in adrenergic axons. *Nature New Biol.* 237, 57-58.

Viveros, O.H. (1975). Mechanism of secretion of catecholamines
from adrenal medulla. In: *Handbook of Physiology* Section 7:
Endocrinology Vol. 6 (eds.) H. Blaschko, G. Sayers & A.D. Smith,
pp. 389-426.

Viveros, O.H., Arqueros, L. & Kirshner, N. (1968). Release of
catecholamines and dopamine-β-oxidase from the adrenal medulla.
Life Sci. 7, 609-618.

Weinshilboum, R. & Axelrod, J. (1971). Serum dopamine beta-
hydroxylase activity. *Circ. Res.* 28, 307-315.

Weinshilboum, R.M., Thoa, N.B., Johnson, D.G., Kopin, I.J. &
Axelrod, J. (1971). Proportional release of norepinephrine
and dopamine-β-hydroxylase from sympathetic nerves. *Science*
174, 1349-1351.

Winkler, H. (1976). The composition of adrenal chromaffin granules: an assessment of controversial results. *Neuroscience*
1, 65-80.

ULTRASTRUCTURAL STUDIES OF THE MECHANISM OF RELEASE

M. Fillenz

I   INTRODUCTION

The bulk of the evidence concerning transmitter release is biochemical; ultrastructural studies have recently made an increasing contribution to this problem. The interpretation of the
ultrastructural findings, however, is often difficult. Although
there are at present few studies of release from noradrenergic
neurons, there is a large amount of work on secretion from glands
and transmitter release from peripheral, mostly cholinergic,,
nerve terminals. Extrapolations have been made to secretory processes in general from experiments on these two kinds of preparation, in spite of the recognition that they differ from each
other in some fundamental respects. Thus it is generally believed
that glands release their secretions by exocytosis and that the
empty vesicles are not immediately reusable for release. In the
case of neurotransmitters there is evidence to suggest that exocytosis is followed by reuse of vesicles involving a process of
membrane recycling confined to the nerve terminal (for review see
Holtzmann, 1977).

The adrenergic neuron occupies a special position: it is embryo-
logically related to the adrenal medullary cell, but being a
neuron, will share some of the characteristics of the most
thoroughly studied synapse - the neuromuscular junction. The
adrenal medulla is a gland and behaves like other glands,
although in tissue culture it grows processes which are morpho-
logically indistinguishable from sympathetic nerve terminals.
Although the adrenal medulla has been very useful as a model,
results obtained on it do not necessarily hold for the noradrenergic neuron.

The present review will examine the problem of release under the
following aspects: storage of noradrenaline, site of release,
mechanism of release, source of transmitter, fate and origin of
vesicles. As much as possible I shall restrict myself to evidence obtained on adrenergic neurons, since my underlying assumption is that release mechanisms may not be the same in glands and
neurons, nor even in neurons releasing different transmitters;
these differences may be the expression of important differences
in function.

II   STORAGE

The application of electron microscopy to biological material
added a powerful tool to the study of the nervous system.
De Robertis and Bennett in 1955 were the first to describe synaptic vesicles; they recognised them as a characteristic feature of
the synapse and suggested that they might represent the storage
organelles of chemical substances active at the synapse.   An
important observation was the close association between synaptic
vesicles and endoplasmic reticulum; it was suggested that the
latter may play a part in the synthesis of vesicular contents.
In 1961 De Robertis and Pellegrino de Iraldi described vesicles
with a dense osmium deposit, later called dense-cored vesicles,
in terminals of sympathetic neurons innervating blood vessels,
the pineal gland and the spleen.   They argued that since sympathetic nerves contain noradrenaline in a particulate form, as shown
by von Euler and Hillarp (1956), the presence of vesicles strongly
reducing osmium tetroxide may mean that they represented the specific storage site of the amine.

In 1962 Richardson in an ultrastructural study of the vas deferens
introduced the terms granular and agranular vesicles.   He suggested that the two kinds of vesicle in sympathetic nerve terminals
may represent stages in the formation of catecholamine storage
components.   Larger dense-cored vesicles found in presynaptic
terminals of autonomic ganglia were described by Hager and Tafuri
(1959) and Taxi (1961).   Grillo and Palay (1962) recognised that
dense-cored vesicles were a heterogeneous group; they identified
three varieties of granular or dense-cored vesicles in the adult
rat: type 1 being vesicles with a mean diameter of 85 nm and type
2 and 3 with a mean diameter of 50 nm but differing from each
other in core size.   The distinction between type 2 and 3 was soon
dropped and later workers classified dense-cored vesicles into
large and small on the basis of vesicle diameter (for a review of
the early work see Grillo, 1966).

Falck and his colleagues (Falck, Hillarp, Thieme & Torp, 1962)
showed that the varicosities of sympathetic fibres, demonstrated
by Hillarp (1946) with methylene blue, showed bright fluorescence
with the histochemical method for catecholamines.   This indicated
that they contained high concentrations of noradrenaline.   Varicosities seen in the light microscope corresponded to axon expansions containing clusters of dense-cored vesicles; this was strong
presumptive evidence that the dense-cored vesicles were the noradrenaline storage particles.   However, a clear demonstration of
the identity of the noradrenaline storage particles required a
histochemical method for catecholamines at the electron microscopic level.

The early studies of sympathetic nerve terminals used osmium fixation;   with this fixative dense-cored vesicles were seen in non-
catecholaminergic neurons, such as the preganglionic terminals in
autonomic ganglia, and many of the vesicles in sympathetic nerve
terminals lacked electron dense cores.   Osmium tetroxide was
clearly not a satisfactory fixative for the demonstration of noradrenaline at the ultrastructural level.

Wood and Barnett (1964) adapted the chromaffin reaction for
electron microscopy by using glutaraldehyde in dichromate.
They showed that oxidation by dichromate at pH 4.1 produced an
electron-dense precipitate in noradrenaline but not adrenaline-
containing cells of the adrenal medulla and stained small dense-
cored vesicles in the hypothalamus. Further modifications of
this fixative were developed by Tranzer (Tranzer & Snipes, 1968)
and Woods (1969). A number of careful studies were carried out
to show that the electron dense core seen in both small and large
vesicles in sympathetic nerve terminals after dichromate oxidation
without osmication is related to their noradrenaline content
(Tranzer & Thoenen, 1967a, 1967b, 1968; Tranzer, Thoenen, Snipes
& Richards, 1969). After osmium fixation the large axonal vesicles have a core whose electron density is unrelated to noradrenaline content (Till & Banks, 1976; Thuresson-Klein, Chen-Yen &
Klein, 1974). Richardson (1966) and Hökfelt and Jonsson (1968)
found that fixation in 3-6% potassium permanganate was an effective fixative for demonstrating dense-cored vesicles in both peripheral and central noradrenergic neurons. The development of
histochemical methods for noradrenaline were followed by further
ultrastructural studies of the noradrenaline storage vesicles.
Bisby and Fillenz (1971) showed that the light and heavy noradrenaline storage particles isolated on density gradients from the
vas deferens corresponded to the small and large dense-cored vesicles seen in electron microscopy of tissue sections. Using both
dichromate and permanganate oxidation, Fillenz and Pollard (1975)
carried out a quantitative analysis of the core size of the small
vesicles in various sympathetic nerve terminals. This study showed that both the mean core volume and the core size distribution
differed in sympathetic nerve terminals to different organs.
Parallel biochemical work (Fillenz, Howe & West, 1976) showed that
core size in the small vesicles reflected the noradrenaline content of the vesicle and the degree to which the maximum noradrenaline storage capacity was saturated. Furthermore, the morphological study showed that the population of small vesicles was heterogenous with respect to noradrenaline content.

The earliest attempts to isolate the noradrenaline storage particles by density gradient centrifugation showed that the distribution of noradrenaline was closely paralleled by that of the enzyme
dopamine-β-hydroxylase (Potter & Axelrod, 1963; Bisby, Fillenz &
Smith, 1973; Nelson & Molinoff, 1976) although De Potter and
Chubb, working with dog spleen, concluded that there was a population of low density noradrenaline storage vesicle which did not
contain dopamine-β-hydroxylase (De Potter, 1971; De Potter &
Chubb, 1977). The study of the localization of dopamine-β-hydroxylase at the ultrastructural level has been only partially suc-
cessful. Pickel, Joh and Reis (1976), using the peroxidase-anti-
peroxidase immunocytochemical method, described the distribution
of dopamine-β-hydroxylase in cell bodies, dendrites and proximal
axons; they found dopamine-β-hydroxylase staining in a reticulum
of interconnecting membranes not parallel to the surface, which
they took to be endoplasmic reticulum. They failed, however, to
get staining for dopamine-β-hydroxylase in nerve terminals.
Lundberg, Bylock, Goldstein, Hansson and Dahlström (1977) using a

different modification of the immunocytochemical method, demonstrated dopamine-β-hydroxylase in synaptic boutons in the hypothalamus: they found extensive staining of vesicles 50-70 nm in
diameter. Both groups of workers reported absence of dopamine-β-
hydroxylase staining on mitochondrial and plasma membrane.

III SITE OF RELEASE

The microscopical study of the nervous system flourished in the
19th century, and was dominated by two rival theories: the reticular and the neuron theory. Cajal put forward the view that functional connections between neurons occur at specialised areas of
close contact and his descriptions of neuronal morphology still
stands unchallenged. It was Sherrington who introduced the term
'synapse' in 1897 in an attempt to explain the characteristic
features of the reflex arc. In 1904 Elliot demonstrated that
electrical stimulation of nerves could be mimicked by the injection of adrenaline, thus laying the foundation of the theory of
chemical synaptic transmission. The application of electron microscopy to biological material in the 1950's opened up a new era
in the study of the nervous system. It was found that there were
extensive areas of contact between neurons, but the precise connections within the nervous system were explained by the hypothesis that only at the synapse did functional interaction between
neurons occur. Two features were taken as essential characteristics of a synapse: vesicle accumulation and membrane thickening.
These two features were found both in the central nervous system
and the neuromuscular junction. Gray (1959, 1963) defined the
nature of the membrane thickenings more precisely and described
the presynaptic dense projections. These were taken as coexten-
sive with the active zone (Couteaux, 1961) where neurotransmission,
i.e., transmitter release, actually takes place.

Microscopy of noradrenergic neurons, both peripheral and central,
has shown that their nerve terminals are characterised by lengths
of varicose fibres (Hökfelt, 1974). Malmfors (1969) produced
evidence which suggested that noradrenaline was released from the
varicosities of sympathetic fibres: electrical stimulation caused
a decrease in the fluorescence intensity of the varicosities and
an increase in the preterminal fibres. At the ultrastructural
level the varicosities are found to correspond to vesicle filled
axon expansions. The axon expansions in the periphery are at
variable distances from the postsynaptic elements which they are
thought to control; membrane thickenings are not seen in varicosities of either peripheral or central neurons (Hökfelt, 1974).
Since noradrenaline is released from these varicose terminals,
presynaptic dense projections cannot be an essential requirement
for transmitter release. That leaves the accumulation of synaptic
vesicles as the only general characteristic of chemically trans-
mitting synapses. There is some evidence for certain differences
in the conductance properties of terminal and non-terminal membranes (Katz & Miledi, 1969) but this may not be demonstrable mor-
phologically. Recent work has cast some doubt on the nature of
the presynaptic dense projections: Gray (1975) suggests on the
basis of EM stereoscopy that presynaptic dense projections, and

other ultrastructural features of the synapse, are a reticulate precipitate which occurs in regions rich in protein complexes when these are fixed and processed for electron microscopy. If the presynaptic densities turn out to be fixation artifacts, vesicle accumulation becomes the characteristic feature of release sites. This raises the question whether release of transmitter occurs from regions of the neuron other than the terminal axon where vesicle accumulations are seen. Hökfelt (1969) and Eränkö (1972) have described the occurrence of clusters of small vesicles in dendrites. There have been a number of reports of possible release from dendrites (Taxi & Sotelo, 1973; Björklund & Lindvall, 1975; Geffen, Jessell, Cuello & Iversen, 1977). Some of these studies have been on the dopaminergic neurons of the substantia nigra. Whether similar release from dendrites occurs in noradrenergic neurons is at present not known.

IV   MECHANISM OF RELEASE

The presence of synaptic vesicles in electronmicroscopy and the discovery of the quantal nature of release gave rise to the hypothesis that one quantum of transmitter represented the contents of one vesicle (Del Castillo & Katz, 1954). The finding that stimulation of the adrenal medulla led to the release into the perfusate of the soluble, but not of the membrane bound constituents of chromaffin granules led to the hypothesis that release occurred by exocytosis, i.e., fusion of the vesicle with the plasma membrane in such a way that the vesicle interior became continuous with the extracellular space.(for review see Smith & Winkler, 1972). De Robertis and Vaz Ferreira (1957) first suggested release by exocytosis on the basis of EM observations.

Four main approaches have been used in the search for morphological evidence of exocytosis:

1. the examination of fixed material for signs of vesicle fusion.
2. the uptake of electron-dense molecules into vesicles during release.
3. the use of freeze-fracture.
4. the study of changes in the number and distribution of vesicles resulting from transmitter release.

All four methods have yielded interesting results, but there are considerable difficulties in their interpretation.

Electron microscopy of fixed adrenal medulla produced a wealth of evidence in support of exocytosis: not only were omega figures found in large numbers, but dense cores were found both inside the vesicles and in the extracellular compartment (Grynszpan-Winograd, 1971). The omega figures were particularly abundant in adrenals of the golden hamster; they were only rarely seen in adrenals of the rat, although there was no parallel biochemical difference in catecholamine release between the two species.

The search for morphological evidence for vesicle fusion in nerve
terminals produced only very few instances in rat vas deferens
(Fillenz, 1971). However, large vesicles fused with the plasma
membrane have been described in bovine splenic nerve and nerve
endings in spleen capsule (Thureson-Klein, 1975; Thureson-Klein &
Klein, 1975) as well as human omental veins and arteries (Thureson-
Klein, Stjärne & Brundin, 1976; Thureson-Klein, Klein & Stjärne,
1976). Whole vesicles outside nerve terminals have also been described (Grillo, 1970).

The difficulty is to decide how many of these appearances represent artefacts. Since the biochemical evidence suggests that
membrane bound components are retained, the appearance of intact
vesicles outside the nerve terminal are almost certainly due to
fixation artefacts. Similarly the appearance of whole cores in
the extracellular space is most probably explained by the mechanical extrusion of a fixed core during processing. That leaves the
question to what extent the omega figures are also fixation
artefacts.

Exocytosis can be of two kinds: irreversible, when the vesicle
membrane becomes incorporated into the plasma membrane, and reversible, when there is only momentary fusion after which the
vesicle detaches itself from the plasma membrane. Irreversible
exocytosis implies similarity in the composition of vesicle and
plasma membrane: it will lead to expansion in the surface area
of the nerve terminal and to reduction in vesicle number unless
exocytosis is exactly paralleled by some form of endocytotic
membrane retrieval. Reversible exocytosis on the other hand will
lead to the appearance of "empty" vesicles, with no change in
surface area of the terminal. Peripheral cholinergic nerve terminals subjected to black widow spider venom (Clark, Hurlbut &
Mauro, 1972) or to intense electrical stimulation (Zimmermann &
Whittaker, 1974) show electron microscopic evidence suggestive
of irreversible exocytosis. On the other hand in the adrenal
medulla the presence of empty vesicles after release (Benedecky
& Somogy, 1974) as well as the difference in composition between
vesicle and plasma membrane (Winkler, Schneider, Rufener, Kakane
& Hortnagl, 1974) suggests that exocytosis is reversible.

There is at present little published work on adrenergic nerve
terminals. The histochemical demonstration of dopamine-β-hydroxylase associated with the vesicle membrane but absent from the
plasma membrane argues against incorporation of the vesicle into
the plasma membrane.

The uptake of electron-dense extracellular markers into vesicles
following increased release has been demonstrated for peripheral
cholinergic nerve endings (Heuser & Reese, 1974; Whittaker, 1977)
and synaptosomes prepared from brain (Friend & Blaustein, 1976).
The problem with electronmicroscopy is that it is difficult to
show the time relationship between the uptake of extracellular
markers and release. In a study in which horseradish peroxidase
uptake into synaptosomes and release of acetylcholine was measured

biochemically, no relation was found between release of acetylcholine and uptake of horseradish peroxidase (Marchbanks, 1977).
In a preliminary note Busbaum and Heuser (1976) have reported
80% depletion of large and small dense-cored vesicles in electrically stimulated mouse vas deferens; when muscles were stimulated
in the presence of horseradish peroxidase, and then given a period
of rest, there was greatly enhanced horseradish peroxidase loading
of synaptic vesicles.

Freeze-fracture or freeze-etching represented an important method-
ological advance as it offered the opportunity of avoiding dis-
tortion due to dehydration and fixation. In practice it was
found that unfixed material showed conspicuous damage (Pfenniger,
Akert, Moor & Sandri, 1972) and most early workers used freeze-
fracture on fixed material. Early interpretations of results
were complicated by conflicting views about the site of fracturing
(Plattner, 1970). Branton's (1966) view that freeze-fracture
separates the two leaflets of the unit membrane is now generally
accepted. Two features studied by freeze-fracture are relevant
to the problem of release: evidence of vesicle attachment suggesting exocytosis and the presence of large particles in the presynaptic membrane at the active zone.

Fixing muscles with aldehydes during or just after electrode
stimulation followed by freeze-fracture shows numerous plasmalemmal deformations suggestive of exocytosis (Heuser, Reese & Landis,
1974; Couteaux & Pecot-Dechavassine, 1970; Dreyer, Peper, Akert,
Sandri & Moor, 1973; Streit, Akert, Sandri, Livingston & Moor,
1972; Pfenninger & Rovainen, 1974). These plasmalemmal deformations, which take the form of dimples in the cytoplasmic leaflet
of the membrane, occur close to the large intramembranous particles, which in turn are in register with the presynaptic thickening seen in tissue sections. These morphological features are
all regarded as characteristics of the active zone or release
site. The number of vesicle attachment sites could be shown to
be correlated with activity, i.e., presence or absence of stimulation and Ca^{++} and Mg^{++} concentration - factors which are known
to affect the rate of transmitter release. However, their number
also varied with the concentration of aldehydes in the fixative,
a dilute aldehyde fixative resulting in the appearance of larger
number of vesicle attachment sites for a given rate of stimulation.
Also, the number of vesicle attachments seen is greater than the
number of quanta calculated to have been released. Recently
Heuser, Reese and Landis (1976) have used a method of much more
rapid freezing, based on the principle suggested by Eränkö (1954)
of pressing tissue against a cold metal block. With this method
good freezing can be obtained without the use of fixatives, and
Heuser et al. have compared the appearance of fixed and unfixed
tissue after freeze-fracture. A number of important findings
emerged: electrically stimulated neuromuscular junctions showed
vesicular attachments in fixed but never in unfixed tissue. This
was true, even though the interval between electrical stimulation
and contact with the freezing block varied from 0-5 msec; the
authors calculated that freezing occurred in less than 10 msec.
Also in unfixed tissue the external leaflet of the plasma membrane
shows none of the characteristics of the active zone.

The implications of these results are very important: morphological signs of exocytosis are seen only in the presence of fixative
and the number of exocytotic figures varies with the aldehyde
concentration. Heuser *et al*. concluded that if exocytosis of
vesicles occurs at all, it must be completed and no longer vis-
ible within 10 msec after it is initiated by the arrival of the
nerve impulse. The effect of the fixative however can be explained in three possible ways: 1. that it causes transmitter
release and that the release initiated by nerve stimulation is
therefore prolonged and the interval between release and freezing
further shortened; 2. that the fixative prolongs the period for
which the vesicle remains attached to the membrane and open to
the exterior; 3. that the fixative, by changing the stickiness
of the plasma membrane, causes adherence of vesicles and opening
at the point of contact, which do not occur under physiological
conditions.

The importance of the rapid freezing technique in the absence of
fixative is that it illustrates a type of artefact which probably
depends not so much on the mere presence of fixative but the rate
at which it acts on different cell components, e.g., plasma membrane versus vesicles. The assessment of the significance of
appearances such as exocytosis in tissue sections, expansion of
the surface area of the terminal with intense stimulation etc.
will have to await further work with rapid freezing in the absence
of fixative.

Although no freeze-fracture studies of noradrenergic neurons
comparable to those on the neuromuscular junction are available,
there is a recent paper on carotid body type I cells, which
store dopamine (Hellström & Kjaergaard, 1976). Stimulation
of the carotid body by hypoxia or metacholine administration leads
to several interesting changes seen by the freeze-fracture technique: a high proportion of the electron-dense vesicles, which
are the storage organelles for dopamine, are located close to the
plasma membrane; exocytotic-like profiles, not seen in unstimulated tissue, appear; and membrane-associated particles on the
plasma membrane are greatly increased as compared with controls.
The intramembrane particles were not arranged in any regular pattern and no specialized regions are seen in these cells normally,
in either tissue sections or freeze-fracture replicas. This suggests that alterations of the particle components of the membrane
can occur as a dynamic phenomenon, and may not be a permanent
structural feature.

Studies on changes in vesicle number as a result of stimulation,
such as are available for the neuromuscular junction and the
electric organ of Torpedo, have not yet been done on noradrenergic neurons.

V   SOURCE OF RELEASED NORADRENALINE

There is evidence which suggests a subdivision of the transmitter
pool into a reserve store and a readily releasable store; the latter contains newly-synthesized transmitter. This two compartment

model is inferred from the finding that after the administration of labelled precursor the specific activity of the released transmitter is higher than that of the total transmitter store. The high specific activity of released transmitter has been demonstrated for both acetylcholine (Dunant, Gautron, Israel, Lesbats & Manaranche, 1972) and noradrenaline released from nerve terminals. In the case of noradrenaline the experiments were carried out on the nerve endings in the spleen of the cat (Kopin, Breese, Krauss & Weise, 1968). These findings provide evidence for a two-compartmental model only if one assumes a functionally homogeneous population of nerve terminals. It is not at all clear at present what the morphological counterpart of the two compartments is; in the cholinergic nerve terminal it has been variously suggested that the readily releasable pool corresponds to either cytoplasmic acetylcholine (Marchbanks, 1975) or to a subpopulation of vesicles which are fragile and are close to the axon membrane to which they tend to adhere on homogenisation (Barker, Dowdall & Whittaker, 1972). In the case of adrenergic nerve terminals there is no evidence for vesicle clustering or the presynaptic specialisation suggesting release sites, such as are found in cholinergic nerve terminals. On the other hand there are two populations of vesicles, the large and the small, and there is further evidence for heterogeneity in the small vesicle population (Fillenz & Pollard, 1976). Both the large and small vesicle populations have been proposed as candidates for the readily releasable pool. The hypothesis that large vesicles are the source of released noradrenaline (Smith, 1973; Dahlström, 1973) is supported by the finding that nerve stimulation causes the appearance of soluble dopamine-β-hydroxylase in plasma or perfusate; in axonal vesicles, which appear to be identical with large terminal vesicles, 20% of the dopamine-β-hydroxylase is soluble. Further support comes from the finding of omega figures involving large but not small vesicles (Thureson-Klein & Klein, 1975). However, density gradient centrifugation of sympathetically innervated organs shows that transmitter release evoked by drugs, electrical stimulation and cold stress is associated with a much greater reduction in the low density than the high density noradrenaline peak (Fillenz & Howe, 1975; Bisby, Cripps & Dearnaley, 1971; Molinoff & Nelson, 1976); this finding has been interpreted as showing that released noradrenaline comes predominantly from the small vesicle population. Hamilton and Robinson (1973) found that red back spider venom, which causes release of noradrenaline, as indicated by loss of fluorescence and loss of biochemically assayed noradrenaline, also causes loss of small vesicles in the nerve terminals of the cat vas deferens; large vesicles are either not affected or are the last to disappear. The heterogeneity of the small vesicle population raises the possibility that it reflects a functional subdivision within this group of vesicles. There is at present only circumstantial evidence for the hypothesis that amongst the small vesicles those with the highest noradrenaline content represent the readily releasable pool of transmitter (Fillenz, 1977).

VI   FATE OF VESICLES AFTER RELEASE

The available evidence suggests that the release of noradrenaline from vesicles does not involve the incorporation of the vesicle membrane into the axon membrane and that the process is one of reversible exocytosis. For the adrenal medulla there is both biochemical and ultrastructural evidence that after intense catecholamine release, such as is produced by insulin, a population of empty vesicles appear in the adrenal medullary cells. Such empty vesicles do not take up catecholamines and therefore cannot be reused for release of catecholamines (Viveros, 1975). They are thought to be taken up into lysosomes for degradation. For noradrenergic neurons there is less evidence available. The uptake of exogenous noradrenaline into the noradrenaline storage vesicles can be used to measure the vesicular noradrenaline storage capacity; in some nerve terminals the normal noradrenaline content of the vesicles is below the maximum storage capacity (Fillenz, Howe & West, 1976). Transmitter release results in a reduction, not only of noradrenaline content but also noradrenaline storage capacity (Fillenz & West, 1976). This suggests that the vesicles in noradrenaline neurons, like those in the adrenal medulla, are not immediately reusable after release.

Extracellular markers, such as horseradish peroxidase, have been used to follow the events accompanying and following release. In the frog neuromuscular junction this method has yielded results which have been interpreted to show recycling and re-use of vesicle membrane in the terminal. Whittaker (1977) in the electric organ of Torpedo has identified a subpopulation of smaller vesicles which contain the extracellular marker dextran and which constitute the readily releasable pool. Apart from a preliminary communication (Busbaum & Heuser, 1976) no equivalent studies have been done on adrenergic neurons. However, Holtzman, Teichberg, Citkowitz, Crain & Kawai (1973) have described the distribution of horseradish peroxidase in explants of embryonic spinal cord, where neurons are whole and the connection between terminals and cell body is not severed, as it is in the case of the lung. Horseradish peroxidase in this preparation was found in multivesicular bodies (MVBs) in axons and perikarya, suggesting that there is retrograde transport from terminals to the cell body. The uptake of horseradish peroxidase by dendrites and axons, unrelated to transmitter release by exocytosis, cannot, however, be excluded. Teichberg and Bloom (1976) have followed the uptake of horseradish peroxidase into sympathetic neurons. They found tracer in MVBs and tubular structures, which were not in continuity with the endoplasmic reticulum. They concluded that retrograde transport of horseradish peroxidase occurs in MVBs and tubular structures but not in endoplasmic reticulum.

Since dopamine-β-hydroxylase is a marker for vesicle membranes it can be used to follow the fate of the vesicles after they have undergone exocytosis. The retrograde transport of dopamine-β-hydroxylase from nerve terminals towards the cell body has been demonstrated by a number of different methods: Brimijoin demonstrated an accumulation of dopamine-β-hydroxylase below both a

ligature and a length of cooled nerve (Brimijoin, 1974; Brimijoin
& Helland, 1976). Dopamine-β-hydroxylase antibody accumulation
in cell bodies after either intravenous administration (Jacobowitz,
Ziegler & Thomas, 1975) or local injection into the vicinity of the
nerve terminals (Fillenz, Gagnon, Stoeckel & Thoenen, 1976) demonstrated that this was not a response to injury but occurred in intact neurons in the living animal. Much of this retrogradely transported dopamine-β-hydroxylase is enzymatically inactive (Nagatsu,
Kondo, Kato & Nagatsu, 1976). All these characteristics would be
compatible with the hypothesis that retrogradely transported
dopamine-β-hydroxylase represents the membranes of vesicles which
have undergone exocytosis and are no longer able to take up noradrenaline. Taken together with the appearance of horseradish
peroxidase in MVB in the cell body it suggests that one of the
functions of the retrograde transport may be the disposal of vesicles no longer able to store and therefore release transmitters.

VII ORIGIN OF VESICLES

Weiss and Hiscoe (1948) produced evidence of transport of material
from the cell body of neurons to their terminals. They offered no
suggestion about the fate or the role of the transported material.
Although there has been a great deal of work in this area in the
intervening 30 years, the answers to these two questions are not
much clearer. Van Breeman, Anderson and Reger (1958) first suggested that synaptic vesicles originated in the cell body and
travelled down to the nerve terminals, although there was little
evidence to support this suggestion since the agranular cholinergic vesicles cannot be distinguished from other vesicular
structures.

Dahlström (1965), using fluorescence microscopy, demonstrated the
accumulation of noradrenaline above a ligature in ligated axons,
and Kapeller and Mayor (1967) using electron microscopy, showed
an accumulation of dense-cored vesicles above a ligature. They
used osmium fixation, and found only large dense-cored vesicles.
The experiments were later repeated by Tomlinson (1975) using
Wood's acrolein-dochromate fixative; with this fixation method,
a considerable proportion of small dense-cored vesicles were seen.
This is interesting in view of the fact that clusters of small
dense-cored vesicles are occasionally seen in intact axons
(Tranzer, 1973), but does not answer the question whether the
small vesicles are formed in the cell body and are transported
down to the tie or are formed locally either in response to the
ligature or the arrested axoplasmic transport. The latter could
provide an explanation for the presence of small vesicles in
nerve terminals. The evidence from density gradient experiments
showing two populations of noradrenaline storage particles in
terminals but only one, high density population, in axons argues
against the presence of small dense-cored vesicles in axons in
any significant number.

There are a variety of published observations showing what looks
like the budding of vesicles from endoplasmic reticulum. Such
appearances have been described for chick sympathetic ganglia in

organ culture (Holtzman *et al.*, 1973) as well as axons and terminals of sympathetic neurons (Fillenz, 1971; Tranzer, 1972;
Hökfelt, 1973). Further support for the hypothesis that vesicles
can be formed from endoplasmic reticulum comes from the finding
of tubular structures giving a histochemical reaction for catecholamines at the ultrastructural level (what Tranzer called the
third storage compartment for catecholamines), from the electron
microscopic histochemical demonstration of dopamine-β-hydroxylase
in the endoplasmic reticulum (see above) and from measurements
of membrane thickness which show the same thickness for vesicles
and endoplasmic reticulum membrane (Holtzman *et al.*, 1973).

A third possibility for the origin of the small terminal vesicles
is that they are formed from the large axonal vesicles. Although
this seems plausible there is little ultrastructural or biochemical evidence to support such a hypothesis.

Recent evidence for the local formation of vesicles in nerve terminals comes from *in vitro* work on human omental veins (Thureson-
Klein, Klein & Stjärne, 1976; Thureson-Klein, Stjärne & Brundin,
1976). Biopsy specimens were fixed immediately after removal and
after a period of superfusion both with and without field stimulation. Superfusion without field stimulation resulted in increased numbers of both small and large dense cored vesicles in
the nerve terminals, with no change in their relative percentages;
this was taken by the authors to indicate continued axoplasmic
transport during the period of superfusion. After field stimulation there was an increase in the number of small vesicles and a
smaller increase in the number of large vesicles, leading to a
change in their relative proportion; there was also an increase
in the number of exocytotic figures involving large vesicles.
This was interpreted as representing local formation of small
vesicles.

Recent work by.Gray (1976) casts doubt on the existence of
vesicles. Whereas normally endoplasmic reticulum seen in axons
stops short of the nerve terminal, after albumin treatment the
endoplasmic reticulum is seen to extend into the nerve terminal,
spirally wrapped round the microtubules; the latter are also very
much better preserved after albumin treatment and they are seen
to extend up to the axoplasmic membrane. Gray suggests (1977)
that the presynaptic thickenings represent the site of insertion
of neurotubules, that their role is to guide the endoplasmic
reticulum down to the plasma membrane and that transmitter release normally occurs from the endoplasmic reticulum. The mechanical trauma of homogenization and the chemical trauma of fixation
causes fragmentation of the endoplasmic reticulum into transmitter storage particles isolated by differential and density
centrifugation or synaptic vesicles seen in fixed tissue sections.

        VIII   CONCLUSION

Ultrastructural studies of nerve terminals of both peripheral and
central noradrenergic neurons have shown that they differ in a
number of respects from other neurons: they have two populations

of noradrenaline containing vesicles, which are distinguishable
by their size as well as the histochemical properties of their
cores. The varicosities, from which transmitter release occurs,
lack the specializations seen in other presynaptic terminals,
such as membrane thickenings and vesicle clustering. The con-
ventionally accepted criteria for exocytosis, such as omega
figures and the presence of extracellular markers in vesicles,
are found in noradrenergic neurons. Exocytosis appears to be
reversible. There is evidence for a rapid bidirectional transport of material between cell body and terminals: the centrifugal
transport consists of noradrenaline-containing vesicles; the
retrograde transport appears to be endogenous dopamine-β-hydroxy-
lase in a particulate form but not associated with noradrenaline,
as well as extracellular markers, such as horseradish peroxidase,
carried in organelles distinct from endoplasmic reticulum. The
source, interrelation and respective function of large and small
vesicles is not clear: there is ultrastructural evidence which
suggests the formation of small vesicles from endoplasmic reticulum, both in the axon and in the terminals.

There have been recent advances in technique the implications of
which have not yet been fully realized; noradrenaline is the only
transmitter for which a reliable histochemical method is available
and which can be used for quantitative studies. The use of stereo-
electronmicroscopy, albumin treatment and rapid freeze-fracture
without fixation has raised the question of how many of the classical appearances are attributable to the effect of fixatives.

IX REFERENCES

Barker, L.A., Dowdall, M.J. & Whittaker, V.P. (1972). Choline
    metabolism in the cerebral cortex of guinea pigs. Stable
    bound acetylcholine. *J. Biochem*. 130, 1063-1080.

Benedecky, I. & Somogy, P. (1974). Ultrastructure of the adrenal
    medulla of normal and insulin-treated hamsters. *Cell Tissue
    Res*. 162, 541-550.

Bisby, M.A., Cripps, H. & Dearnaley, D.P. (1971). Effects of
    nerve stimulation on the subcellular distribution of noradren-
    aline in the cat spleen. *J. Physiol*. 214, 13-14P.

Bisby, M.A. & Fillenz, M. (1971). The storage of endogenous nor-
    adrenaline in sympathetic nerve terminals. *J. Physiol*. 215,
    163-179.

Bisby, M.A., Fillenz, M. & Smith, A.D. (1973). Evidence for the
    presence of dopamine-β-hydroxylase in both populations of nor-
    adrenaline storage vesicles in sympathetic nerve terminals of
    the rat vas deferens. *J. Neurochem*. 20, 245-248.

Björklund, A. & Lindvall, O. (1975). Dopamine in dendrites of
    substantia nigra neurons: suggestions for a role in dendritic
    terminals. *Brain Res*. 83, 531-537.

Branton, D. (1966). Fracture faces in frozen membranes. *Proc. Natl. Acad. Sci.* [*U.S.A.*] 55, 1048-1056.

Brimijoin, S. (1974). Local changes in subcellular distribution of dopamine-β-hydroxylase after blockade of axonal transport. *J. Neurochem.* 22, 347-353.

Brimijoin, S. & Helland, L. (1976). Rapid retrograde transport of dopamine-β-hydroxylase as examined by the stop-flow technique. *Brain Res.* 102, 217-228.

Busbaum, C.B. & Heuser, J.E. (1976). Ultrastructure of stimulated adrenergic nerve terminals. *J. Cell Biol.* 70, 404A.

Clark, A.W., Hurlburt, W.P. & Mauro, A. (1972). Changes in the fine structure of the neuromuscular junction of the frog caused by black widow spider venom. *J. Cell. Biol.* 52, 1-14.

Couteaux, R. (1961). Principaux criteres morphologiques et citochimiques utilisables aujourd'hui pour definir les divers types de synapses. *Act. Neurophysiol.* 3, 145-173.

Couteaux, R. & Pecot-Dechavassine, M. (1970). Vesicules synaptiques et poches au niveau des "zones actives" de la jonction neuromusculaire. *C.R. Acad. Sci. D.* 271, 2346-2349.

Dahlström, A. (1965). Observations on the accumulation of noradrenaline in the proximal and distal parts of peripheral adrenergic nerves after compression. *J. Anat.* 99, 677-689.

Dahlström, A. (1973). Aminergic transmission. Introduction and short review. *Brain Res.* 62, 441-460.

Del Castillo, J. & Katz, B. (1954). Quantal components of the end-plate potential. *J. Physiol.* 124, 560-573.

De Robertis, E.D.P. & Bennett, H.S. (1955). Some features of the submicroscopic morphology of synapses in frog and earthworm. *J. Biophys. Biochem. Cytol.* 1, 47-58.

De Robertis, E. & Pellegrino de Iraldi, A. (1961). A plurivesicular component in adrenergic nerve endings. *Anat. Res.* 139, 299.

De Robertis, E. & Vaz Ferreira, A. (1957). Electron microscope studies of the excretion of catechol-containing droplets in the adrenal medulla. *Exp. Cell Res.* 12, 568-574.

De Potter, W.P. (1971). Noradrenaline storage particles in splenic nerve. *Phil. Trans. Roy. Soc. B.* 261, 313-317.

De Potter, W.P. & Chubb, I.W. (1977). Biochemical observations on the formation of small noradrenergic vesicles in the splenic nerve of the dog. *Neuroscience* 2, 167-174.

Dreyer, F., Peper, K., Akert, K., Sandri, C. & Moor, H. (1973). Ultrastructure of the active zone in the frog neuromuscular junction. *Brain Res.* 62, 373-380.

Dunant, Y., Gautron, J., Israel, M., Lesbats, B. & Manaranche, R. (1972). Les compartiments d'Acetylcholine de l'organe electrique de la torpille et leurs modifications par la stimulation. *J. Neurochem.* 19, 1987-2002.

Eränkö, O. (1954). Quenching of tissues for freeze-drying. *Acta Anat.* 22, 331-336.

Eränkö, O. (1972). Light and electronmicroscopic evidence of granular and non-granular storage of catecholamines in the sympathetic ganglion of the rat. *Histochem. J.* 4, 213-224.

Euler, U.S. von & Hillarp, N.A. (1956). Evidence for the presence of noradrenaline in submicroscopic structures of adrenergic axons. *Nature* 177, 44-45.

Falck, B., Hillarp, N.A., Thieme, G. & Torp, A. (1962). Fluorescence of catecholamines and related compounds condensed with formaldehyde. *J. Histochem. Cytochem.* 10, 348-354.

Fillenz, M. (1971). The structure of noradrenaline storage vesicles in nerve terminals of the rat vas deferens. *Phil. Trans. Roy. Soc. B.* 261, 319-323.

Fillenz, M. (1977). The factors which provide short-term and long-term control of transmitter release. *Progr. Neurobiol.* 8, 251-278.

Fillenz, M., Gagnon, C., Stoeckel, K. & Thoenen, H. (1976). Selective uptake and retrograde axonal transport of dopamine-β-hydroxylase antibodies in peripheral adrenergic neurons. *Brain Res.* 114, 293-304.

Fillenz, M. & Howe, P.R.C. (1975). Depletion of noradrenaline stores in sympathetic nerve terminals. *J. Neurochem.* 24, 683-688.

Fillenz, M., Howe, P.R.C. & West, D.P. (1976). Vesicular noradrenaline in nerve terminals of rat heart following inhibition of monoamine-oxidase and administration of noradrenaline. *Neuroscience* 1, 113-116.

Fillenz, M. & Pollard, R.M. (1976). Quantitative differences between sympathetic nerve terminals. *Brain Res.* 109, 443-454.

Fillenz, M. & West, D.P. (1976). Fate of noradrenaline storage vesicles after release. *Neuroscience Letters* 2, 285-287.

Friend, R.C. & Blaustein, M.P. (1976). Synaptic vesicle recycling in synaptosomes *in vitro*. *Nature* 261, 255-256.

Geffen, L.B., Hunter, C. & Rush, R.A. (1969). Is there bidirectional transport of noradrenaline in sympathetic nerves? *J. Neurochem*. 16, 469-474.

Geffen, L.B., Jessell, T.M., Cuello, A.C. & Iversen, L.L. (1977). Release of dopamine from dendrites in rat substantia nigra. *Nature* 260, 258-260.

Gray, E.G. (1959). Axosmatic and axodendritic synapses of the cerebral cortex: an electron microscope study. *J. Anat*. 93, 420-433.

Gray, E.G. (1963). Electron microscopy of presynaptic organelles of the spinal cord. *J. Anat*. 97, 101-106.

Gray, E.G. (1975). Synaptic fine structure and nuclear cytoplasmic and extracellular networks. The stereoframework concept. *J. Neurocytol*. 4, 315-339.

Gray, E.G. (1976). Microtubules in synapses of the retina. *J. Neurocytol*. 5, 361-370.

Gray, E.G. (1977). Presynaptic microtubules, agranular reticulum and synaptic vesicles. In: *Synapses*, eds., G.A. Cottrell and P.N.N.R. Usherwood, Blackie, pp. 6-18.

Grillo, M. (1966). Electron microscopy of sympathetic tissues. *Pharmacol. Rev*. 18, 387-400.

Grillo, M. (1970). Extracellular synaptic vesicles in the mouse heart. *J. Cell. Biol*. 47, 547-553.

Grillo, M. & Palay, S.L. (1962). Granule-containing vesicles in the autonomic nervous system. In: *Electron Microscopy*, Vol. II (ed.) S.S. Breese, Jr., 5th Int. Congr. for E.M., U, 1.

Grynszpan-Winograd, O. (1971). Morphological aspects of exocytosis in the adrenal medulla. *Phil. Trans. Roy. Soc. B*. 261, 291-298.

Hager, H. & Tafuri, W.L. (1959). Elektronoptische Untersuchungen über die Feinstruktur des Plexus myenterieus (Auerbach) im Colon des Meerschweinchens (Cavia Cobaya). *Arch. Psychiat. Nervenkr*. 199, 437-471.

Hamilton, R.C. & Robinson, P.M. (1973). Disappearance of small vesicles from adrenergic nerve endings in the cat vas deferens caused by red black spider venom. *J. Neurocytol*. 2, 465-480.

Hellström, S. & Kjaergaard, J. (1976). Exocytosis in the carotid body type I cell. *J. Cell. Biol*. 70, 274a.

Heuser, J.E. & Reese, I.S. (1974). Morphology of synaptic vesicle discharge and reformation at the frog neuromuscular junction. In: *Synaptic Transmission and Neuronal Interaction* (ed.) M.V.L. Bennett, Raven Press, N.Y., pp. 59-78.

Heuser, J.E., Reese, T.S. & Landis, D.M.D. (1974). Functional changes in frog neuromuscular junctions studied with freeze-fracture. *J. Neurocytol.* 3, 109-131.

Heuser, J.E., Reese, T.S. & Landis, D.M.D. (1976). Preservation of synaptic structure by rapid freezing. *Cold Spr. Harb. Symp.* 49, 17-24.

Hillarp, N.-Å. (1946). Structure of the synapse and the peripheral innervation apparatus of the autonomic nervous system. *Acta Anat. Suppl.* IV, 153.

Hökfelt, T. (1969). Distribution of noradrenaline storing particles in peripheral adrenergic neurons as revealed by electron microscopy. *Acta Physiol. Scand.* 76, 427-440.

Hökfelt, T. (1973). On the origin of small adrenergic storage vesicles: Evidence for local formation in nerve endings after chronic reserpine treatment. *Experientia* 29, 580-582.

Hökfelt, T. (1974). Morphological contributions to monoamine pharmacology. *Fed. Proc.* 33, 2177-2186.

Hökfelt, T. & Jonsson, G. (1968). Studies on reaction and binding of monoamines after fixation and processing for electron-microscopy with special reference to fixation with potassium permanganate. *Histochemic.* 16, 45-47.

Holtzmann, E. (1977). The origin of secretory packages, especially synaptic vesicles. *Neuroscience* 2, 327-356.

Holtzmann, E., Teichberg, S., Citkowitz, E., Crain, S. de & Kawai, N. (1973). Notes on synaptic vesicles and related structures, endoplasmic reticulum, lysosomes and peroxisomes in nervous tissue and the adrenal medulla. *J. Histochem. Cytochem.* 21, 349-385.

Jacobowitz, D.M., Ziegler, M.G. & Thomas, J.A. (1975). *In vivo* uptake of antibody to dopamine-β-hydroxylase into sympathetic elements. *Brain Res.* 91, 165-170.

Kapeller, K. & Mayor, D. (1967). The accumulation of noradrenaline in constricted sympathetic nerves as studied by fluorescence and electron microscopy. *Proc. Roy. Soc. B.* 167, 282-292.

Katz, B. & Miledi, R. (1969). Tetrodotoxin-resistant electric activity in presynaptic terminals. *J. Physiol.* 203, 459-487.

Kopin, I.J., Breese, G.R., Krauss, K.R. & Weise, V. (1968). Selective release of newly synthesised norepinephrine from the cat spleen during sympathetic nerve stimulation. *J. Pharmacol. Exp. Ther.* 161, 271-278.

Lundberg, T., Bylock, A., Goldstein, M., Hansson, H.A. &
    Dahlström, A. (1977). Ultrastructural localisation of
    dopamine-β-hydroxylase in nerve terminals of the rat brain.
    Brain Res. 120, 549-552.

Malmfors, T. (1969). Histochemical studies on the release of
    adrenergic transmitter by nerve impulses in combination with
    drugs, especially adrenergic neuron blocking agents.
    Pharmacology 2, 138-150.

Marchbanks, R.M. (1975). The subcellular origin of the acetyl-
    choline released at synapses. *J. Biochem*. 6, 303-312.

Marchbanks, R.M. (1977). The relationship of the uptake of horse-
    radish peroxidase and release of acetylcholine from isolated
    nerve terminals. *Proc. I.U.P.S.* 12, 184.

Mollinoff, P.B. & Nelson, D.L. (1976). Effects of physiological
    and pharmacological stress on the subcellular distribution of
    adrenergic storage vesicles in rat heart. In: *Catecholamines
    and Stress* (eds.) I.J. Kopin and E. Usdin, Raven Press, N.Y.,
    pp. 401-406.

Nagatsu, I., Kondo, Y., Kato, T. & Nagatsu, T. (1976). Retrograde
    axoplasmic transport of inactive dopamine-β-hydroxylase in
    sciatic nerves. *Brain Res*. 116, 277-285.

Nelson, D.L. & Molinoff, P.B. (1976). Distribution and properties
    of adrenergic storage vesicles in nerve terminals. *J. Pharmacol.
    Exp. Ther*. 196, 346-359.

Pfenniger, K., Akert, K., Moor, H. & Sandri, C. (1972). The fine
    structure of freeze-fractured presynaptic membranes. *J. Neuro-
    cytol*. 1, 129-149.

Pfenniger, K.H. & Rovainen, C.M. (1974). Stimulation and calcium
    dependence of vesicle attachment sites in the presynaptic mem-
    brane, a freeze-cleave study on the lamprey spinal cord.
    Brain Res. 72, 1.

Pickel, V.M., Joh, T.H. & Reis, D.J. (1976). Monoamine synthe-
    sising enzymes in central dopaminergic, noradrenergic and sero-
    tonergic neurons. Immunocytochemical localization by light
    and electron microscopy. *J. Histochem. Cytochem*. 24, 792-806.

Plattner, H. (1970). A study on the interpretation of freeze-
    etched animal tissues and cell organelles. *Mikroskopie* 26,
    233-250.

Potter, L.T. & Axelrod, J. (1963). Properties of norepinephrine
    storage particles of the rat heart. *J. Pharmacol. Exp. Ther*.
    142, 299-305.

Richardson, K.C. (1962). The fine structure of autonomic nerve
    endings in smooth muscle of the rat vas deferens. *J. Anat*.
    96, 427-442.

Richardson, K.C. (1966). Electron microscopic identification of autonomic nerve endings. *Nature* 210, 756.

Smith, A.D. (1973). Mechanisms involved in the release of noradrenaline from sympathetic nerves. *Br. Med. Bull.* 29, 123-129.

Smith, A.D. & Winkler, H. (1972). Fundamental mechanisms in the release of catecholamines. In: *Catecholamines: Handbook of Experimental Pharmacology*, Vol. 33 (eds.) H. Blaschko and E. Muscholl, Springer-Verlag, Berlin, Heidelberg, New York, pp. 538-617.

Streit, P., Akert, K., Sandri, C., Livingston, R.B. & Moor, A. (1972). Dynamic ultrastructure of presynaptic membranes at nerve terminals in the spinal cord of rats. Anaesthetized and unanaesthetized preparations compared. *Brain Res.* 48, 11-26.

Taxi, J. (1961). Etude de l'ultrastructure des zones synaptiques dans les ganglions sympathiques de la grenouille. *C.R. Acad. Sci.* 252, 174-176.

Taxi, J. & Sotelo, C. (1973). On the dynamics of catecholamines storage structures in sympathetic neurons of the rat as studied by radioautography. In: *Frontiers of Catecholamine Research* (eds.) E. Usdin and S. Snyder, Pergamon Press, N.Y., pp. 509-511.

Teichberg, S. & Bloom, D. (1976). Uptake and fate of horseradish peroxidase in axons and terminals of sympathetic neurons. *J. Cell. Biol.* 70, 285a.

Thureson-Klein, A. (1975). Release of contents from noradrenergic vesicles by exocytosis. *J. Rep. Biol. Med.* 33, 365.

Thureson-Klein, A., Chen-Yen, S.H. & Klein, R.L. (1974). Retention of matrix density in adrenergic vesicles after extensive norepinephrine depletion. *Experientia* 30, 935-937.

Thureson-Klein, A. & Klein, R.L. (1975). Evidence for exocytosis from large dense core vesicles in noradrenergic neurons. *6th Int. Congr. Pharmacol.* p. 488.

Thureson-Klein, A., Klein, R.L. & Stjärne, L. (1976). Increased numbers of noradrenergic vesicles and exocytotoc profiles in nerves of human veins after field stimulation. *Neuroscience Abst.* 2, 997.

Thureson-Klein, A., Stjärne, L. & Brundin, J. (1976). Effects of field stimulation on nerve terminals in human blood vessels. *34th Ann. Proc. E.M. Soc. Amer.* (ed.) G.W. Bailey,

Till, R. & Banks, P. (1976). Pharmacological and ultrastructural studies on the electron dense cores of the vesicles that accumulate in noradrenergic axons constricted *in vitro*. *Neuroscience* 1, 49-55.

Tomlinson, D. (1975). Two populations of granular vesicles in constricted postganglionic sympathetic nerves. *J. Physiol.* 245, 727-735.

Tranzer, J.P. (1972). A new amine storing compartment in adrenergic axons. *Nature New Biol.* 237, 57-58.

Tranzer, J.P. (1973). New aspects of the localization of catecholamines in adrenergic neurons. In: *Frontiers of Catecholamine Research* (eds.) E. Usdin and S. Snyder, Pergamon Press, N.Y., pp. 453-458.

Tranzer, J.P. & Snipes, R. (1968). The structural localisation of noradrenaline in sympathetic nerve terminals. *Proc. 4th Eur. Reg. Conf. Elect. Microcop. Rome* 2, 519-520.

Tranzer, J.P. & Thoenen, H. (1967a). Electronmicroscopic localization of 5-hydroxydopamine (3,4,5-trihydroxy-phenyl-ethylamine) a new "false" sympathetic transmitter. *Experientia* 23, 743-745.

Tranzer, J.P. & Thoenen, H. (1967b). Significance of "empty vesicles" in postganglionic sympathetic nerve terminals. *Experientia* 24, 484-486.

Tranzer, J.P., Thoenen, H., Snipes, R.L. & Richards, J.G. (1969). Recent developments on the ultrastructural aspect of adrenergic nerve endings in various experimental conditions. *Progr. in Brain Res.* 31, 33-46.

Van Breemen, V.L., Anderson, E. & Reger, J.F. (1958). An attempt to determine the origin of synaptic vesicles. *Exp. Cell Res. Suppl.* 5, 153-167.

Viveros, O.H. (1975). Mechanisms of secretion of catecholamines from adrenal medulla. In: *Handbook of Physiology*, Section 7, Vol. 6 (eds.) H. Blaschko, G. Sayers and A.D. Smith, American Physiological Society, pp. 389-426.

Weiss, P. & Hiscoe, H.B. (1948). Experiments on the mechanism of nerve growth. *J. Exp. Zool.* 107, 315-395.

Whittaker, V.P. (1977). Acetylcholine storage and release in electromotor synapses of Torpedo. *Proc. I.U.P.S.* 12, 185.

Winkler, H. Schneider, F.H., Rufener, C., Nakane, P.K. & Hortnagl, H. (1974). Membranes of adrenal medulla: Their role in exocytosis. *Advances in Cytopharmacology* Vol. 2 (eds.) Cecarelli, B., Meldolesi, J. and Clementi, F., Raven Press, N.Y., pp. 127-139.

Wood, J.G. & Barnett, R.J. (1964). Histochemical demonstration of norepinephrine at a fine structural level. *J. Histochem. Cytochem.* 12, 197-209.

Woods, R.I. (1969). Acrylic aldehyde in sodium dichromate as a fixative for identifying catecholamine storage sites with the electron microscope. *J. Physiol.* 203, 35-36P.

Zimmermann, H. & Whittaker, V.P. (1974). Effect of electrical stimulation on the yield and composition of synaptic vesicles from the cholinergic synapses of the electric organ of Torpedo: A combined biochemical electrophysiological and morphological study. *J. Neurochem.* 22, 435-450.

THE ROLE OF CALCIUM IN CATECHOLAMINE RELEASE FROM ADRENERGIC NERVE TERMINALS

M. P. Blaustein

I   INTRODUCTION

It is now generally accepted that an increase in the intracellular calcium concentration is the signal which initiates secretion of neurotransmitter substances, although the precise mechanism of calcium's action has not yet been elucidated. There is also widespread, but not universal, acceptance of the idea that the transmitters are secreted in multi-molecular packets, or "quanta". The morphological correlates of these quanta are the synaptic vesicles, found in abundance in the presynaptic terminals of chemical synapses. Calcium-dependent release of the vesicular contents apparently occurs by exocytosis.

The available data show that secretory activity in many exocrine and endocrine glands and neurosecretory organs bears a striking resemblance to neurotransmitter release in terms of its calcium dependence and quantal nature. The convergent observations lead to the conclusion that all of these secretory processes are fundamentally similar. Thus, information about the secretory process obtained from any one type of preparation may provide useful insights into the mechanism of secretion in other secretory systems as well. This is particularly important under circumstances where different types of preparations are not all equally suitable for certain types of experimental manipulations. With these considerations in mind, the experimental observations on the frog neuromuscular junction, the squid giant synapse, and the mammalian adrenal medulla, all of which may have a bearing on transmitter release mechanisms at sympathetic nerve terminals, will be briefly reviewed. The authoritative reviews by Heuser & Reese (1977) and by Martin (1977) should be consulted for more detailed information on general aspects of synaptic morphology and physiology, respectively. The subsequent sections of this chapter are concerned primarily with the metabolism of calcium at presynaptic terminals and speculation about the role of calcium in the secretory process.

II   REVIEW OF THE EVIDENCE THAT CALCIUM
        PLAYS A ROLE IN EXOCYTOSIS

  A. Neuromuscular Junction

The seminal study of Harvey & MacIntosh (1940), on a sympathetic ganglion, was the first to establish the fact that Ca ions are required for neurotransmitter (acetylcholine) release. Electrophysiological studies, primarily by Katz and his colleagues, demonstrated that transmitter (acetylcholine) release at the frog neuromuscular junction is quantal (Fatt & Katz, 1952; Del Castillo & Katz, 1954a). Subsequently, Katz & Miledi (1965; 1967a) showed that transmitter release could be triggered in the absence of nerve impulses, provided that Ca was present when the nerve terminal was depolarized (by focal current pulses). This led to the enunciation of the "Calcium Hypothesis", viz.: depolarization causes an increase in the calcium permeability of the presynaptic terminal plasmalemma. Ca then enters the terminal, moving down its electrochemical gradient. The consequent rise in the intra-terminal calcium concentration then, by an unknown mechanism, induces the fusion of the synaptic vesicle membrane with the plasma membrane so that the vesicular contents are extruded into the synaptic cleft.

The morphological studies of De Robertis & Bennett (1955) provided the first evidence of structural correlates for the transmitter quanta: they named the small vesicles, found in abundance in the presynaptic terminals, "synaptic vesicles", and suggested that these vesicles might be filled with neurotransmitter. Biochemical data from nerve terminal fractionation studies (De Robertis, Pellegrino de Iraldi, Rodriquez de Lores Arnaiz & Salganicoff, 1962; Gray & Whittaker, 1962), showed that some synaptic vesicles did, indeed, contain acetylcholine. Moreover, extracellular marker uptake and vesicle membrane recycling studies (especially by Heuser & Reese, 1973) have provided strong support for the hypothesis that acetylcholine is released by exocytosis of vesicular contents.

B. Adrenal Medulla

Douglas and his colleagues carried out a number of pioneering studies on the role of calcium in the secretion of catecholamines by the adrenal medulla. In particular, Douglas & Rubin (1961; 1963) showed that extracellular Ca (or Sr or Ba; Douglas & Rubin, 1964) is required for secretion, and that Ca-dependent secretion can be triggered by either acetylcholine or a potassium-rich medium. Both of these treatments depolarize the chromaffin cells and induce them to take up Ca from the bathing medium (Douglas & Poisner, 1961 and 1962). The sequence of events: depolarization → Ca uptake → catecholamine release, was termed, "Stimulus-Secretion Coupling" by Douglas & Rubin (1961) to emphasize the analogy to excitation-contraction coupling in muscle (Sandow, 1952; and cf. Costantin, 1977). This sequence is, of course, essentially identical to the "Calcium Hypothesis" of Katz & Miledi, mentioned above.

The evidence that the contents of adrenal chromaffin cell secretory granules are secreted by exocytosis is quite strong. In addition to catecholamines, the secretory granules contain ATP and the soluble proteins chromogranin A and dopamine-β-hydroxylase. Stimulation of secretion in the adrenal medulla induces the release of these substances in approximate proportion to their respective concentrations within the secretory granules

(see the review by Kirshner & Viveros, 1970); the contents of
each secretory granule appears to be released in all-or-none
fashion (Viveros, Arqueros & Kirshner, 1969).

Recent electrophysiological experiments on adrenal medullary
chromaffin cells provide evidence for a previously unrecognized
similarity between these cells and neurons. Brandt, Hagiwara,
Kidoroko & Miyazaki (1976) studied the electrical properties of
disaggregated rat adrenal chromaffin cells, while Biales, Dichter
& Tischler (1976) examined cultured human and gerbil chromaffin
cells. Both groups were able to elicit regenerative, overshoot-
ing action potentials in the cells by passing depolarizing current pulses. These action potentials appeared to be due primarily
to an inward Na current because they were markedly reduced when
Na was omitted from the bathing medium, or when 1 μM tetrodotoxin
was added. In addition, Brandt *et al.* obtained evidence that the
action potentials also had a Ca conductance component: a small regenerative spike was observed in Na-free media, and this action
potential (which presumably involves divalent ion-selective channels; see section IV) was prolonged when external Ca was replaced
by Ba. Both groups found that acetylcholine depolarized the chromaffin cells; this depolarization could either trigger action
potentials or enhance spontaneous spike activity in the cells.
The implication, from these studies, is that secretion is normally
triggered by the following sequence of events in adrenal chromaffin cells: acetylcholine (released by the neurons which in-
nervate the adrenal medulla) depolarizes the cells, thereby inducing spike activity. This increases the Ca conductance of the
plasma membrane, and Ca enters the cells and triggers secretion
by exocytosis.

C.   Squid Giant Synapse

Some of the strongest evidence in support of the calcium hypothesis has been obtained from a series of elegant experiments on the
squid giant synapse by Katz & Miledi (1967b); 1969a) and by
Kusano and his colleagues (Kusano, Livengood & Werman, 1967;
Kusano, 1970). These investigators showed that depolarization of
tetrodotoxin-blocked terminals is sufficient to trigger an increase in Ca conductance, and release of neurotransmitter: the
magnitude of the depolarization-induced inward current depended
upon the Ca concentration in the bathing medium, and depolarization to about + 130 mV (i.e., in the neighborhood of the Ca equilibrium potential) suppressed both the inward current and transmitter release. The association between the increase in the intracellular Ca concentration and transmitter release was directly
demonstrated by Llinas & Nicholson (1975); they injected the Ca-
sensitive photoprotein, aequorin, into the presynaptic terminals,
and detected the depolarization-induced rise in the ionized Ca^{2+}
concentration by an increase in light output. Furthermore,
Miledi (1973) showed that iontophoresis of Ca, but not Mg, into
the presynaptic terminal triggers transmitter release without depolarization. These experiments provide clear-cut evidence that
an increase in the intraterminal free Ca^{2+} concentration($[Ca^{2+}]_i$)
is necessary and sufficient to induce transmitter release.

    D. Sympathetic Nerve Terminals

The spectrum of properties reviewed in the preceding three sub-
sections are also characteristic of sympathetic nerve terminals
(e.g., see the review by Smith, 1972). Burn & Gibbons (1964)
employed a rabbit ileum preparation to demonstrate that release
of noradrenaline from postganglionic sympathetic fibers requires
Ca in the bathing medium. Subsequently, Huković & Muscholl (1962)
showed that the amount of noradrenaline released from cardiac
sympathetic neurons, per impulse, is reduced when the Ca concentration in the bathing medium is reduced. Kirpekar & Misu (1967)
explored the effects of alkali metal ions on transmitter release
from the electrically-stimulated splenic nerve; they showed that
Sr and Ba could substitute for Ca in supporting noradrenaline release. On the other hand, increasing the concentration of Mg in
the bathing medium reduced the transmitter output, an effect comparable to the inhibition by Mg of acetylcholine release at the
frog neuromuscular junction (Del Castillo & Katz, 1954b).

Baldessarini & Kopin (1966; and see Katz & Kopin 1969) showed that
electric field stimulation of brain and heart slices triggered the
Ca-dependent release of noradrenaline from these tissues; although
K-rich media also enhanced noradrenaline release, the Ca dependence of this effect was not tested. Toxin from the scorpion,
Leiurus quinquestriatus, which depolarizes neurons by a Na-depen-
dent, tetrodotoxin-sensitive mechanism (Narahashi, Shapiro,
Deguchi, Scuka & Wang, 1972), has also been shown to stimulate
noradrenaline release from peripheral adrenergic neurons; the
toxin-induced release is blocked by tetrodotoxin, and reduced
when Ca is omitted from the bathing medium (Moss, Thoa & Kopin,
1974).

Another preparation which has recently become popular for the
study of presynaptic function is the pinched-off nerve terminal
("synaptosome") preparation of De Robertis *et al*. (1962) and Gray
& Whittaker (1962). Many of the pinched-off terminals have membrane potentials (Blaustein & Goldring, 1975) and depolarizing
agents stimulate Ca uptake and transmitter release in these preparations (Blaustein, 1975). For example, the catecholaminergic
terminals (in the heterogeneous population) release noradrenaline
when treated with veratridine, scorpion toxin or K-rich media;
the evoked release can be prevented by omitting Ca from the media
or, in the case of veratridine or scorpion toxin stimulation, by
adding tetrodotoxin (Blaustein, Johnson & Needleman, 1972;
Blaustein, 1975; Raiteri, Levi & Federico, 1975; Mulder, Van Den
Berg & Stoof, 1975; Cotman, Haycock & Frost, 1976). The transmitter may be released by exocytosis because these terminals show
evidence of synaptic vesicle recycling (Fried & Blaustein, 1976).
[Of course, since the terminal population is heterogenous, one
cannot be certain that the catecholaminergic terminals take up Ca
or demonstrate vesicle recycling, when stimulated.]

All of the preceding observations are consistent with the calcium
hypothesis of stimulus-secretion coupling. In addition, the
electrophysiological behavior of the sympathetic nerve-smooth

muscle junction may be similar to that of many other types of
chemical synapses. One important observation, by Burnstock &
Holman (1961; 1966) is that sympathetic nerve-smooth muscle junctions exhibit spontaneous junction potentials, analogous to the
miniature endplate potentials observed at cholinergic neuromuscular junctions (Del Castillo & Katz, 1954a). Moreover, the amplitude of the evoked excitatory junction potential at the sympathetic endings is reduced by Mg (Bennett, 1973), as is the case at
the motor nerve-skeletal muscle junction (Del Castillo & Katz,
1954b). These junction potentials also show facilitation and
fatigue in response to trains of stimuli to the adrenergic nerve
axons (Burnstock & Kuriyama, 1964; Holman, 1970; Bennett, 1973),
again, analogous to the effects observed at cholinergic junctions
(Eccles & McFarlane, 1949; Mallart & Martin, 1967 and 1968) as
well as other synapses. Calcium ions play a critical role in
facilitation at the motor nerve-skeletal muscle junction (Katz &
Miledi, 1968), and it will be of considerable interest to determine whether or not this is also the case at the sympathetic
neuron-smooth muscle junction.

A variety of studies on tissues with sympathetic nerve innervation
have demonstrated that, as in the adrenal medulla, secretion of
noradrenaline is accompanied by the secretion of the soluble intra-
vesicular proteins, chromogranin A and dopamine-β-hydroxylase
(e.g., De Potter, de Schaepdryver, Moerman & Smith, 1969; Gewirtz
& Kopin, 1970); the amount of protein released is proportional to
the amount of catecholamine released (Smith, 1971; Weinshilboum,
Thoa, Johnson, Kopin & Axelrod, 1972). The release of both noradrenaline and dopamine-β-hydroxylase from sympathetic neurons is
augmented when the Ca concentration in the bathing medium is elevated (Johnson, Thoa, Weinshilboum, Axelrod & Kopin, 1971). Moreover, dopamine-β-hydroxylase, alone, is released when sympathetic
neurons are stimulated following reserpine-induced depletion of
noradrenaline stores (Thoa, Wooten, Axelrod & Kopin, 1975). In
sum, these experiments imply that the release of noradrenaline
from sympathetic nerve endings involves a Ca-dependent exocytotic
mechanism which is normally triggered by depolarization. However,
there remains some controversy over the question of whether the
entire content of each secretory vesicle is released in all-or-
none fashion, or whether only a small fraction is released at a
time. The latter possibility has been proposed to explain apparent discrepancies between the calculated amount of catecholamine
contained in one vesicle, and the amount released per impulse
(Folkow & Häggendal, 1970; Stjärne, 1970).

III   CALCIUM-DEPENDENT VERSUS CALCIUM-INDEPENDENT
       NORADRENALINE RELEASE

The aforementioned observations on sympathetic nerve terminals
provide overwhelming evidence that these terminals can, when depolarized, release transmitter by a Ca-dependent mechanism
(presumably as a consequence of Ca entry into the terminals). In
addition, however, noradrenaline may be released by mechanisms
which do not require Ca. One typical example is tyramine-induced

noradrenaline release (cf. Thoa, Wooten, Axelrod & Kopin, 1975):
tyramine is transported into the terminals and accumulated in the
secretory vesicles, thereby displacing noradrenaline which then
leaks into the cytosol and is transported out of the terminals
(perhaps on a "carrier").

Although K-stimulated noradrenaline release is inhibited when external Ca is removed (see section II-D), Bogdanski & Brodie (1969)
have also observed a Ca-independent K-promoted noradrenaline release. Reaccumulation of noradrenaline by the presynaptic terminals appears to involve the carrier-mediated cotransport of Na
with noradrenaline; net accumulation of noradrenaline, against a
concentration gradient, is driven by energy derived from the Na
electrochemical gradient across the plasmalemma (White, 1976).
Since the transport of Na + noradrenaline involves the movement
of net charge across the membrane, a reduction in the Na electrochemical gradient (either by depolarization or alteration of the
Na concentrations) should favor noradrenaline efflux via the
carrier-mediated transport system (cf. Blaustein & King, 1977).
This mechanism may also explain why depletion of extracellular
Na enhances norepinephrine release (Kirpekar & Wakade, 1968;
Paton, 1973), but not dopamine-β-hydroxylase release (Garcia &
Kirpekar, 1975), and why inhibition of metabolism (Chang, von
Euler & Lishajko, 1972) or of the Na pump (Paton, 1973) also enhances noradrenaline release; in these instances, the release
would be non-vesicular. Alternatively, since Ca efflux from nerve
terminals appears also to be coupled to Na influx via Na-Ca exchange (Blaustein & Ector, 1976; and see below), it is possible
that reducing the Na electrochemical gradient may, by enhancing
net Ca entry, also promote some vesicular transmitter release by
(Ca-dependent) exocytosis.

It is quite clear that several different mechanisms may mediate
transmitter efflux from the nerve terminals; consequently, the Ca
dependency, among other parameters, must be carefully tested.

IV   HOW DOES Ca ENTER THE TERMINALS?

The as yet unproven assumption, which follows from the preceding
discussion, is that the depolarization-evoked, Ca-dependent noradrenaline release at catecholaminergic endings involves exocytosis of vesicular contents, triggered by a rise in $[Ca^{2+}]_i$. It is
clear that future efforts should be directed toward the preparation and study of isolated adrenergic nerve terminals, in an
effort to unequivocally demonstrate Ca entry and vesicle recycling
in these terminals. Despite this uncertainty, the circumstantial
evidence is very strong. It therefore appears worthwhile to examine the available data on Ca metabolism at nerve terminals in
general, on the assumption that this information will help provide
insight into the mechanisms underlying noradrenaline release at
catecholaminergic endings.

As noted above, depolarization of the terminals induces an increase in Ca conductance; Ca then enters the terminals, moving

(passively) down its electrochemical gradient. The first question
to be answered, then, is: what is the mechanism responsible for
this Ca entry?

At the squid synapse, this process is manifested as an external
Ca-dependent net inward current (Katz & Miledi, 1969; and see
Llinas, 1977) associated with a rise in $[Ca^{2+}]_i$ (Llinas, Blinks &
Nicholson, 1972; Llinas & Nicholson, 1975) while in synaptosomes,
the net Ca entry has been measured chemically (Blaustein, 1975).
The available evidence indicates that the depolarization triggers
the opening of "Ca-selective channels", analogous to the "Na-selective channels" observed in many excitable cells. The Ca-selective channels differ from Na-selective channels in that the latter
are blocked by tetrodotoxin, and normally inactivate (i.e., close)
within a few milliseconds when depolarization is maintained (cf.,
Hille, 1977). The Ca channels, on the other hand, are not affected by tetrodotoxin (Katz & Miledi, 1969a; Blaustein, 1975) and inactivate only slowly, if at all (Katz & Miledi, 1971; Blaustein,
1975); they are blocked by other divalent cations (e.g., Mg^{2+} and
Mn^{2+}; Katz & Miledi, 1969b; Blaustein, 1975) and by verapamil and
D-600 (Kohlhardt, Bauer, Krause & Fleckenstein, 1972; Baker &
Glitsch, 1975).

At the squid giant synapse, the Ca channels appear to be confined
primarily to the presynaptic terminal membrane near the active
zone (Katz & Miledi, 1969a). Heuser (1977) has suggested that the
large intramembranous particles seen in freeze-fracture electron
micrographs of the neuromuscular junction active zone membrane may
be Ca channels. Venzin, Sandri, Akert & Wyss (1977) have observed
similar structures at mammalian central synapses, and have also
speculated that these particles may be Ca channels.

In order to understand how Ca triggers transmitter release, we may
begin by determining how much Ca is required to evoke secretion;
i.e., to what level is the ionized Ca^{2+} raised? Llinas (1977) has
obtained a value of about 35 µA for the Ca current density at the
squid synapse. If the interval between depolarization and transmitter release is about 200 µsec (Hubbard & Schmidt, 1963), and
the mean displacement of Ca is about 1500 A from the plasmalemma
(Parsegian, 1977), the Ca^{2+} concentration in the cytoplasm, within
1500 A of the plasmalemma, will increase (in 200 µsec) to about 3-
4 µM (starting from an initial level of about 0.1 µM; see below).
In synaptosomes, the K-stimulated Ca uptake, ~2-3 µmoles/gm protein x min (Blaustein, 1975) corresponds to about 4×10^{-24} moles/
synaptosome x msec (cf., Blaustein, 1975); if all the Ca enters
the terminals at the active zone (~4×10^{-10} cm^2) and remains within 1500 A of the plasma membrane for 200 µsec, $[Ca^{2+}]_i$ would increase by about 0.2 µM. [This value may be an underestimate if the
Ca channels inactivate during a 60 sec depolarization, or if a significant fraction of the resealed terminals are non-functional.]

V   WHAT IS THE ROLE OF CALCIUM IN VESICULAR EXOCYTOSIS?

Available evidence (see below) indicates that the level of free
(ionized) Ca^{2+} in the cytosol of resting neurons is probably on
the order of $10^{-7}M$. Moreover, as noted in the preceding section,
the amount of Ca which enters during a normal transient depolarization may only increase $[Ca^{2+}]_i$ to 10^{-6} or $10^{-5}M$ (at most).
This implies that the mechanism which regulates exocytosis is
probably activated by Ca^{2+} concentrations in the range between
10^{-7} and $10^{-5}M$. In addition, the intracellular ionized Mg^{2+} concentration ($[Mg^{2+}]_i$) may be on the order of $10^{-3}M$ (e.g., see De
Weer, 1976); consequently, the regulatory mechanism must have a
very high selectivity for Ca^{2+} over Mg^{2+}.

Several types of mechanisms have been proposed to explain Ca-dependent exocytosis. One hypothesis is that vesicles may move
randomly in the cytoplasm near the plasma membrane. A rise in
$[Ca^{2+}]_i$ might, for example, increase the fluidity of the cytoplasm (cf., Hodgkin & Katz, 1949) near the plasmalemma, so that
the chances of collision between vesicles and the plasmalemma may
be increased (e.g., Mathews, 1970). Two important criticisms
have been leveled against this hypothesis: 1. Rather high Ca^{2+}
concentrations ($\sim 10^{-3}M$) may be required to increase significantly
the fluidity of the cytosol (Hodgkin & Katz, 1949), and; 2. It is
unlikely that the activation energy for fusion will often be exceeded because of electrostatic repulsion between vesicles and
plasmalemma (Mathews, 1970; Parsegian, 1977).

A hypothesis which may circumvent the latter criticism is that the
Ca^{2+} ions bind to the vesicle membrane and intracellular surface
of the plasmalemma, thereby neutralizing the surface charges on
these membranes, so that electrostatic repulsion is reduced
(Blioch, Glagoleva, Liberman & Nenashev, 1968; Matthews, 1970;
Matthews & Nordmann, 1976). However, it seems unlikely that small
changes in $[Ca^{2+}]_i$ will significantly influence surface charge in
the presence of an ambient $[Mg^{2+}]_i$ on the order of $10^{-3}M$ (cf.,
Parsegian, 1977). Heuser (1977) has observed that a high concentration of Mg in the bathing medium greatly increases the contact
between vesicles and plasmalemma, at the neuromuscular junction,
so that the plasmalemma actually bulges over the vesicles; fusion
is not observed, however. This implies that fusion involves another type of process.

Parsegian (1977) has calculated that, on energetic grounds, fusion
mechanisms involving purely physical forces are highly improbable.
An alternative hypothesis invokes Ca-activated systems which pull
the vesicles up to the plasmalemma and/or displace the polar
groups on the surfaces of the vesicles and plasmalemma. The latter effect may be particularly important. Parsegian (1977) has
shown that, when the separation between membranes is less than
about 30 A, electrostatic forces are much smaller than hydration
forces. Considerable work is required to strip the water molecules from the phospholipid polar head-groups, or to displace the
polar groups, so that the hydrophobic regions from the two membranes can coalesce.

Examples of suggested Ca-activated systems include those involving microtubules, microfilaments (Lacy, Howell, Young & Funk,
1968; Thoa, Wooten, Axelrod & Kopin, 1972; but see Douglas &
Sorimachi, 1972) or contractile proteins (Berl, Puszkin & Nicklas,
1973), all of which appear to be present in nerve terminals. Alternatively, the Ca may be required to activate a biochemical reaction, such as ATP hydrolysis or cleavage of phospholipid polar
headgroups, in order to initiate vesicle-plasmalemma fusion. The
attraction of these hypotheses is that they invoke the specific
binding of Ca to proteins - presumably at high-affinity binding
sites; this is consistent with the sensitivity and selectivity of
the exocytosis mechanism for Ca^{2+}. Unfortunately, crucial data
are still lacking, and it remains to be seen whether or not one
of these Ca-regulated systems does, indeed, participate in neurotransmitter release.

VI   CALCIUM BUFFERING IN NERVE TERMINALS

In the preceding sections, reference was made to the fact that
$[Ca^{2+}]_i$ in the cytoplasm of resting neurons (including terminals)
may be on the order of $10^{-7}M$. What is the evidence for this
statement? The evidence is most direct and convincing for squid
giant axons and synapses. Katz & Miledi (1967b) have shown that,
when the presynaptic terminals are depolarized to about + 130 mV,
transmitter release is suppressed - presumably because this volt-
age corresponds to the Ca equilibrium potential (E_{Ca}), and there
will be no net Ca entry even though the Ca channels are open.
With an E_{Ca} of + 130 mV and an external Ca^{2+} concentration of 11
mM, $[Ca^{2+}]_i$ should be about $4 \times 10^{-7}M$. In the giant axon, more
direct measurements, employing the Ca-sensitive photoprotein,
aequorin, have provided estimates of about $0.3 - 5 \times 10^{-7}M$ (Baker,
Hodgkin & Ridgeway, 1971; DiPolo, Requena, Brinley, Mullins,
Scarpa & Tiffert, 1976).

Data regarding $[Ca^{2+}]_i$ in vertebrate neurons and nerve terminals
is much more indirect. One type of evidence is purely circumstantial, and is based on the known ability of mitochondria, including
those from brain (Lazarewicz, Haljamae & Hamberger, 1974), to accumulate Ca or phosphorylate ADP at the expense of energy derived
from electron transport. At ambient Ca^{2+} concentrations of a few
micromolar or more, most of the energy obtained from electron
transport will be used to take up Ca, in preference to ADP phosphorylation (Rossi & Lehninger, 1964). Since this is hardly likely to be the prevailing condition in most neurons, $[Ca^{2+}]_i$ is
most probably about $10^{-6}M$ or less.

Studies from our laboratory (Kendrick, Blaustein, Ratzlaff &
Fried, 1976; Blaustein, Ratzlaff & Kendrick, 1977) have indicated
that there is another Ca sequestering system in nerve terminals -
perhaps associated with the smooth endoplasmic reticulum. This
system, which requires ATP, has a higher affinity for Ca^{2+} than
does the mitochondrial transport system: the non-mitochondrial
transport is half-saturated at a Ca^{2+} concentration of about 0.35
μM (Blaustein *et al.*, 1977). If this transport system helps to

buffer intracellular Ca^{2+} in order to keep $[Ca^{2+}]_i$ low enough so that mitochondria can phosphorylate ADP, we would not expect the system to be saturated in resting neurons; the implication is that $[Ca^{2+}]_i$ may therefore be on the order of 0.5 µM or less. In fact, data from our laboratory (Schweitzer & Blaustein, unpublished) indicate that disrupted synaptosomes (with the intraterminal organelles exposed) can buffer Ca^{2+} to a level of about 0.3-0.5 µM when Ca^{2+} (up to about 50 µmoles Ca/mg protein - or 8-10 times the normal tissue Ca level) is added to the suspensions; in these experiments the Ca-sensitive dye, arsenazo III, was used to measure ionized Ca^{2+} (Kendrick, Ratzlaff & Blaustein, 1977).

In addition to the aforementioned Ca sequestration mechanisms (involving mitochondria and, perhaps, the smooth endoplasmic reticulum), it seems possible that intracellular Ca may also be buffered by soluble cytoplasmic high-affinity Ca-binding proteins. One example is the Ca-binding protein from squid axoplasm described by Baker & Schlaepfer (1975). However, no such protein has yet been identified in vertebrate neuronal cytoplasm.

These Ca-buffering mechanisms may play an important role in terminating evoked, Ca-dependent secretion at the nerve terminals - by rapidly (within a couple of milliseconds) buffering the Ca which enters during depolarization. It is clear these systems have a limited capacity, however, and cannot account for the long-term regulation of cell Ca.

VII   EXTRUSION OF CALCIUM FROM NERVE TERMINALS

The Ca which enters during depolarization must eventually be extruded, in order for the terminals to return to the normal resting condition. This Ca must be moved out against a very large electrochemical gradient: the resting membrane potential is about -60 mV, inside negative, and the $[Ca^{2+}]out/[Ca^{2+}]in$ ratio is on the order of 10^{-4} in mammalian neurons. Thus some type of energy-linked transport system is required.

When synaptosomes are loaded with Ca, net extrusion of Ca requires the presence of Na in the external medium (Blaustein & Ector, 1976); furthermore, an increase in intracellular Na and/or a decrease in extracellular Na tends to promote Ca entry into the terminals (Blaustein & Oborne, 1975). These observations have led to the suggestion (Blaustein & Ector, 1976) that Ca extrusion from the nerve terminals may be mediated by a Na-Ca counter-transport mechanism powered by energy from the Na electrochemical gradient, rather than directly from ATP. This Ca transport system may therefore be similar to the one observed in squid axons and a variety of other types of cells (Blaustein, 1974 and 1977).

The Ca entry, buffering and extrusion mechanisms are summarized in the diagram in Fig. 1. The main point is that when Ca enters the terminals, and raises $[Ca^{2+}]_i$ acutely, some Ca may be rapidly re-extruded; however, most of the entering Ca is presumably buffered by Ca-binding proteins, smooth endoplasmic reticulum and mitochond-

ria. Then, as the extrusion mechanism tends to lower $[Ca^{2+}]_i$
further, the buffers release some of the bound Ca. This process
maintains $[Ca^{2+}]_i$ at a slightly elevated level until all the Ca
which entered the terminals during depolarization is extruded,
and the normal resting Ca balance is re-established. An interesting possibility is that facilitation, which appears to result from
Ca retention by the terminals (Katz & Miledi, 1968), may be explained by this Ca buffering and delayed extrusion.

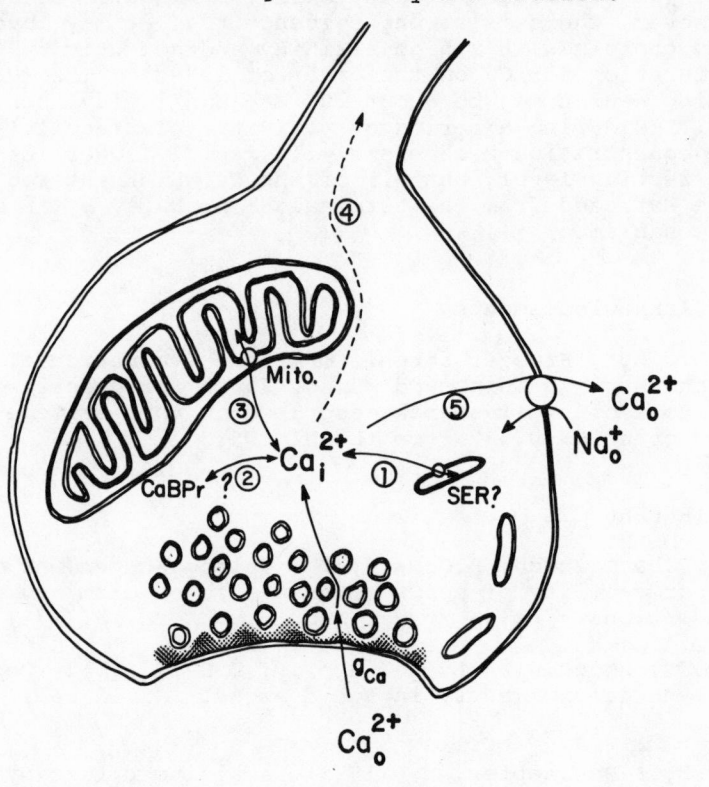

Fig. 1.   Diagram of presynaptic nerve terminal illustrating intra-
          terminal Ca compartmentation and the main routes of Ca
          entry and exit. A large (net) influx of Ca occurs when
          the terminal is depolarized, as a result of a transient
          increase in the Ca conductance (g_{Ca}). The rise in
          $[Ca^{2+}]_i$ triggers transmitter release. Some of the Ca
          which enters may be rapidly bound to cytoplasmic Ca bind-
          ing proteins (BPr; reaction number 2); some Ca may be se-
          questered, by energy-dependent reactions, in vesicles
          (perhaps smooth endoplasmic reticulum, or SER; reaction
          number 1) and in mitochondria (reaction number 3). A
          small fraction may diffuse into the axon (reaction num-
          ber 4). Eventually, all the Ca which entered must be ex-
          truded; Na-Ca exchange appears to play an important role
          here (reaction number 5). See text for further details
          (from Blaustein, Ratzlaff & Kendrick, 1977).

VIII SUMMARY AND CONCLUSION

Evidence has been reviewed which implicates the following sequence of events in catecholaminergic nerve terminals: depolarization of the terminal (by an invading action potential) $\rightarrow$ increased membrane Ca conductance $\rightarrow$ net Ca entry $\rightarrow$ rise in $[Ca^{2+}]_i$ $\rightarrow$ transmitter release by exocytosis of synaptic vesicle contents. The mechanism by which the exocytosis is triggered remains uncertain; however, there is strong evidence that it may involve a Ca-modulated protein with a high affinity and selectivity for Ca (half-saturation for Ca on the order of $10^{-6}M$). The $[Ca^{2+}]_i$ in the resting neuron may be about $10^{-7}M$; $[Ca^{2+}]_i$ may increase to 10^{-6} or $10^{-5}M$ during a period of activity. Intracellular Ca binding and sequestration mechanisms will rapidly lower $[Ca^{2+}]_i$ toward the resting level, but all of the Ca which entered must eventually be extruded from the terminals - probably by an Na-Ca exchange mechanism.

Acknowledgements

I thank Dr. B.K. Krueger for his critical evaluation of the manuscript, and Mrs. A. Guinn and Ms. J. Jones for preparing the typescript. Some of the research described in this article was supported by grant NS-08442 from the NINCDS.

IX   REFERENCES

Baker, P.F. & Glitsch, H.G. (1975). Voltage-dependent changes in the permeability of nerve membranes to calcium and other divalent cations. *Phil. Trans. Roy. Soc. Lond. B.* 270, 389-409.

Baker, P.F., Hodgkin, A.L. & Ridgeway, E.B. (1971). Depolarization and calcium entry in squid axons. *J. Physiol.* 218, 709-755.

Baker, P.F. & Schlaepfer, W. (1975). Calcium uptake by axoplasm extruded from giant axons of *Loligo*. *J. Physiol.* 249, 37P-38P.

Baldessarini, R.J. & Kopin, I.J. (1966). Tritiated norepinephrine: release from brain slices by electrical stimulation. *Science* 152, 1630-1631.

Bennett, M.R. (1973). An electrophysiological analysis of the storage and release of noradrenaline at sympathetic nerve terminals. *J. Physiol.* 229, 515-531.

Berl, S., Puszkin, S. & Nicklas, W.J. (1973). Actomyosin-like protein in brain. *Science* 179, 441-446.

Biales, B., Dichter, M. & Tischler, A. (1976). Electrical excitability of cultured adrenal chromaffin cells. *J. Physiol.* 262, 743-753.

Blaustein, M.P. (1974). The interrelationship between sodium and calcium fluxes across cell membranes. *Rev. Physiol. Biochem. Pharmacol.* 70, 33-82.

Blaustein, M.P. (1975). Effects of potassium, veratridine and scorpion venom on calcium accumulation and transmitter release by nerve terminals *in vitro*. *J. Physiol.* 247, 617-655.

Blaustein, M.P. (1977). Sodium ions, calcium ions, blood pressure regulation and hypertension: a reassessment and a hypothesis. *Am. J. Physiol.* 232, C165-C173.

Blaustein, M.P. & Ector, A.C. (1976). Carrier-mediated sodium-dependent and calcium-dependent calcium efflux from pinched-off presynaptic nerve terminals (synaptosomes) *in vitro*. *Biochim. Biophys. Acta* 419, 295-308.

Blaustein, M.P. & Goldring, J.M. (1975). Membrane potentials in pinched-off presynaptic nerve terminals monitored with a fluorescent probe: evidence that synaptosomes have diffusion potentials. *J. Physiol.* 247, 589-615.

Blaustein, M.P., Johnson, E.M., Jr. & Needleman, P. (1972). Calcium-dependent norepinephrine release from presynaptic nerve endings *in vitro*. *Proc. Natl. Acad. Sci.* [*U.S.A.*] 69, 2237-2240.

Blaustein, M.P. & King, A.C. (1976). Influence of membrane potential on the sodium-dependent uptake of gamma-aminobutyric acid by presynaptic nerve terminals: experimental observations and theoretical considerations. *J. Membr. Biol.* 30, 153-173.

Blaustein, M.P. & Oborne, C.J. (1975). The influence of sodium on calcium fluxes in pinched-off nerve terminals *in vitro*. *J. Physiol.* 247, 657-686.

Blaustein, M.P., Ratzlaff, R.W. & Kendrick, N.C. (1977). The regulation of intracellular calcium in presynaptic nerve terminals. *Ann. N.Y. Acad. Sci.*, in press.

Blioch, Z.L., Glagoleva, I.M., Liberman, E.A. & Nenashev, V.A. (1968). A study of the mechanism of quantal transmitter release at a chemical synapse. *J. Physiol.* 199, 11-35.

Bagdanski, D.F. & Brodie, B.B. (1969). The effects of inorganic ions on the storage and uptake of H^3-norepinephrine by rat heart slices. *J. Pharmacol. Exp. Ther.* 165, 181-189.

Brandt, B.L., Hagiwara, S., Kidoroko, Y. & Miyazaki, S. (1976). Action potentials in the rat chromaffin cell and the effects of acetylcholine. *J. Physiol.* 263, 417-439.

Burn, J.H. & Gibbons, W.R. (1964). The part played by calcium in determining the response to stimulation of sympathetic postganglionic fibres. *Br. J. Pharmacol.* 22, 540-548.

M. P. Blaustein

Burnstock, G. & Holman, M.E. (1961). The transmission of excita-
    tion from autonomic nerve to smooth muscle. *J. Physiol.* 155,
    115-133.

Burnstock, G. & Holman, M.E. (1966). Junction potentials at ad-
    renergic synapses. *Pharmacol. Rev.* 18, 481-493.

Burnstock, G. & Kuriyama, H. (1964). Facilitation of transmission
    from autonomic nerve to smooth muscle of guinea-pig vas defer-
    ens. *J. Physiol.* 172, 31-49.

Chang, P., von Euler, V.S. & Lishajko, F. (1972). Effects of 2,
    -4-dinitrophenol on release and uptake of noradrenaline in
    guinea pig heart. *Acta Physiol. Scand.* 85, 501-505.

Costantin, L.L. (1977). Activation in striated muscle. In:
    Handbook of Physiology Section 1: *The Nervous System* Vol. I,
    Part 1 (Section eds.) J.M. Brookhart & V.B. Mountcastle
    (Volume ed.) E.R. Kandel, American Physiological Society,
    Bethesda, MD, pp. 215-259.

Cotman, C.W., Haycock, J.W. & White, W.F. (1976). Stimulus-secre-
    tion coupling processes in brain: analysis of noradrenaline
    and gamma-aminobutyric and release. *J. Physiol.* 254, 475-505.

Del Castillo, J. & Katz, B. (1954a). Quantal components of the
    endplate potential. *J. Physiol.* 124, 560-573.

Del Castillo, J. & Katz, B. (1954b). The effect of magnesium on
    the activity of motor nerve endings. *J. Physiol.* 124, 553-559.

De Potter, W.P., de Schaepdryver, A.F., Moerman, E.J. & Smith,
    A.D. (1969). Evidence for the release of vesicle-proteins to-
    gether with norepinephrine upon stimulation of the splenic
    nerve. *J. Physiol.* 204, 102P-104P.

De Robertis, E.D.P. & Bennett, H.S. (1955). Some features of the
    submicroscopic morphology of synapses in frog and earthworm.
    J. Biophys. Biochem. Cytol. 1, 47-58.

De Robertis, E., Pellegrino de Irqldi, A., Rodriquez de Lores
    Arnaiz, G.,& Salganicoff, L. (1962). Cholinergic and non-
    cholinergic endings in rat brain. I. Isolation and subcellu-
    lar distribution of acetylcholine and acetylcholinesterase.
    J. Neurochem. 9, 23-35.

De Weer, P. (1976). Axoplasmic free magnesium levels and magnes-
    ium extrusion from squid giant axons. *J. Gen. Physiol.* 67,
    433-467.

Douglas, W.W. & Poisner, A.M. (1961). Stimulation of uptake of
    calcium-45 in the adrenal gland by acetylcholine. *Nature*
    192, 1299.

Douglas, W.W. & Poisner, A.M. (1962). On the mode of action of acetylcholine in evoking adrenal medullary secretion: increased uptake of calcium during the secretory response. *J. Physiol.* 162, 385-392.

Douglas, W.W. & Rubin, R.P. (1961). The role of calcium in the secretory response of the adrenal medulla to acetylcholine. *J. Physiol.* 159, 40-57.

Douglas, W.W. & Rubin, R.P. (1963). The mechanism of catechol-amine release from the adrenal medulla and the role of calcium in stimulus-secretion coupling. *J. Physiol.* 167, 288-310.

Douglas, W.W. & Rubin, R.P. (1964). The effects of alkaline earths and other divalent cations on adrenal medullary secretion. *J. Physiol.* 175, 231-241.

Douglas, W.W. & Sorimachi, M. (1972). Colchicine inhibits adrenal medullary secretion evoked by acetylcholine without affecting that evoked by potassium. *Br. J. Pharmacol.* 45, 129-132.

Eccles, J.C. & MacFarlane, W.V. (1949). Actions of anticholin-esterases on endplate potential of frog muscle. *J. Neuro-physiol.* 12, 59-80.

Fatt, P. & Katz, B. (1952). Spontaneous subthreshold activity at motor nerve endings. *J. Physiol.* 117, 109-128.

Folkow, B. & Häggendal, J. (1970). Some aspects of the quantal release of the adrenergic transmitter. In: *Bayer-Symposium. II. New Aspects of Storage and Release Mechanisms of Catecho-lamines* (eds.) H.J. Schumann & G. Kroneberg, Springer-Verlag, N.Y., pp. 91-97.

Fried, R.C. & Blaustein, M.P. (1976). Synaptic vesicle recycling in synaptosomes *in vitro*. *Nature* 261, 255-256.

Garcia, A.G. & Kirpekar, S.M. (1975). On the mechanism of re-lease of norepinephrine from cat spleen slices by sodium de-privation and calcium pretreatment. *J. Pharmacol. Exp. Ther.* 192, 343-350.

Gewirtz, P.G. & Kopin, I.J. (1970). Release of dopamine-β-hydr-oxylase with norepinephrine during cat splenic nerve stimu-lation. *Nature* 227, 406-407.

Gray, E.G. & Whittaker, V.P. (1962). The isolation of nerve end-ings from brain: an electron-microscopic study of cell frag-ments derived by homogenization and centrifugation. *J. Anat.* 96, 79-88.

Harvey, A.M. & MacIntosh, F.C. (1940). Calcium and synaptic transmission in a sympathetic ganglion. *J. Physiol.* 97, 408-416.

Heuser, J.E. (1977). Synaptic vesicle exocytosis revealed in quick-frozen frog neuromuscular junctions treated with 4-aminopyridine and given a single electrical shock. In: *Society for Neuroscience Symposia* Vol. II. *Approaches to the Cell Biology of Neurons* (eds.) W.M. Cowan & J.A. Ferrendelli, Society for Neuroscience, Bethesda, MD, pp. 215-239.

Heuser, J.E. & Reese, T.S. (1973). Evidence for recycling of synaptic vesicle membrane during transmitter release at the frog neuromuscular junction. *J. Cell Biol.* 57, 315-344.

Heuser, J.E. & Reese, T.S. (1977). Structure of the synapse. In: *Handbook of Physiology* Section 1. *The Nervous System* Vol. I, Part 1 (Section eds.) J.M. Brookhart & V.B. Mountcastle (Vol. ed.) E.R. Kandel, American Physiological Society, Bethesda, MD, pp. 261-294.

Hille, B. (1977). Ionic basic of resting and action potentials. In: *Handbook of Physiology* Section 1. *The Nervous System* Vol. I, Part 1 (Section eds.) J.M. Brookhart & V.B. Mountcastle (Vol. ed.) E.R. Kandel, American Physiological Society, Bethesda, MD., pp. 99-136.

Hodgkin, A.L. & Katz, B. (1949). The effect of calcium on the axoplasm of giant nerve fibers. *J. Exp. Biol.* 26, 292-294.

Holman, M.E. (1970). Junction potentials in smooth muscle. In: *Smooth Muscle* (eds.) E. Bulbring, A.F. Brading, A.W. Jones & T. Tomita, Williams & Wilkins Co., Baltimore, pp. 244-288.

Hubbard, J.I. & Schmidt, R.F. (1963). The electrophysiological investigation of mammalian motor nerve terminals. *J. Physiol.* 166, 145-167.

Huković, S. & Muscholl, E. (1962). Die Noradrenalin-Abgebe aus dem isolierten Kaninchenherzen bei sympathisher Nervenreizung und ihre pharmakologische Beeinflussung. *Naunyn-Schmiedeberg's Arch. Exp. Path. Pharmak.* 244, 81-96.

Johnson, D.G., Thoa, N.B., Weinshilboum, R., Axelrod, J. & Kopin, I.J. (1971). Enhanced release of dopamine-β-hydroxylase from sympathetic nerves by calcium and phenoxybenzamine and its reversal by prostaglandins. *Proc. Natl. Acad. Sci. [U.S.A.]* 68, 2227-2230.

Katz, B. & Miledi, R. (1965). The effect of calcium on acetylcholine release from motor nerve terminals. *Proc. Roy. Soc. Lond. B.* 161, 496-503.

Katz, B. & Miledi, R. (1967a). The release of acetylcholine from nerve endings by graded electric pulses. *Proc. Roy. Soc. Lond. B.* 167, 23-38.

Katz, B. & Miledi, R. (1967b). A study of synaptic transmission in the absence of nerve impulses. *J. Physiol.* 192, 407-436.

Katz, B. & Miledi, R. (1968). The role of calcium in neuromuscu-
    lar facilitation. *J. Physiol.* 195, 481-492.

Katz, B. & Miledi, R. (1969a). Tetrodotoxin-resistant electrical
    activity in presynaptic terminals. *J. Physiol.* 203, 459-487.

Katz, B. & Miledi, R. (1969b). The effect of divalent cations on
    transmission in the squid giant synapse. *Pubbl. Staz. Zool.
    Napoli.* 37, 303-310.

Katz, B. & Miledi, R. (1971). The effect of prolonged depolari-
    zation on synaptic transfer in the stellate ganglion of the
    squid. *J. Physiol.* 216, 503-512.

Katz, R.I. & Kopin, I.J. (1969). Release of norepinephrine-[3]H
    and serotonin-^{3}H evoked from brain slices by electrical-field
    stimulation - calcium dependency and the effects of lithium,
    ouabain and tetrodotoxin. *Biochem. Pharmacol.* 18, 1935-1939.

Kendrick, N.C., Blaustein, M.P., Ratzlaff, R.W. & Fried, R.C.
    (1976). ATP-dependent calcium storage in presynaptic nerve
    terminals. *Nature* 265, 246-248.

Kendrick, N.C., Ratzlaff, R.W. & Blaustein, M.P. (1977). Arsenazo
    III as an indicator for ionized calcium in physiological salt
    solutions: its use for determination of the CaATP dissociation
    constant. *Analyt. Biochem.* 83, in press.

Kirpekar, S.M. & Misu, Y. (1967). Release of noradrenaline by
    splenic nerve stimulation and its dependence on calcium.
    J. Physiol. 188, 219-234.

Kirpekar, S.M. & Wakade, A.R. (1968). Release of noradrenaline
    from the cat spleen by potassium. *J. Physiol.* 194, 595-608.

Kirshner, N. & Viveros, O.H. (1970). Quantal aspects of the sec-
    retion of catecholamines and dopamine-β-hydroxylase from the
    adrenal medulla. In: *Bayer-Symposium II. New Aspects of
    Storage and Release Mechanisms of Catecholamines* (eds.)
    H.J. Schumann & G. Kroneberg, Springer-Verlag, N.Y., pp. 78-
    88.

Kohlhardt, M., Bauer, B., Krause, H. & Fleckenstein, A. (1972).
    Differentiation of the transmembrane Na and Ca channels in
    mammalian cardiac fibres by the use of specific inhibitors.
    Pfleuger's Arch. 335, 309-322.

Kusano, K. (1970). Influence of ionic environment on the relation-
    ship between pre- and postsynaptic potentials. *J. Neurobiol.*
    1, 437-457.

Kusano, K., Livengood, D.R. & Werman, R. (1967). Correlation of
    transmitter release with membrane properties of the presynap-
    tic fiber of the squid giant synapse. *J. Gen. Physiol.* 50,
    2579-2601.

Lacy, P.E., Howell, S.L., Young, D.A. & Fink, C.J. (1968). A new hypothesis of insulin secretion. *Nature* 219, 1177-1179.

Lazarewicz, J.W., Haljamae, H. & Hamberger, A. (1974). Calcium metabolism in isolated brain cells and subcellular fractions. *J. Neurochem.* 22, 33-45.

Llinas, R.R. (1977). Calcium and transmitter release in squid synapse. In: *Society for Neuroscience Symposia* Vol. II *Approaches to the Cell Biology of Neurons* (eds.) W.M. Cowan & J.A. Ferrendelli, Society for Neuroscience, Bethesda, MD, pp. 139-160.

Llinas, R., Blinks, J.R. & Nicholson, C. (1972). Calcium transient in presynaptic terminal of squid giant synapse: detection with aequorin. *Science* 176, 1127-1129.

Llinas, R. & Nicholson, C. (1975). Calcium role in stimulus-secretion coupling: an aequorin study in squid giant synapse. *Proc. Natl. Acad. Sci.* [*U.S.A.*] 72, 187-190.

Mallart, A. & Martin, A.R. (1967). An analysis of facilitation of transmitter release at the neuromuscular junction of the frog. *J. Physiol.* 193, 679-694.

Mallart, A. & Martin, A.R. (1968). The relation between quantum content and facilitation at the neuromuscular junction of the frog. *J. Physiol.* 196, 593-604.

Martin, A.R. (1977). Junctional transmission. II. Presynaptic mechanisms. In: *Handbook of Physiology* Section 1. *The Nervous System* Vol. I, Part 1 (Section eds.) J.M. Brookhart & V.B. Mountcastle (Vol. ed.) E.R. Kandel, American Physiological Society, Bethesda, MD., pp. 329-355.

Matthews, E.K. (1970). Calcium and hormone release. In: *Calcium and Cellular Function* (ed.) A.W. Cuthbert, St. Martins Press, Inc., N.Y., pp. 163-182.

Matthews, E.K. & Nordmann, J.J. (1976). The synaptic vesicle: calcium ion binding to the vesicle membrane and its modification by drug action. *Mol. Pharmacol.* 12, 778-788.

Miledi, R. (1973). Transmitter release induced by injection of calcium ions into nerve terminals. *Proc. Roy. Soc. Lond. B.* 183, 421-425.

Moss, J., Thoa, N.B. & Kopin, I.J. (1974). On the mechanism of scorpion toxin-induced release of norepinephrine from peripheral adrenergic neurons. *J. Pharmacol. Exp. Ther.* 190, 39-48.

Mulder, A.H., Van Den Berg & Stoof, J.C. (1975). Calcium-dependent release of radiolabelled catecholamines and serotonin from rat brain synaptosomes in a superfusion system. *Brain Res.* 99, 419-424.

Narahashi, T., Shapiro, B.I., Deguchi, T., Scuka, M. & Wang, C.M. (1972). Effects of scorpion venom on squid axon membranes. *Am. J. Physiol.* 222, 850-857.

Parsegian, V.A. (1977). Considerations in determining the mode of influence of calcium on vesicle-membrane interactions. In: *Society for Neuroscience Symposia* Vol. II. *Approaches to the Cell Biology of Neurons* (eds.) W.M. Cowan & J.A. Ferrendelli, Society for Neuroscience, Bethesda, MD, pp. 161-171.

Paton, D.M. (1973). Mechanism of efflux of noradrenaline from adrenergic nerves in rabbit atria. *Br. J. Pharmacol.* 49, 614-627.

Raiteri, M., Levi, G. & Federico, R. (1975). Stimulus-coupled release of unmetabolized ^{3}H-norepinephrine from rat brain synaptosomes. *Pharmacol. Res. Commun.* 7, 181-187.

Rossi, C.S. & Lehninger, A.L. (1964). Stoichiometry of respiratory stimulation, accumulation of Ca^{++} and phosphate, and oxidative phosphorylation in rat liver mitochondria. *J. Biol. Chem.* 239, 3971-3980.

Sandow, A. (1952). Excitation-contraction coupling in muscular response. *Yale J. Biol. Med.* 25, 176-201.

Smith, A.D. (1971). Secretion of proteins (chromogranin A and dopamine-β-hydroxylase) from a sympathetic neuron. *Phil. Trans. Roy. Soc. B.* 261, 363-370.

Smith, A.D. (1972). Cellular control of the uptake, storage and release of noradrenaline in sympathetic neurons. *Biochem. Soc. Symp.* 36, 103-131.

Stjärne, L. (1970). Quantal or graded secretion of adrenal medullary hormone and sympathetic neurotransmitter. In: *Bayer-Symposium* II. *New Aspects of Storage and Release Mechanisms of Catecholamines* (eds.) H.J. Schumann & G. Kroneberg, Springer-Verlag, N.Y., pp. 112-127.

Thoa, N.B., Wooten, G.F., Axelrod, J. & Kopin, I.J. (1972). Inhibition of release of dopamine-β-hydroxylase and norepinephrine from sympathetic nerves by colchicine, vinblastine, or cytochalasin-B. *Proc. Natl. Acad. Sci. [U.S.A.]* 69, 520-522.

Thoa, N.B., Wooten, G.F., Axelrod, J. & Kopin, I.J. (1975). On the mechanism of release of norepinephrine from sympathetic nerves induced by depolarizing agents and sympathomimetic drugs. *Mol. Pharmacol.* 11, 10-18.

Venzin, M., Sandri, C., Akert, K. & Wyss, V.R. (1977). Membrane associated particles of the presynaptic active zone in rat spinal cord. A morphometric analysis. *Brain Res.* 130, 393-404.

Viveros, O.H., Arqueros, L. & Kirshner, N. (1969). Quantal secretion from adrenal medulla: all or none release of storage vesicle content. *Science* 165, 911-913.

Weinshilboum, R.M., Thoa, N.B., Johnson, D.B., Kopin, I.J. & Axelrod, J. (1972). Proportional release of norepinephrine and dopamine-β-hydroxylase from sympathetic nerves. *Science* 174, 1349-1351.

White, T.D. (1976). Models for neuronal noradrenaline uptake. In: *The Mechanism of Neuronal and Extraneuronal Transport of Catecholamines* (ed.) D.M. Paton, Raven Press, N.Y., pp. 175-193.

PRESYNAPTIC ADRENOCEPTORS AND REGULATION OF RELEASE

S. Z. Langer

I   INTRODUCTION

For almost three decades it has been well established that noradrenaline is the neurotransmitter released from adrenergic nerve
terminals in the peripheral nervous system. It was von Euler in
1946 who found that the sympathomimetic substance in purified extracts of sympathetic nerves and effector organs bore a strong
resemblance to noradrenaline by all criteria used. The first observation on release of noradrenaline during stimulation of sympathetic nerves was made by Peart (1949).

The terminal varicosities of noradrenergic neurons in the peripheral nervous system have been the focus of extensive studies
during the last two decades. Such investigations were carried
out at the biochemical, physiological and pharmacological level.
Considerable information was obtained from these studies, regarding the synthesis, storage, release, effects on the postsynaptic
receptors and subsequent inactivation of the neurotransmitter,
noradrenaline.

Upon arrival of nerve impulses, noradrenaline is released from the
varicosities through a calcium-dependent exocytotic·process. The
released transmitter then activates specific adrenoceptors located
in the membrane of the postsynaptic effector cell producing the
characteristic response of the effector organ : positive chronotropic and inotropic effects, contraction or relaxation of a
smooth muscle, secretion from salivary glands, etc.

It is only during the past few years that the evidence became
available for the presence of adrenoceptors in the outer surface
of the membrane of the noradrenergic varicosities. These receptor which were called presynaptic, because of their location and
their activation can modify the release of the neurotransmitter
upon arrival of nerve impulses.

II   PRESYNAPTIC ALPHA-ADRENOCEPTORS

The first observation regarding the effects of alpha-adrenoceptor
blockade on the release of noradrenaline was reported in 1957 by
Brown and Gillespie. These authors found that phenoxybenzamine,
an alpha-adrenoceptor blocking agent, increased the stimulation-
induced overflow of noradrenaline in the perfused cat spleen.
These results were interpreted as being due to the blockade of

the postsynaptic alpha-adrenoceptors by phenoxybenzamine, preventing released noradrenaline from combining with the receptors and
thus increasing the transmitter collected in the venous effluent.
A similar hypothesis was postulated several years later by
Häggendal (1970); namely that the postsynaptic alpha-adrenoceptors
are involved in a transsynaptic regulatory mechanism for transmitter release. In other words, blockade of the postsynaptic
alpha-adrenoceptors would decrease the response of the effector
organ and lead to an increase in noradrenaline release from the
presynaptic nerve endings (Häggendal, 1970; Farnebo and Malmfors,
1971).

Since phenoxybenzamine in low concentrations can inhibit neuronal
uptake of noradrenaline (Hertting, 1965; Iversen, 1965) and in
higher concentrations is also able to inhibit extraneuronal uptake of noradrenaline (Iversen, 1967; Eisenfeld et al., 1967;
Iversen & Langer, 1969), it was postulated that the increase in
noradrenaline overflow obtained in the presence of this drug
could be causally related to the blockade of one or both of these
sites of loss for the released transmitter.

However, when complete inhibition of neuronal uptake of noradrenaline is achieved with agents which do not block the alpha-adrenoceptors like cocaine or desipramine, little or no increase in
transmitter overflow was obtained during nerve stimulation
(Blakeley et al., 1963; Geffen, 1965; Boullin et al., 1967;
Dubocovich & Langer, 1973, 1976; Langer & Enero, 1974).

The possible significance of the inhibition by phenoxybenzamine
of extraneural uptake of noradrenaline became apparent when it
was reported in studies on stimulation-induced transmitter release
carried out with [^{3}H]noradrenaline that a significant fraction of
the ^{3}H-transmitter released by nerve stimulation was collected as
tritiated metabolites of noradrenaline (Langer, 1970; Langer et
al., 1972a; Langer, 1974a; Cubeddu et al., 1974; Langer & Enero,
1974; Luchelli-Fortis & Langer, 1975; Dubocovich & Langer, 1976).
Although phenoxybenzamine is able to prevent entirely the metabolism of [^{3}H]noradrenaline released by nerve stimulation, this effect does not fully account for the increase in transmitter overflow elicited by phenoxybenzamine (Langer, 1970; Langer & Vogt,
1971; Langer, 1974b; 1977; Starke, 1977).

Consequently the increase in stimulation-induced overflow of noradrenaline obtained in the presence of phenoxybenzamine is due
to an actual increase in transmitter release and cannot be explained as the consequence of the inhibition of neuronal and extraneuronal uptake of noradrenaline (Langer, 1970; Langer & Vogt,
1971). In support of this view it was reported that both phentolamine and phenoxybenzamine increase the stimulation-induced
release of noradrenaline in concentrations which do not inhibit
either neuronal or extraneuronal uptake (Langer et al., 1971;
Starke et al., 1971; Enero et al., 1972). In addition, it was
reported that the release of dopamine-β-hydroxylase was increased
when neurotransmission in the perfused spleen was studied in the
presence of phenoxybenzamine or phentolamine (De Potter et al.,

.1971; Cubeddu *et al.*, 1974). Since dopamine-β-hydroxylase is a large molecule which is not taken up by noradrenergic nerve endings or inactivated by the tissue after its exocytotic release, an increase in overflow of the enzyme does in fact represent an actual increase in release.

It is of interest to note that the increase in noradrenaline release observed in the presence of alpha-receptor blocking agents was obtained in the range of drug concentrations which elicit postsynaptic alpha-adrenoceptor blockade (Enero *et al.*, 1972; Dubocovich & Langer, 1974). Yet, a causal relationship between the block of the responses of the effector organ and the increase in stimulation-induced noradrenaline release can be excluded because in tissues like guinea-pig atria, the perfused rabbit heart and the perfused cat heart where the postsynaptic adrenoceptors that mediate the response of the effector organ are of the beta type, alpha-receptor blocking agents produce the same increase in the stimulation-evoked release of noradrenaline (Langer *et al.*, 1971; Starke *et al.*, 1971; McCulloch *et al.*, 1972; Farah & Langer, 1974; Langer *et al.*, 1977).

These results led to the hypothesis which postulates the presence of alpha-adrenoceptors in the outer surface of the noradrenergic nerve terminals. As shown schematically in Fig. 1 these presynaptic alpha-adrenoceptors are involved in the regulation of noradren adrenaline release through a negative feedback mechanism mediated by the neurotransmitter itself. Consequently, noradrenaline released by nerve stimulation once it reaches a threshold concentration in the synaptic gap activates presynaptic alpha-adrenoceptors triggering a negative feedback mechanism which inhibits further release of the transmitter (Langer *et al.*, 1971; Farnebo & Hamberger, 1971; Enero *et al.*, 1972; Starke, 1972a; Rand *et al.*, 1973; Langer, 1973).

In support of this hypothesis it has been demonstrated that α-adrenoceptor agonists inhibit noradrenaline release during nerve stimulation, independently of the alpha or beta nature of the postsynaptic adrenoceptor that mediates the response of the effector organ (Langer *et al.*, 1972b; Starke, 1972b; Kirpekar *et al.*, 1973; Starke *et al.*, 1974; Starke *et al.*, 1975a; Rand *et al.*, 1975; Langer *et al.*, 1975a). It is of interest to note that the magnitude of the inhibition of transmitter release during exposure to alpha-adrenoceptor agonists is inversely related to the frequency of nerve stimulation (Langer *et al.*, 1975a; Starke *et al.*, 1975a). In other words, the reduction in stimulation-evoked noradrenaline release is the more pronounced the lower the frequency of nerve stimulation. In addition in the high range of frequencies of nerve stimulation alpha-adrenoceptor agonists fail to reduce the output of noradrenaline induced by nerve stimulation.

The frequency-dependence of the inhibition of noradrenaline release elicited by alpha-adrenoceptor agonists differs from the effects of neuron blocking agents which also reduce the output of noradrenaline at high frequencies of nerve stimulation (Armstrong & Boura, 1973).

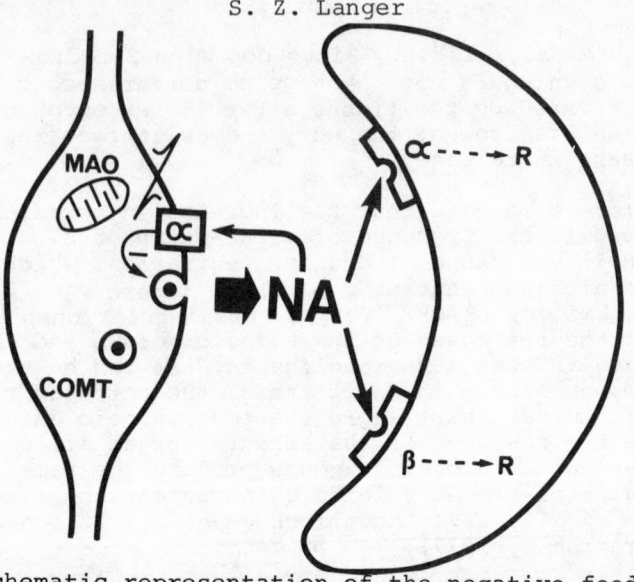

Fig. 1.   Schematic representation of the negative feedback mechanism for noradrenaline released by nerve stimulation, mediated
by presynaptic α-adrenoceptors.   Noradrenaline (NA) released by
nerve stimulation once it reaches a threshold concentration in
the synaptic cleft activates presynaptic α-adrenoceptors leading
to inhibition of transmitter release.   The presynaptic negative
feedback mechanism is present both in tissues where the response
(R) of the effector organ is mediated through α- or through β-adrenoceptors.   MAO : monoamine oxidase; COMT : catechol-O-methyl-
transferase.

The frequency-dependence of the inhibition of transmitter release
by alpha-receptor agonists like clonidine has also been observed
under *in vivo* conditions in the rat and in the dog (Armstrong &
Boura, 1973; Scriabine & Stavorski, 1973; Robson & Antonaccio,
1974; Yamaguchi *et al.*, 1977).

Further support for the hypothesis that noradrenaline release is
regulated through a negative feedback mechanism mediated by presynaptic alpha-adrenoceptors was obtained in experiments in which
an increase in stimulation-evoked transmitter release was obtained
in the presence of alpha-receptor blocking agents.   Again, the enhancement in noradrenaline release obtained by alpha-receptor
blockade was observed regardless of the alpha or beta-type of the
postsynaptic adrenoceptor that mediates the response of the effector organ (for reviews see Langer, 1974b, 1977; Starke, 1977).

The negative feedback mechanism for noradrenaline release by nerve
stimulation should be expected to operate most effectively when
the transmitter released by nerve impulses reaches a threshold
concentration in the synaptic cleft.   In support of this view, it
has been shown that when the endogenous noradrenaline stores are
depleted either by pretreatment with reserpine or by the inhibition of synthesis with α-methyl-*p*-tyrosine the effectiveness of

phenoxybenzamine in increasing the stimulation-induced release of
[^{3}H]noradrenaline and dopamine-β-hydroxylase is almost completely
lost (Enero & Langer, 1973; Cubeddu & Weiner, 1975). Therefore,
when the concentration of released noradrenaline in the synaptic
gap fails to attain a certain threshold it does not trigger the
presynaptic negative feedback mechanism that regulates noradrenaline release. In support of this view, Rand et al. (1975) demonstrated that phenoxybenzamine does not increase the stimulation-
induced release of [^{3}H]noradrenaline from isolated guinea-pig
atria elicited by a single pulse. Under the same experimental
conditions phenoxybenzamine produced a 4.5-fold increase in [^{3}H]-
noradrenaline release when a train of 16 pulses was applied.

As previously discussed for the inhibition of transmitter release
induced by alpha-receptor agonists there is also a relationship
between the frequency of nerve stimulation and the magnitude of
the increase in the stimulation-evoked release of noradrenaline
in the presence of alpha-receptor blocking agents. As the frequency of nerve stimulation is increased the effectiveness of
alpha-receptor blocking agents in enhancing noradrenaline release
during nerve stimulation is progressively reduced (Brown &
Gillespie, 1957; Kirpekar & Cervoni, 1963; Haefely et al., 1965;
Langer, 1970; Langer et al., 1975a; Dubocovich & Langer, 1976).

It appears that at high frequencies of nerve stimulation the negative feedback regulatory mechanism which is mediated by presynaptic alpha-adrenoceptors, does not play an important role in the
regulation of transmitter release (Dubocovich & Langer, 1974;
Langer et al., 1975a).

In contrast to the release of noradrenaline elicited by nerve
stimulation or by potassium, tyramine releases noradrenaline by
displacing the transmitter from vesicular binding sites by a
mechanism which is not calcium-dependent. The presynaptic feedback mechanism that regulates noradrenaline release is operative
for the release elicited by nerve stimulation or by potassium
while this presynaptic mechanism is not involved in the regulation
of transmitter release elicited by tyramine (Starke & Montel,
1973a; Pelayo et al., 1977; Dubocovich et al., 1978). It is possible that the negative feedback mechanism modifies the availability of calcium ions for the release process and consequently the
calcium-independent release induced by tyramine is not influenced
by this regulatory mechanism.

In support of the view that the activation of presynaptic alpha-
adrenoceptors reduces the availability of calcium for the excitation-secretion coupling, the inhibition of transmitter release
obtained by exposure to exogenous noradrenaline was found to be
more pronounced when the calcium concentration in the medium is
reduced from 2.6 mM to 0.65 mM (Langer et al., 1975a). The
potentiation of the inhibitory effects of alpha-adrenoceptor
agonists on neurotransmission by a reduction in the external calcium concentration indicates that the negative feedback mechanism
mediated by presynaptic alpha-adrenoceptors may operate by reducing the availability of calcium for the exocytotic release of the
neurotransmitter.

Recently a possible link between activation of presynaptic alpha-
adrenoceptors and an increase in the levels of cyclic guanosine
monophosphate (cGMP) in noradrenergic nerve terminals has been
postulated by several authors. In the rat pineal gland depolarization by potassium or exposure to noradrenaline produces an increase in the levels of cGMP which is prevented by alpha-receptor
blocking agents (O'Dea & Zatz, 1976). Since these effects are
observed in the innervated but not in the surgically denervated
pineal gland, these authors postulated the existence of an alpha-
adrenoceptor located in the noradrenergic nerve endings of the
pineal gland and linked to the stimulation of neuronal guanylate
cyclase activity (O'Dea & Zatz, 1976).

Recently it was reported the alpha-presynaptic negative feedback
mechanism for the stimulation-evoked release of noradrenaline is
present in the rat pineal gland (Pelayo *et al.*, 1977). In addition these authors reported that dibutyryl cGMP mimicked the effects of the alpha receptor agonist oxymetazoline in reducing the
potassium-induced release of [^{3}H]noradrenaline. The concentrations
of dibutyryl cGMP which reduced the potassium-evoked release of
[^{3}H]noradrenaline did not affect the release of the labelled transmitter elicited by tyramine (Dubocovich *et al.*, 1978). These results are compatible with the view that stimulation of presynaptic
alpha-adrenoceptors is linked with an increase in cGMP levels in
noradrenergic nerve endings. Additional experiments are required
to verify the hypothesis that neuronal cGMP may be involved in
the sequence of events starting with the stimulation of presynaptic alpha-adrenoceptors and leading to inhibition of the stimulation-evoked release of the neurotransmitter.

III   DIFFERENCES BETWEEN THE PRESYNAPTIC AND
THE POSTSYNAPTIC ALPHA-ADRENOCEPTORS

Although both the pre- and the postsynaptic alpha-adrenoceptors
are stimulated by alpha-receptor agonists and blocked by alpha-
receptor antagonists, it appears that the postsynaptic alpha-
adrenoceptors that mediate the responses of the effector organ
are not identical with the presynaptic alpha-adrenoceptors which
regulate the release of noradrenaline during nerve stimulation.

The first observation regarding the differences between pre- and
postsynaptic alpha-adrenoceptors was made for the alpha-adrenoceptor agonists in the cat spleen (Langer, 1973). Subsequently
it was shown in the perfused cat spleen that phenoxybenzamine is
at least 30 times more potent in blocking the postsynaptic alpha-
receptors that mediate the responses of the effector organ than
it is in blocking the presynaptic alpha-receptors that regulate
the release of noradrenaline during nerve stimulation. These results led to the postulate that the pre- and the postsynaptic
alpha-adrenoceptors are not identical (Dubocovich & Langer, 1974;
Langer, 1974b).

In support of this view it was found that in experiments in which
the overflow of dopamine-β-hydroxylase was determined in the

perfused cat spleen, phenoxybenzamine was 30 to 100 times more
potent in blocking the postsynaptic alpha-receptors than the presynaptic receptors (Cubeddu.et al., 1974). On the other hand
these authors found only a very small difference for the potency
of phentolamine in blocking the pre- and the postsynaptic alpha-
adrenoceptors in the perfused cat spleen.

These results led to the concept (Langer, 1974b) that there were
actually two types of alpha-adrenoceptors, the postsynaptic receptors which mediate on the whole excitatory responses (e.g.,
vasoconstriction) and which should be referred to as α_1 and the
presynaptic alpha-receptors which mediate an inhibitory effect
(reduction of noradrenaline release during nerve stimulation)
which were referred to as α_2.

In further support of the concept that there are differences between the presynaptic and the postsynaptic alpha-adrenoceptors in
their affinities for agonists and for antagonists, it was subsequently shown that the alpha-receptor blocking agent, yohimbine
is more potent in blocking the presynaptic or α_2-adrenoceptor
than in blocking the postsynaptic or α_1-adrenoceptor (Starke et
al., 1975b). It was also shown that the alpha-receptor agonist
clonidine is more potent in reducing noradrenaline release during
nerve stimulation than in stimulating the postsynaptic alpha-
adrenoceptors (Starke et al., 1974).

Table 1 summarizes the differences between the postsynaptic (α_1)
and presynaptic (α_2) adrenoceptors based on the relative order of
potency of agonists and of antagonists.

The affinity for the α_1 and α_2 adrenoceptors is similar when agonists like naphazoline, adrenaline and noradrenaline are considered.
Tramazoline, alphamethylnoradrenaline, clonidine and oxymetazoline
have a higher affinity for the presynaptic or α_2 than for the postsynaptic or α_1 adrenoceptor. Finally phenylephrine and methoxamine have a high affinity for the α_1-adrenoceptor and little or
no affinity for the presynaptic or α_2-adrenoceptor.

Differences exist in relative affinities for the pre- and postsynaptic alpha-adrenoceptors when several alpha-receptor blocking
agents are considered (Table 1). Phentolamine has the same potency in blocking the α_1 or α_2-adrenoceptors. On the other hand
yohimbine, piperoxane and tolazoline are more potent in blocking
the α_2 or presynaptic adrenoceptor when compared with the α_1-ad-
renoceptors. Prazosin has a high affinity for the blockade of
postsynaptic alpha receptors and it is practically devoid of alpha-
receptor blocking properties on the presynaptic alpha-adrenoceptors (Doxey & Everitt, 1977; Drew, 1977; Dubocovich & Langer, unpublished observations).

Recent results point to the possibility that there might be species differences between the α_2-adrenoceptors. While prazosin
fails to block the α_2-receptors in the rat, it was recently shown
that this alpha-adrenoceptor antagonist can block the α_2-receptors
in the dog's heart (Cavero et al., 1977; Roach et al., 1978).

Table 1.   Subclassification of Alpha-Adrenoceptors : Presynaptic
or α_2 and Postsynaptic or α_1.

Shown are the relative order of potencies of different alpha-agon-
ists and antagonists on the postsynaptic (α_1) receptors that mediate the responses of the effector organ and on the presynaptic
(α_2) receptors which mediate the inhibition of noradrenaline release during nerve stimulation.   The results shown were obtained
in noradrenergically innervated tissues of the peripheral nervous
system.

PRE AND POSTSYNAPTIC ALPHA ADRENOCEPTORS

RELATIVE ORDER OF POTENCY OF AGONISTS

TRAMAZOLINE $>$ αCH$_3$NORADRENALINE $>$ CLONIDINE $>$ OXYMETAZOLINE $>$ α_2

$>$ NAPHAZOLINE $>$ ADRENALINE $>$ NORADRENALINE $>$ $\alpha_2 = \alpha_1$

$>$ PHENYLEPHRINE $>$ METHOXAMINE α_1

RELATIVE ORDER OF POTENCY OF ANTAGONISTS

YOHIMBINE $>>$ PIPEROXAN $>$ TOLAZOLINE $>$ α_2

$>$ PHENTOLAMINE $>$ $\alpha_2 = \alpha_1$

$>$ PHENOXYBENZAMINE $>$ $>>$ PRAZOSIN α_1

Another factor which appears to be of importance for the relative
potencies of the pre- and postsynaptic effects of alpha-receptor
agonists, is the time course of their effects under *in vivo* conditions.   In the pithed rat, after the *in vivo* administration of
clonidine (1 and 5 µg per Kg), the duration of the presynaptic
effects was nearly 10 times longer than that of the postsynaptic
pressor effects (Cavero *et al.*, 1978).

It is of interest to note that there is an intrarenal alpha-adrenoceptor which mediates inhibition of renin release (Pettinger
et al., 1976).   Clonidine is more potent than methoxamine in reducing serum renin activity, indicating that this alpha-receptor
is probably of the α_2-type (Pettinger *et al.*, 1976).

IV   EVIDENCE FOR THE PRESYNAPTIC LOCATION OF THE ALPHA-
     ADRENOCEPTOR INVOLVED IN THE NEGATIVE FEEDBACK
     MECHANISM THAT REGULATES NORADRENALINE RELEASE DURING
     NERVE STIMULATION.

Although some authors suggested that the negative feedback mechanism for noradrenaline release during nerve stimulation might
be of a transsynaptic nature (Häggendal, 1970; Farnebo & Malmfors,
1971), the evidence accumulated during the last few years appears
to favour the view that the alpha-adrenoceptor involved in the
regulation of transmitter release is located in noradrenergic
nerve endings.

In recently formed nerve endings from cultured rat superior cervical ganglia, phenoxybenzamine enhances the release of [^{3}H]nor-
adrenaline evoked by potassium-depolarization (Vogel *et al.*,
1972). Under these experimental conditions alpha-receptor blockade enhanced the stimulation-evoked release of [^{3}H]noradrenaline
in the absence of an effector postsynaptic cell.

In the rat submaxillary gland there is an atrophy of the secretory
cells 15 days after duct ligation (Standish & Shafer, 1957). In
these atrophied salivary glands the secretory responses to adrenoceptor or cholinoceptor agonists are abolished although neither
the cholinergic nor the noradrenergic innervation are affected
(Filinger *et al.*, 1978). Under these experimental conditions exposure to phentolamine produced a 3-fold increase in the potassium-
evoked release of [^{3}H]noradrenaline from slices of the normal and
the atrophied gland as well (Filinger *et al.*, 1978). Consequently
the alpha-receptor blocking agent was equally effective in
increasing the stimulation-induced transmitter release in normal
as well as in atrophied salivary glands. These results support
the view that the effects of phentolamine were mediated through
a presynaptic mechanism since it could be demonstrated independently of the presence of a postsynaptic effector cell.

Langer and Luchelli-Fortis (1977) reported that after short-term
denervation of the cat nictitating membrane there are marked
changes in the sensitivity of the presynaptic alpha-adrenoceptors
that regulate noradrenaline release during nerve stimulation.
These authors found that 18 hours after surgical denervation of
the cat nictitating membrane, phentolamine failed to significantly
increase the stimulation-induced release of [^{3}H]noradrenaline and
clonidine was significantly less effective in reducing ^{3}H-trans-
mitter release. Under these experimental conditions, the postsynaptic changes in sensitivity are not yet developed (Langer,
1975) and the ability of phentolamine to block and of clonidine
to stimulate the postsynaptic alpha-adrenoceptors does not differ
from the corresponding controls (Langer & Luchelli-Fortis, 1977).
These authors concluded that the changes observed in neurotransmission after short term denervation are due to subsensitivity of
the presynaptic alpha-adrenoceptors. This phenomenon may be due
to the leakage of noradrenaline from degenerating nerve endings
at the onset of the "degeneration contraction" of the cat nictitating membrane (Langer, 1966; Langer & Trendelenburg, 1966).

The subsensitivity of the presynaptic alpha-adrenoceptors observed
after short-term surgical denervation is selective for this presynaptic receptor since it was not observed for the presynaptic
inhibitory opiate or muscarinic receptors (Luchelli-Fortis &
Langer, unpublished observations).

It is of interest to note that the sensitivity of the presynaptic
alpha-adrenoceptor can be modified after exposure to an effective
concentration of an alpha-adrenoceptor agonist. In the cat spleen
perfused with cocaine there is a nearly 2-fold increase in ^{3}H-
transmitter release during nerve stimulation after a 60 minute exposure to 0.59 μM noradrenaline (Langer & Dubocovich, 1977).
This effect is probably due to a short-lasting subsensitivity of
the presynaptic alpha-adrenoceptors resulting from the previous
exposure to the agonist, noradrenaline. Compatible with this
interpretation is the fact that this phenomenon is not observed
in the presence of phentolamine (Langer & Dubocovich, 1977).
Consequently, it is possible that, as already demonstrated for
the postsynaptic receptor, chronic stimulation or blockade of the
presynaptic alpha-adrenoceptors may lead to changes in their sensitivity to the neurotransmitter. This phenomenon might be involved in the rebound hypertension which is observed after the
sudden withdrawal of clonidine in hypertensive patients (Hansson
et al., 1973).

In addition, attention should be drawn to the fact that chronic
stimulation or blockade of the presynaptic alpha-adrenoceptors
may lead to changes in their sensitivity which may affect the
regulation of neurotransmission.

V.   PHYSIOLOGICAL AND PHARMACOLOGICAL SIGNIFICANCE OF THE
      NEGATIVE FEEDBACK MECHANISM MEDIATED BY PRESYNAPTIC
      ALPHA-ADRENOCEPTORS

If the negative feedback mechanism mediated by presynaptic alpha-
adrenoceptors plays a physiological role in the regulation of
neurotransmission, the enhancement in transmitter release observed in the presence of alpha-receptor blocking agents should be
reflected in an increase in the response of the effector organ to
nerve stimulation. In tissues in which the postsynaptic responses
are mediated through alpha-adrenoceptors (e.g., blood vessels,
nictitating membrane, spleen), the responses to nerve stimulation
are reduced by alpha-receptor blocking agents. Nonetheless,
yohimbine, which is more potent in blocking the presynaptic (α_2)
than the postsynaptic (α_1) adrenoceptors, increased both the overflow of [^{3}H]noradrenaline and the responses to nerve stimulation
of the rabbit pulmonary artery in the low range of concentrations
(Starke *et al.*, 1975b).

In tissues in which the response of the effector organ is mediated
through beta adrenoceptors, exposure to alpha-receptor blocking
agents should enhance the responses to nerve stimulation as a result of the increase in transmitter release observed under these
experimental conditions. When the responses to accelerans nerve

stimulation at low frequencies were determined in guinea-pig
atria, exposure to phentolamine produced a significant increase
in the positive chronotropic responses to nerve stimulation.
Under these experimental conditions the alpha-receptor blocking
agent produced a significant increase in ^{3}H-transmitter release
during nerve stimulation (Langer *et al.*, 1977).

The causal relationship between the increase in stimulation-evoked
release of noradrenaline and the enhancement in the positive
chronotropic responses to nerve stimulation obtained in the presence of phentolamine, supports the view that the negative feedback mechanism mediated by presynaptic alpha-adrenoceptors plays
a major physiological role in noradrenergic neurotransmission.

Similar results were obtained under *in vivo* experimental conditions : clonidine reduced the positive chronotropic responses to
cardioaccelerator nerve stimulation (Armstrong & Boura, 1973;
Yamaguchi *et al.*, 1977) while alpha-receptor blocking agents potentiated the positive chronotropic effects of cardioaccelerator
nerve stimulation (Hokhandwala & Buckley, 1976; Yamaguchi *et al.*,
1977).

Evidence is now available for the presence of presynaptic alpha-
adrenoceptors in human vasoconstrictor nerves (Stjärne & Gripe,
1973; Stjärne & Brundin, 1975). These authors performed their
experiments in isolated superfused biopsy specimens of human peripheral arteries and veins. Under these experimental conditions
there was a decrease in [^{3}H]noradrenaline release in the presence
of alpha-adrenoceptor agonists and an increase in the stimulation-
evoked release of the labelled transmitter in the presence of
alpha-receptor blocking agents (Stjärne & Gripe, 1973; Stjärne &
Brundin, 1977).

VI   INFLUENCE OF NEURONAL UPTAKE OF NORADRENALINE ON THE
      NEGATIVE FEEDBACK MECHANISM MEDIATED BY PRESYNAPTIC
      ALPHA-ADRENOCEPTORS

Neuronal uptake of noradrenaline is the main mechanism for the
inactivation of the transmitter released by nerve stimulation
(Langer, 1974a, 1977). This active transport mechanism for noradrenaline across the membrane of the nerve ending effectively reduces the concentration of the transmitter in the synaptic cleft.
It follows then that neuronal uptake, by decreasing the effective
concentration of the transmitter in the outer surface of the nerve
terminal can modulate the presynaptic feedback mechanism since it
regulates the fraction of the transmitter released by stimulation
which is available to activate presynaptic alpha-adrenoceptors
(Langer, 1974b). In support of this view, it has been reported
that when neuronal uptake is inhibited by cocaine a higher fraction of the noradrenaline released by nerve stimulation becomes
available for activation of the presynaptic inhibitory alpha-
adrenoceptors (Langer & Enero, 1974; Cubeddu *et al.*, 1974;
Dubocovich & Langer, 1976). In addition, in the presence of 3
and 30 µM cocaine, a concentration-dependent reduction in the

overflow of dopamine-β-hydroxylase during nerve stimulation was
reported (Cubeddu *et al.*, 1974).'

Consequently, it appears that inhibition of neuronal uptake by
cocaine leads to a decrease in transmitter output because of enhanced feedback inhibition by the higher concentration of the
transmitter achieved in the vicinity of the nerve ending (Enero
et al., 1972; Langer, 1974b; Langer & Enero, 1974; Langer, 1977).

The physiological importance of neuronal uptake in regulating the
concentration of noradrenaline in the biophase is inversely related to the distance of the neuromuscular interval : the narrower
the neuroeffector gap, the more important is neuronal uptake in
the regulation of the concentration of the neurotransmitter in
the biophase. The width of the neuromuscular distance would also
be expected to modify the presynaptic negative feedback mechanism
because it influences the concentration of the released transmitter achieved in the synaptic cleft. In support of this view,
the analysis of results obtained in different tissues with known
neuromuscular distances showed that the magnitude of the increase
in transmitter release elicited by nerve stimulation in the presence of phentolamine was the more pronounced the smaller the
neuromuscular interval of the tissue (Langer *et al.*, 1975b;
Langer, 1977). Therefore it appears that in organs with narrow
neuromuscular gaps, the presynaptic feedback inhibition for noradrenaline release during nerve stimulation plays a more important role as a regulatory mechanism than in tissues with wide
synaptic gaps.

VII EVIDENCE FOR THE PRESENCE OF PRESYNAPTIC BETA-ADRENOCEPTORS IN NORADRENERGIC NERVE ENDINGS

In addition to the negative feedback mechanism for noradrenaline
released by nerve stimulation which is mediated by presynaptic
alpha-adrenoceptors, a positive feedback mechanism exists in noradrenergic nerve endings which is triggered through the activation
of presynaptic beta-adrenoceptors (Langer *et al.*, 1974; Adler-
Graschinsky & Langer, 1975; Langer *et al.*, 1975a; Stjärne &
Brundin, 1975; Dahlöf *et al.*, 1975; Langer, 1976; Stjärne &
Brundin, 1976a; Yamaguchi *et al.*, 1977; Weinstock *et al.*, 1978;
Celuch *et al.*, 1978; Dubocovich *et al.*, 1978). In support of this
view, it has been reported that exposure to low concentrations of
isoprenaline enhances the release of noradrenaline during low-
frequency nerve stimulation in several noradrenergically innervated organs : guinea-pig atria, cat thoracic aorta and perfused
spleen and rat pineal glands. It is of interest to note that the
presence of presynaptic facilitatory beta-adrenoceptors was also
reported in the human oviduct (Hedqvist & Moawad, 1975) and in
human vasoconstrictor nerves (Stjärne & Brundin, 1976a,b). In
addition presynaptic beta-adrenoceptors are present in recently
formed noradrenergic nerve endings when rat superior cervical
ganglia are cultured (Weinstock *et al.*, 1978). Under these experimental conditions, the authors are dealing only with presynaptic nerve endings and their preparation is devoid of postsynaptic

structures.

The increase in stimulation-evoked noradrenaline release obtained
in the presence of isoprenaline is antagonized by preincubation
with 0.1 μM propranolol (Adler-Graschinsky & Langer, 1975; Celuch
et $al.$, 1978). However, acute exposure to 0.1 μM propranolol
does not always reduce stimulation-evoked noradrenaline release.
A small, but statistically significant reduction of transmitter
release elicited by nerve stimulation was obtained in isolated
guinea-pig atria (Adler-Graschinsky & Langer, 1975), in the perfused cat spleen (Celuch et $al.$, 1978) and in the calf muscle of
the cat pretreated with phenoxybenzamine (Dahlöf et $al.$, 1975).
On the other hand, exposure to 0.1 μM propranolol did not reduce
[^{3}H]noradrenaline release from human omental arteries and veins
(Stjärne & Brundin, 1975) and from the rat pineal gland
(Dubocovich et $al.$, 1978). Considerably higher concentrations of
propranolol reduce noradrenaline release during nerve stimulation
in several tissues. However, this effect is not due to the beta-
receptor blocking properties of the drug but rather appears to be
related to its local anaesthetic and membrane stabilizing effects
(Barret & Nunn, 1970; Hughes & Kneen, 1976).

While all the results discussed so far were obtained under in
$vitro$ conditions, the physiological significance of presynaptic
beta-adrenoceptors in sympathetic neurotransmission under in $vivo$
conditions remained an open question. Recently however, it was
shown that in the anaesthetized dog, an infusion of isoprenaline
enhanced the release of noradrenaline elicited by right cardioaccelerator nerve stimulation at low frequencies (Yamaguchi et $al.$,
1977). These authors also reported that the administration of the
beta-receptor blocking agent, sotalol, reduced significantly the
release of noradrenaline at stimulation frequencies between 1 and
5 Hz. These experiments carried out under in $vivo$ conditions are
compatible with the view that presynaptic beta-adrenoceptors may
play a physiological role in peripheral noradrenergic neurotransmission.

It is of interest to note that as already shown for the presynaptic alpha-adrenoceptor (Stjärne, 1974; Farah et $al.$, 1978), the
presynaptic beta-adrenoceptor is also stereospecific. The enhancement in transmitter release observed with (-)-isoprenaline
was not obtained when (+)-isoprenaline was added to the perfusion
medium in the cat spleen (Celuch et $al.$, 1978).

The effects of chronic beta-adrenoceptor blockade on noradrenergic
neurotransmission has been explored by several authors. Ljung et
$al.$ (1975) reported that prolonged administration of propranolol
or metoprolol to spontaneously hypertensive rats resulted in a
reduction in the responses to postganglionic nerve stimulation in
the portal vein preparation without concomitant changes in sensitivity to exogenous noradrenaline. In addition, Lewis (1974)
reported that in the pithed rat preparation chronic but not acute
administration of practolol reduced the pressor responses to preganglionic sympathetic stimulation.

More recently, Chubb and Raine (1976) demonstrated that long-term treatment with propranolol reduced tyrosine hydroxylase activity in the superior cervical ganglia of the rabbit. These authors attributed their results to a decreased release of noradrenaline in response to chronic beta-blockade. In addition, Äblad *et al.* (1977) reported that long-term treatment with propranolol leads to a reduction in adrenal tyrosine hydroxylase activity in spontaneously hypertensive rats. Consequently, it is possible that long-term beta-receptor blockade may be more effective than the acute administration in reducing the amount of transmitter released per impulse from noradrenergic nerves.

Stjärne and Brundin (1975) showed that low concentrations of adrenaline increase the release of [^{3}H]noradrenaline elicited by field stimulation from human omental arteries and veins. When the concentration of adrenaline in the medium was increased an inhibition of stimulation-evoked transmitter release was obtained, due to stimulation of presynaptic alpha-adrenoceptors. Stjärne and Brundin (1975) suggested that the presynaptic beta-adrenoceptors can be activated by the levels of circulating catecholamines and may subserve the function of enhancing the secretion of sympathetic transmitter during conditions of increased secretion of adreno-medullary hormone.

The results discussed so far are compatible with the existence of beta-adrenoceptors in noradrenergic nerve endings. Activation of this mechanism by beta-adrenoceptor agonists leads to an increase in transmitter release during nerve stimulation (Fig. 2). The increase in noradrenaline release elicited by activation of presynaptic beta-adrenoceptors is more pronounced at low frequencies of nerve stimulation (Langer *et al.*, 1975b; Yamaguchi *et al.*, 1977; Celuch *et al.*, 1978).

It is possible that the presynaptic beta-adrenoceptors mediate a positive feedback mechanism for noradrenaline released at low frequencies of nerve stimulation (Fig. 2). The transmitter released at low frequencies would then trigger a facilitatory mechanism for its own release through the activation of presynaptic beta-adrenoceptors.

The β_1 or β_2 nature of the presynaptic beta-adrenoceptors is not sufficiently clear. According to Dahlöf *et al.* (1975) the presynaptic beta-adrenoceptors are of the β_1-type because they are blocked by metoprolol, a selective β_1-receptor blocking agent. Yet Stjärne and Brundin (1976a) conclude that the presynaptic beta-adrenoceptors involved in the facilitation of noradrenaline release are of the β_2-type because terbutaline and salbutamol enhanced stimulation-evoked transmitter release, while a β_1-agonist, H 110/38 was without effect. More recently, Dubocovich *et al.* (1978) found that terbutaline enhanced the potassium-evoked release of [^{3}H]noradrenaline from the rat pineal gland.

It is possible that the different results reflect species and tissue differences. On the other hand, it is also possible that the presynaptic beta-adrenoceptors which mediate the facilitation of

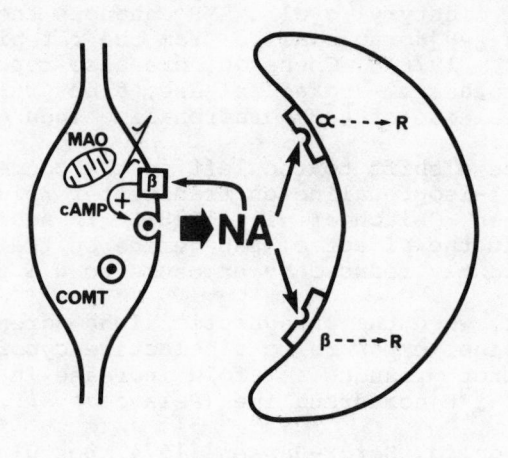

Fig. 2. Schematic representation of the positive feedback mechanism for noradrenaline released by nerve stimulation, mediated
by presynaptic β-adrenoceptors. Noradrenaline (NA) released by
low frequencies of nerve stimulation activates presynaptic β-adrenoceptors, leading to an increase in transmitter release. This
effect appears to be mediated through an increase in the levels
of cyclic AMP (cAMP) in noradrenergic nerve endings. The presynaptic positive feedback mechanism is present both in tissues
where the response (R) of the effector organ is mediated through
α- or through β-adrenoceptors. MAO : monoamine oxidase; COMT :
catechol-O-methyltransferase.

transmitter release during low frequency nerve stimulation differ
from the classical β_1 and β_2 postsynaptic adrenoceptors which mediate the responses of the effector organ. If one extrapolates
the evidence available for the presynaptic alpha-adrenoceptors
(α_2) which clearly differ from the postsynaptic (α_1) adrenoceptors
it follows that the presynaptic beta-adrenoceptors might themselves also differ from the classical postsynaptic beta-receptors.

The facilitation of transmitter release triggered by the activation of presynaptic beta-adrenoceptors may be mediated through an
increase in the levels of cyclic adenosine 3',5'-monophosphate
(cyclic AMP) in noradrenergic nerve endings (Fig. 2). Wooten *et
al*. (1973) reported that dibutyryl cyclic AMP and theophylline
increase the release of noradrenaline and of dopamine-β-hydroxylase elicited by nerve stimulation in the guinea-pig vas deferens.
Papaverine and other phosphodiesterase inhibitors enhance noradrenaline release during nerve stimulation (Langer, 1973; Langer,
et al., 1975a; Cubeddu *et al*., 1975; Celuch *et al*., 1978).

In the perfused cat spleen several cyclic nucleotide analogs enhance both noradrenaline and dopamine-β-hydroxylase release during nerve stimulation (Cubeddu et al., 1975). More recently, it
was reported that dibutyryl cyclic AMP enhances the potassium-
evoked release of [3H]noradrenaline from the rat pineal gland
(Dubocovich et al., 1978). These authors also reported that in
contrast to the potassium-evoked release, dibutyryl cAMP failed
to increase the release of [3H]noradrenaline induced by tyramine.

Papaverine induces a shift to the left in the concentration-ef-
fect curve for (-)-isoprenaline on transmitter release in the
perfused cat spleen (Celuch et al., 1978). In addition, these
authors found that the effect of papaverine on transmitter release is significantly reduced by exposure to 0.1 μM propranolol.

In the rat pineal, when the presynaptic alpha-adrenoceptors are
blocked by yohimbine, exposure to a selective cyclic AMP-phospho-
diesterase inhibitor produces a 2-fold increase in the potassium-
evoked release of [3H]noradrenaline (Pelayo et al., 1978).

In the adrenal medulla, Serck-Hansen (1974) postulated a beta-
adrenergic system confined to the adrenaline storing cell, which
enhances the release of the catecholamine and which appears to be
mediated by an increase in the cellular concentration of cyclic
AMP. The possible involvement of adenylate cyclase present in
noradrenergic nerve endings in the activation of tyrosine hydroxylase activity resulting from nerve stimulation was suggested by
Roth et al. (1975). However, it is not yet clear as to whether
a common presynaptic site of action is involved in the facilitation of noradrenaline release mediated by presynaptic beta-adrenoceptors and the increase in tyrosine hydroxylase activity that
occurs during and after sympathetic nerve stimulation. Both
phenomena appear to be mediated through an increase in cAMP levels
in nerve endings.

The increase in [3H]noradrenaline release observed in human omental blood vessels during exposure to isoprenaline was present
even after the local production of prostaglandins was inhibited
by the addition of 5,8,11,14-eicosatetranoic acid (Stjärne &
Brundin, 1976b).

    VIII WORKING HYPOTHESIS FOR THE PARTICIPATION OF THE PRE-
         SYNAPTIC ALPHA AND BETA-ADRENOCEPTORS IN THE REGULATION
         OF NORADRENALINE RELEASE DURING NERVE STIMULATION

Of the two presynaptic mechanisms which are involved in the auto-
regulation of noradrenaline release during nerve stimulation, the
one mediated by alpha-adrenoceptors appears to be the most
important.

The mechanism mediated by presynaptic beta-adrenoceptors is activated by low concentrations of noradrenaline (i.e., in the range
of low frequencies of nerve stimulation) leading to an increase
in transmitter release. When higher concentrations of noradrenaline are reached in the synaptic cleft, the regulatory mechanism

mediated by presynaptic alpha-adrenoceptors is triggered, leading
to inhibition of transmitter release (Fig. 3).

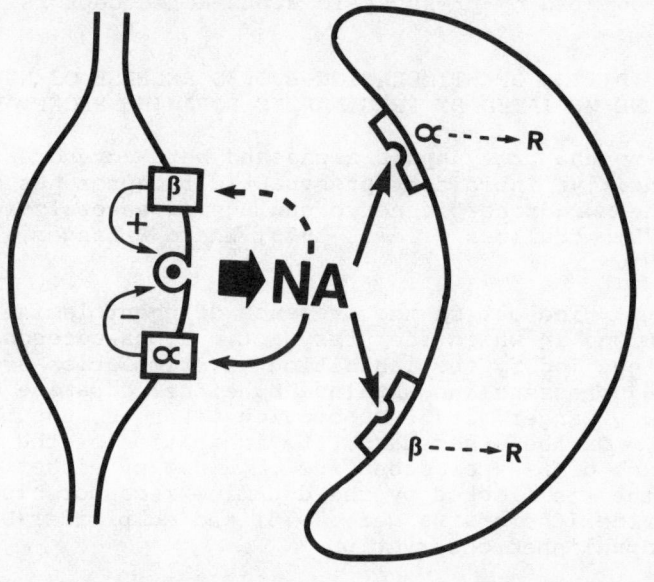

Fig. 3.   Role of the presynaptic α and β-adrenoceptors in the regulation of noradrenaline release during nerve stimulation.   During noradrenaline (NA) release at low frequencies of nerve stimulation (when the concentration of the released transmitter in the
synaptic cleft is rather low) the positive feedback mechanism mediated by presynaptic β-adrenoceptors is activated leading to an
increase in transmitter release. As the concentration of released
noradrenaline increases, a threshold is reached at which the negative feedback mechanism mediated by presynaptic α-adrenoceptors
is triggered, leading to inhibition of transmitter release.   Both
presynaptic feedback mechanisms are present in nerves, irrespective of the α or β nature of the receptors that mediate the response (R) of the effector organ.

The positive feedback mechanism which facilitates transmitter release appears to be mediated through an increase in the cyclic
AMP levels in noradrenergic nerve endings. On the other hand,
the negative feedback mechanism which leads to inhibition of noradrenaline release operates by restricting the calcium available
for the excitation-secretion coupling.

In the rat pineal gland it appears that an increase in the levels
of cyclic GMP in the noradrenergic nerve endings is somehow linked to events triggered by the activation of presynaptic alpha-
adrenoceptors and leading to a decrease in transmitter release
(Dubocovich *et al.*, 1978; Pelayo *et al.*, 1978). The fact that
the most pronounced increases in transmitter release are obtained
when the presynaptic alpha-adrenoceptors are blocked by drugs

supports the view that the major regulatory mechanism for noradrenaline release by nerve stimulation under physiological conditions is mediated by presynaptic alpha-adrenoceptors.

IX   INHIBITION OF STIMULATION-EVOKED RELEASE OF NORADREN-
      ALINE MEDIATED BY PRESYNAPTIC DOPAMINE RECEPTORS

In addition to the presynaptic alpha and beta-adrenoceptors, a
dopamine sensitive inhibitory presynaptic receptor has been described in the noradrenergic nerve endings of several tissues
(Langer, 1973; McCulloch *et al.*, 1973; Enero & Langer, 1975; Long
et al., 1975).

Experiments carried out in the presence of phentolamine (i.e.,
under conditions in which the presynaptic alpha-adrenoceptors are
blocked) do not modify the inhibition of stimulation-evoked release of [^{3}H]noradrenaline obtained by either dopamine or apomorphine (Enero & Langer, 1975; Dubocovich & Langer, unpublished observations). On the other hand, the inhibition of the stimulation-
evoked release of [^{3}H]noradrenaline obtained by either dopamine
or apomorphine was blocked by the dopamine receptor blocking
agents pimozide (Enero & Langer, 1975) and sulpiride (Dubocovich
& Langer, unpublished observations).

In contrast with the presynaptic alpha-adrenoceptors, which have
been found to be present in every tissue in which they were studied (for reviews, see Langer, 1974, 1977; Starke, 1977), the
presynaptic inhibitory dopamine receptors have not been found in
all the tissues in which they were looked for. So far, the presence of presynaptic inhibitory dopamine receptors has been demonstrated in the perfused cat spleen (Langer, 1973), in the cat
nictitating membrane (Enero & Langer, 1975), in the rabbit ear
artery (McCulloch *et al.*, 1973), and in the cat and dog heart
(Long *et al.*, 1975). It appears that the presynaptic dopamine
receptors are of pharmacological rather than physiological importance in peripheral noradrenergic neurotransmission because exposure to dopamine blocking agents does not increase the stimulation-evoked release of noradrenaline as it is the case with alpha-
adrenoceptor blocking agents.

X   REFERENCES

Åblad, B., Almgren, O., Carlsson, A., Henning, M., Jonasson, J. &
    Ljung, B. (1977). Reduced adrenal amine synthesis in spontan-
    eously hypertensive rats after long-term treatment with prop-
    ranolol. *Br. J. Pharmacol.* 61, 318-320.

Adler-Graschinsky, E. & Langer, S.Z. (1975). Possible role of a
    β-adrenoceptor in the regulation of noradrenaline release by
    nerve stimulation through a positive feedback mechanism. *Br.
    J. Pharmacol.* 53, 43-50.

Armstrong, J.M. & Boura, A.L.A. (1973). Effects of clonidine and guanethidine on peripheral sympathetic nerve function in the pithed rat. *Br. J. Pharmacol.* 47, 850-852.

Barret, A.M. & Nunn, B. (1970). Adrenergic neuron blocking properties of (±)-propranolol and (+)-propranolol. *J. Pharm. Pharmacol.* 22, 806-810.

Blakeley, A.G.H., Brown, G.L. & Ferry, C.B. (1963). Pharmacological experiments on the release of the sympathetic transmitter. *J. Physiol. Lond.* 167, 505-514.

Boullin, D.J., Costa, E. & Brodie, B.B. (1967). Evidence that blockade of adrenergic receptors causes overflow of norepinephrine in cat's colon after nerve stimulation. *J. Pharmacol. Exp. Ther.* 157, 125-134.

Brown, G.L. & Gillespie, J.S. (1957). The output of sympathetic transmitter from the spleen of the cat. *J. Physiol. Lond.* 138, 81-102.

Cavero, I., Lefevre, F. & Roach, A.G. (1977). Differential effects of prazosin on the pre- and postsynaptic α-adrenoceptors in the rat and dog. *Br. J. Pharmacol.* 61, 469P.

Cavero, I., Gomeni, R., Lefevre & Roach, A.G. (1978). Time-course analysis of the cardiovascular effects of clonidine resulting from the activation of cardiac pre and vascular postsynaptic α-adrenoceptors in the pithed rat. *Br. J. Pharmacol.* 62, 468P.

Celuch, S.M., Dubocovich, M.L. & Langer, S.Z. (1978). Stimulation of presynaptic β-adrenoceptors enhances ^{3}H-noradrenaline release during nerve stimulation in the perfused cat spleen. *Br. J. Pharmacol.*, in press.

Chubb, I.W. & Raine, A.E.G. (1976). Long term effects of propranolol on tyrosine hydroxylase and dopamine-β-hydroxylase in the superior cervical ganglia of the rabbit. *Br. J. Pharmacol.* 58, 430P.

Cubeddu, L.X., Barnes, E.M., Langer, S.Z. & Weiner, N. (1974). Release of norepinephrine and dopamine-β-hydroxylase by nerve stimulation. I. Role of neuronal and extraneuronal uptake and of alpha-presynaptic receptors. *J. Pharmacol. Exp. Ther.* 190, 431-450.

Cubeddu, L.X., Barnes, E. & Weiner, N. (1975). Release of norepinephrine and dopamine-β-hydroxylase by nerve stimulation. IV. An evaluation of a role for cyclic adenosine monophosphate. *J. Pharmacol. Exp. Ther.* 193, 105-127.

Cubeddu, L.X. & Weiner, N. (1975). Nerve-stimulation mediated overflow of norepinephrine and dopamine-β-hydroxylase. III. Effects of norepinephrine depletion on the alpha presynaptic regulation of release. *J. Pharmacol. Exp. Ther.* 192, 1-14.

Dahlöf, C., Äblad, B., Borg, K.O., Ek, L. & Waldeck, B. (1975).
Prejunctional inhibition of adrenergic nervous vasomotor con-
trol due to β-receptor blockade. *Proceeds. Symposium on
Chemical Tools in Catecholamine Research*, Vol. II (eds.)
O. Almgren, A. Carlsson & J. Engel, pp. 201-210, Amsterdam:
North Holland Publishing Co.

De Potter, W.P., Chubb, I.W., Put, A. & De Schaepdryver, A.F.
(1971). Facilitation of the release of noradrenaline and
dopamine-β-hydroxylase at low stimulation frequencies by
α-blocking agents. *Arch. Int. Pharmacodyn. Ther.* 193, 191-
197.

Doxey, J.C. & Everitt, J. (1977). Inhibitory effects of clonidine on responses to sympathetic nerve stimulation in the
pithed rat. *Br. J. Pharmacol.* 61, 559-566.

Drew, M.G. (1977). Pharmacological characterisation of the presynaptic α-adrenoceptor in the rat vas deferens. *Eur. J.
Pharmacol.* 42, 123-130.

Dubocovich, M.L. & Langer, S.Z. (1973). Effects of flowstop on
the metabolism of ^{3}H-noradrenaline released by nerve stimulation in the perfused cat's spleen. *Naunyn-Schmiedeberg's Arch.
Pharmacol.* 278, 179-194.

Dubocovich, M.L. & Langer, S.Z. (1974). Negative feedback regulation of noradrenaline release by nerve stimulation in the
perfused cat's spleen : differences in potency of phenoxybenzamine in blocking the pre- and post-synaptic adrenergic
receptors. *J. Physiol. Lond.* 237, 505-519.

Dubocovich, M.L. & Langer, S.Z. (1976). Influence of the frequency of nerve stimulation on the metabolism of ^{3}H-norepinephrine
released from the perfused cat spleen : differences observed
during and after the period of stimulation. *J. Pharmacol. Exp.
Ther.* 198, 83-101.

Dubocovich, M.L., Langer, S.Z., Pelayo, F. (1978). Effect of
cyclic nucleotides on ^{3}H-neurotransmitter release induced by
potassium stimulation in the rat pineal gland. *Br. J. Pharmacol.* 62, 383P.

Eisenfeld, A.J., Axelrod, J. & Krakoff, L. (1967). Inhibition of
the extraneuronal accumulation and metabolism of norepinephrine
by adrenergic blocking agents. *J. Pharmacol. Exp. Ther.* 156,
107-113.

Enero, M.A. & Langer, S.Z. (1973). Influence of reserpine-induced
depletion of noradrenaline on the negative feedback mechanism
for transmitter release during nerve stimulation. *Br. J.
Pharmacol.* 49, 214-225.

Enero, M.A. & Langer, S.Z. (1975). Inhibition by dopamine of ^{3}H-noradrenaline release elicited by nerve stimulation in the isolated cat's nictitating membrane. *Naunyn-Schmiedeberg's Arch. Pharmacol.* 289, 179-203.

Enero, M.A., Langer, S.Z., Rothlin, R.P. & Stefano, F.J.E. (1972). Role of the α-adrenoceptor in regulating noradrenaline overflow by nerve stimulation. *Br. J. Pharmacol.* 52, 549-557.

Farah, M.B. & Langer, S.Z. (1974). Protection by phentolamine against the effects of phenoxybenzamine on transmitter release elicited by nerve stimulation in the perfused cat heart. *Br. J. Pharmacol.* 52, 549-557.

Farah, M.B., Langer, S.Z. & Patil, P.N. (1978). Stereoselectivity of prejunctional alpha-adrenoceptors of the rat vas deferens and hypothalamus. *J. Pharmacol. Exp. Ther.*, in press.

Farnebo, L.O. & Malmfors, T. (1971). ^{3}H-noradrenaline release and mechanical response in the field stimulated mouse vas deferens. *Acta Physiol. Scand.* Suppl. 371, 1-18.

Filinger, E.J., Langer, S.Z., Perec, C.J. & Stefano, F.J.E. (1978). Evidence for the presynaptic location of the alpha-adrenoceptors which regulate noradrenaline release in the rat submaxillary gland. *Naunyn-Schmiedeberg's Arch. Pharmacol.*, in press.

Geffen, L.B. (1965). The effect of desmethylimipramine upon the overflow of sympathetic transmitter from the cat's spleen. *J. Physiol. Lond.* 181, 69-70P.

Haefely, W., Hurlimann, A. & Thoenen, H. (1965). Relation between the rate of stimulation and the quantity of noradrenaline liberated from sympathetic nerve endings in the isolated perfused spleen of the cat. *J. Physiol. Lond.* 181, 48-58.

Häggendal, J. (1970). Some further aspects on the release of the adrenergic transmitter. In: *New Aspects of Storage and Release Mechanisms of Catecholamines* (eds.) H.J. Schümann & G. Kroneberg, pp. 100-109, Berlin, Heidelberg:Springer-Verlag.

Hansson, L., Hunyor, S.N., Julius, S. & Hoobler, S.W. (1973). Blood pressure crisis following withdrawal of clonidine (Catapres, Catapresan) with special reference to arterial and urinary catecholamine levels, and suggestions for acute management. *Am. Heart J.* 85, 605-610.

Hedqvist, P. & Moawad, A. (1975). Presynaptic α- and β-adrenoceptor mediated control of noradrenaline release in human oviduct. *Acta Physiol. Scand.* 95, 494-496.

Hertting, G. (1965). Effects of drugs and sympathetic denervation on noradrenaline uptake and binding in animal tissues. In: *Pharmacology of Cholinergic and Adrenergic Transmission* (eds.) W.W. Douglas & A. Carlsson, pp. 277-288, Pergamon Press, Oxford.

Hughes, I.E. & Kneen, B. (1976). The effect of propranolol on sympathetic nerve stimulation in isolated vasa deferentia. *J. Pharm. Pharmacol.* 28, 200-205.

Iversen, L.L. (1965). The inhibition of noradrenaline uptake by drugs. *Adv. Drug Res.* 2, 5-23.

Iversen, L.L. (1967). In: *The Uptake and Storage of Noradrenaline in Sympathetic Nerves.* Cambridge University Press.

Iversen, L.L. & Langer, S.Z. (1969). Effect of phenoxybenzamine on the uptake and metabolism of noradrenaline in the rat heart and vas deferens. *Br. J. Pharmacol.* 37, 627-637.

Kirpekar, S.M. & Cervoni, P. (1963). Effect of cocaine, phenoxybenzamine and phentolamine on the catecholamine output from spleen and adrenal medulla. *J. Pharmacol. Exp. Ther.* 142, 59-70.

Kirpekar, S.M., Furchgott, R.F., Wakade, A.R. & Prat, J.C. (1973). Inhibition by sympathomimetic amines of the release of norepinephrine evoked by nerve stimulation in the cat spleen. *J. Pharmacol. Exp. Ther.* 187, 529-538.

Langer, S.Z. (1966). The degeneration contraction of the nictitating membrane in the anaesthetized cat. *J. Pharmacol. Exp. Ther.* 151, 66-72.

Langer, S.Z. (1970). The metabolism of ^{3}H-noradrenaline released by electrical stimulation from the isolated nictitating membrane of the cat and from the vas deferens of the rat. *J. Physiol. Lond.* 208, 515-546.

Langer, S.Z. (1973). The regulation of transmitter release elicited by nerve stimulation through a presynaptic feedback mechanism. In: *Frontiers in Catecholamine Research* (eds.) E. Usdin & S. Snyder, pp. 543-549, Pergamon Press, New York.

Langer, S.Z. (1974a). Selective metabolic pathways for noradrenaline in the peripheral and in the central nervous system. *Med. Biol.* 52, 372-383.

Langer, S.Z. (1974b). Presynaptic regulation of catecholamine release. *Biochem. Pharmacol.* 23, 1973-1800.

Langer, S.Z. (1975). Denervation supersensitivity. In: *Handbook of Psychopharmacology* Vol. 2, pp. 245-279, Plenum Publ. Corp, New York.

Langer, S.Z. (1976). The role of α- and β-presynaptic receptors in the regulation of noradrenaline release elicited by nerve stimulation. *Clin. Sci. Mol. Med.* 51, 423-426.

Langer, S.Z. (1977). Presynaptic receptors and their role in the regulation of transmitter release. *Sixth Gaddum Memorial Lecture. Br. J. Pharmacol.* 60, 481-497.

Langer, S.Z., Adler, E., Enero, M.A. & Stefano, F.J.E. (1971).
The role of the α-receptor in regulating noradrenaline over-
flow by nerve stimulation. *XXVth International Congress of
Physiological Sciences*, p. 335, Munich.

Langer, S.Z., Adler-Graschinsky, E. & Enero, M.A. (1974). Positive feed-back mechanism for the regulation of noradrenaline
released by nerve stimulation. Abstract of: Jerusalem Satel-
lite Symposia. *XXVIth International Congress of Physiological
Sciences*, p. 81.

Langer, S.Z., Adler-Graschinsky, E. & Giorgi, O. (1977). Physiological significance of the alpha-adrenoceptor mediated negative feed-back mechanism that regulates noradrenaline release
during nerve stimulation. *Nature* 265, 648-650.

Langer, S.Z. & Dubocovich, M.L. (1977). Subsensitivity of presynaptic α-adrenoceptors after exposure to noradrenaline.
Eur. J. Pharmacol. 41, 87-88.

Langer, S.Z., Dubocovich, M.L. & Celuch, S.M. (1975a). Prejunctional regulatory mechanisms for noradrenaline release elicited by nerve stimulation. In: *Chemical Tools in Catecholamine
Research*, Vol. II (eds.) C. Almgren, A. Carlsson & J. Engel,
pp. 183-191, Amsterdam:Elsevier, North Holland/USA.

Langer, S.Z. & Enero, M.A. (1974). The potentiation of responses
to adrenergic nerve stimulation in the presence of cocaine :
its relationship to the metabolic fate of released norepinephrine. *J. Pharmacol. Exp. Ther.* 191, 431-443.

Langer, S.Z., Enero, M.A., Adler-Graschinsky, E., Dubocovich, M.L.
& Celuch, S.M. (1975b). Presynaptic regulatory mechanisms for
noradrenaline release by nerve stimulation. In: *Proc. Symp.
Central Action of Drugs in the Regulation of Blood Pressure*
(eds.) D.S. Davies & J.L. Reid, pp. 133-151, Pitman Medical,
London.

Langer, S.Z., Enero, M.A., Adler-Graschinsky, E. & Stefano, F.J.E.
(1972b). The role of the α-receptor in the regulation of transmitter overflow elicited by stimulation. *Vth Int. Cong.
Pharmacology*, p. 134, San Francisco.

Langer, S.Z. & Luchelli-Fortis, M.A. (1977). Subsensitivity of
the presynaptic alpha-adrenoceptors after short term surgical
denervation of the cat nictitating membrane. *J. Pharmacol.
Exp. Ther.* 202, 610-621.

Langer, S.Z., Stefano, F.J.E. & Enero, M.A. (1972a). Pre and
post-synaptic origin of the norepinephrine metabolites formed
during transmitter release elicited by nerve stimulation.
J. Pharmacol. Exp. Ther. 183, 90-102.

Langer, S.Z. & Trendelenburg, U. (1966). The onset of denervation
supersensitivity. *J. Pharmacol. Exp. Ther.* 151, 73-86.

Langer, S.Z. & Vogt, M. (1971). Noradrenaline release from isolated muscles of the nictitating membrane of the cat. *J.
   Physiol. Lond.* 214, 159-171.

Lewis, M.J. (1974). Effect of acute and chronic treatment with
   practolol on cardiovascular responses in the pithed rat.
   J. Pharm. Pharmacol. 26, 783-788.

Ljung, B., Äblad, B., Dahlöf, C., Henning, M. & Hultberg, E.
   (1975). Impaired vasoconstrictor nerve function in spontaneously hypertensive rats after long-term treatment with propranolol and metoprolol. *Blood Vessels* 12, 311-315.

Lokhandwala, M.F. & Buckley, J.P. (1976). Effect of presynaptic
   α-adrenoceptor blockade on responses to cardiac nerve stimulation in anesthetized dogs. *Eur. J. Pharmacol.* 40, 183-186.

Long, J.P., Heintz, S., Cannon, J.G. & Kim, J. (1975). Inhibition
   of the sympathetic nervous system by 5,6-dihydroxy-2-dimethyl-
   amino tetralin (M-7), apomorphine and dopamine. *J. Pharmacol.
   Exp. Ther.* 192, 336-342.

Luchelli-Fortis, M.A. & Langer, S.Z. (1975). Selective inhibition
   by hydrocortisone of ^{3}H-normetanephrine formation during ^{3}H-
   transmitter release elicited by nerve stimulation in the isolated nerve-muscle preparation of the cat nictitating membrane.
   Naunyn-Schmiedeberg's Arch. Pharmacol. 287, 261-275.

McCulloch, M.W., Rand, M.J. & Story, D.F. (1972). Inhibition of
   ^{3}H-noradrenaline release from sympathetic nerves of guinea pig
   atria by a presynaptic α-adrenoceptor mechanism. *Br. J. Pharmacol.* 46, 523-524P.

McCulloch, M.W., Rand, M.J. & Story, D.F. (1973). Evidence for a
   dopaminergic mechanism for modulation of adrenergic transmission in the rabbit ear artery. *Br. J. Pharmacol.* 49, 41P.

O'Dea, R.F. & Zatz, M. (1976). Catecholamine stimulated cyclic
   GMP accumulation in the rat pineal : apparent presynaptic site
   of action. *Proc. Nat. Acad. Sci. USA* 73, 3398-3402.

Peart, W.S. (1949). The nature of splenic sympathin. *J. Physiol.
   Lond.* 108, 491-501.

Pelayo, F., Dubocovich, M.L. & Langer, S.Z. (1977). Regulation
   of noradrenaline release in the rat pineal through a negative
   feedback mechanism mediated by presynaptic alpha-adrenoceptors.
   Eur. J. Pharmacol. 45, 317-318.

Pelayo, F., Dubocovich, M.L. & Langer, S.Z. (1978). Regulation
   of noradrenaline release from the rat pineal through presynaptic adrenoceptors : possible involvement of cyclic nucleotides.
   Nature, in press.

Pettinger, W.A., Keeton, T.K., Campbell, W.B. & Harper, D.C. (1976). Evidence for a renal α-adrenergic receptor inhibiting renin release. *Circ. Res.* 38, 338-346.

Rand, M.J., McCulloch, M.W. & Story, D.F. (1975). Pre-junctional modulation of noradrenergic transmission by noradrenaline, dopamine and acetylcholine. In: *Central Action of Drugs in Blood Pressure Regulation* (eds.) D.S. Davies & J.L. Reid, pp. 94-132, Pitman Medical, London.

Rand, M.J., Story, D.F., Allen, G.S., Glover, A.B. & McCulloch, M.W. (1973). Pulse-to-pulse modulation of noradrenaline release through a prejunctional α-receptor auto-inhibitory mechanism. In: *Frontiers in Catecholamine Research* (eds.) E. Usdin & S. Snyder, pp. 579-581, Pergamon Press, New York.

Roach, A.G., Lefevre, F. & Cavero, I. (1978). Effects of prazosin and phentolamine on cardiac presynaptic α-adrenoceptors in the cat, dog and rat. *Clin. Exp. Hypert.*, 1, 87-101.

Robson, R.D. & Antonaccio, M.J. (1974). Effect of clonidine on responses to cardiac nerve stimulation as a function of impulse frequency and stimulus duration in vagotomized dogs. *Eur. J. Pharmacol.* 29, 182-186.

Roth, R.H., Walters, J.R., Murrin, L.C. & Morgenroth, V.H. (1975). Dopamine neurons : Role of impulse flow and presynaptic receptors in the regulation of tyrosine hydroxylase. In: *Pre- and Post-Synaptic Receptors* (eds.) E. Usdin & W.E. Bunney, pp. 5-46, Marcel Dekker, New York.

Scriabine, A. & Stavorski, J.M. (1973). Effect of clonidine on cardiac acceleration in vagotomized dogs. *Eur. J. Pharmacol.* 24, 101-104.

Serck-Hanssen, G. (1974). Effects of theophylline and propranolol on acetylcholine induced release of adrenal medullary catecholamines. *Biochem. Pharmacol.* 23, 2225-2235.

Standish, S.M. & Shafer, W.G. (1957). Serial histologic effects of rat submaxillary and sublingual salivary gland duct and blood vessel ligation. *J. Dental Res.* 36, 866-879.

Starke, K. (1972a). Alpha sympathomimetic inhibition of adrenergic and cholinergic transmission in the rabbit heart. *Naunyn-Schmiedeberg's Arch. Pharmacol.* 274, 18-45.

Starke, K. (1972b). Influence of extracellular noradrenaline on the stimulation-evoked secretion of noradrenaline from sympathetic nerves : Evidence for an alpha-receptor mediated feed-back inhibition of noradrenaline release. *Naunyn-Schmiedeberg's Arch. Pharmacol.* 275, 11-23.

Starke, K. (1977). Regulation of noradrenaline release by presynaptic receptors systems. *Rev. Physiol. Biochem. Pharmacol.* 77, 1-124.

Starke, K., Borowski, E. & Endo, T. (1975b). Preferential blockade of presynaptic α-adrenoceptors by yohimbine. *Eur. J.
Pharmacol.* 34, 385-388.

Starke, K., Endo, T. & Taube, H.D. (1975a). Relative pre- and
postsynaptic potencies of α-adrenoceptor agonists in the rabbit pulmonary artery. *Naunyn-Schmiedeberg's Arch. Pharmacol.*
291, 55-78.

Starke, K. & Montel, H. (1973). Influence of drugs with affinity
for alpha-adrenoceptors on noradrenaline release by potassium
and tyramine. *Proc. 2nd Ann. Mtg. - Adrenergic Mechanisms,*
pp. 53-54, Porto.

Starke, K., Montel, H., Gay, K.W. & Merker, R. (1974). Comparison of the effects of clonidine on pre and postsynaptic adrenoceptors in the rabbit pulmonary artery. *Naunyn-Schmiedeberg's
Arch. Pharmacol.* 285, 133-150.

Starke, K., Montel, H. & Schumann, J.J. (1971). Influence of
cocaine and phenoxybenzamine on noradrenaline uptake and release. *Naunyn-Schmiedeberg's Arch. Pharmacol.* 270, 210-214.

Stjärne, L. (1974). Stereoselectivity of presynaptic α-adrenoceptors involved in feedback control of sympathetic neurotransmitter secretion. *Acta Physiol. Scand.* 90, 286-288.

Stjärne, L. & Brundin, J. (1975). Dual adrenoceptor-mediated control of noradrenaline secretion from human vasoconstrictor nerves : facilitation by β-receptors and inhibition by α-receptors.
Acta Physiol. Scand. 94, 139-141.

Stjärne, L. & Brundin, J. (1976a). β_2-adrenoceptors facilitating
noradrenaline secretion from human vasoconstrictor nerves.
Acta Physiol. Scand. 97, 88-93.

Stjärne, L. & Brundin, J. (1976b). Additive stimulating effects
of inhibitor of prostaglandin synthesis and of β-adrenoceptor
agonist on sympathetic neuroeffector function in human omental
blood vessels. *Acta Physiol. Scand.* 97, 267-269.

Stjärne, L. & Brundin, J. (1977). Frequency-dependence of ^{3}H-nor-
adrenaline secretion from human vasoconstrictor nerves : modification by factors interfering with α- or β-adrenoceptor or
prostaglandin E2 mediated control. *Acta Physiol. Scand.* 101,
199-210.

Stjärne, L. & Gripe, K. (1973). Prostaglandin-dependent and -in-
dependent feedback control of noradrenaline secretion in vasoconstrictor nerves of normotensive human subjects. A preliminary report. *Naunyn-Schmiedeberg's Arch. Pharmacol.* 280, 441-
446.

Vogel, S.A., Silberstein, S.D., Berv, K.R. & Kopin, I.J. (1972).
Stimulation-induced release of norepinephrine from rat superior cervical ganglia *in vitro*. *Eur. J. Pharmacol.* 20, 308-311.

Von Euler, U.S. (1946). A specific sympathomimetic ergone in adrenergic nerve fibres (sympathin) and its relationship to ad-
-enaline and noradrenaline. *Acta Physiol. Scand.* 12, 73-97.

Weinstock, M., Thoa, N.B. & Kopin, I.J. (1978). β-adrenoceptors
modulate noradrenaline release from axonal sprouts in cultured
rat superior cervical ganglia. *Eur. J. Pharmacol.* 47, 297-302.

Wooten, G.F., Thoa, N.B., Kopin, I.J. & Axelrod, J. (1973). Enhanced release of dopamine-β-hydroxylase and norepinephrine
from sympathetic nerves by dibutyryl adenosine 3'5'-monophos-
phate and theophylline. *Mol. Pharmacol.* 9, 178-183.

Yamaguchi, N., De Champlain, J. & Nadeau, R.A. (1977). Regulation
of norepinephrine release from cardiac sympathetic fibers in
the dog by presynaptic alpha and beta receptors. *Circ. Res.*
41, 108-117.

PRESYNAPTIC MUSCARINE RECEPTORS AND INHIBITION OF RELEASE

E. Muscholl

I   INTRODUCTION

The concept of the muscarinic inhibitory mechanism originated from the observation on the perfused rabbit heart that atropine facilitated the noradrenaline release evoked by acetylcholine but not that by dimethylphenylpiperazinium (DMPP) (Löffelholz, Lindmar & Muscholl, 1967). It was soon realized (Lindmar, Löffelholz & Muscholl, 1968) that atropine blocked not only the classical end-organ (or postsynaptic) receptors but also receptors inhibiting release of the transmitter, and it was suggested that the latter were situated on the terminal adrenergic nerve fibre (or presynaptically, as expressed in current terminology).

Reviewing the work that led to the hypothesis of presynaptic muscarinic inhibition a tribute has to be made to the investigations and ideas of Burn and Rand (1962) which attracted the interest of a great many students of the autonomic nervous system. Subsequently, and with the advance in techniques allowing quantitative determination of the release of transmitters, it was possible to differentiate between presynaptic and postsynaptic actions of acetylcholine and other cholinomimetic drugs, and to circumvent the diffculty that atropine-like agents are unsuitable tools for a selective blockade of either pre- or postsynaptic receptors. When the effect of acetylcholine on noradrenaline overflow evoked by electrical stimulation of the sympathetic nerves of the rabbit heart was studied (Löffelholz & Muscholl, 1969) it was found that the inhibitory action persisted in the presence of hexamethonium. Thus, for the terminal adrenergic neuron a clear distinction between the two recognized autonomic cholinergic receptor sites was achieved.

There are several reviews in which cholinergic-adrenergic interactions occurring at the presynaptic level are discussed (Kosterlitz & Lees, 1972; Muscholl, 1970, 1973a, 1973b; Vanhoutte, 1976) but the reader is also referred to publications dealing with presynaptic modulatory systems in general, including the muscarinic inhibition (Bacq, 1976; Baldessarini, 1975; Kirpekar, 1975; Starke, 1977; Stjärne, 1975a).

II   MUSCARINIC INHIBITION OF NORADRENALINE RELEASE EVOKED BY
      ELECTRICAL STIMULATION OF SYMPATHETIC NERVES

Heart. In extension of the experiments (see section III) demonstrating a muscarinic inhibition of noradrenaline release caused
by the nicotinic drug, DMPP, Löffelholz and Muscholl (1969)
investigated the action of acetylcholine (6 nM - 55 μM) on the
noradrenaline output evoked by electrical stimulation (10 Hz) of
the postganglionic sympathetic nerves of the perfused rabbit
heart. The lowest concentration of acetylcholine did not significantly alter the noradrenaline output but 55 nM - 5.5 μM decreased
it in a concentration-dependent manner. With the latter concentration the inhibition was 81% and maximal, 55 μM producing an
identical effect. The inhibition caused by acetylcholine was
fully antagonized by atropine, unaffected by hexamethonium, rapid
in onset (≤ 1 min), reversed by perfusion with drug-free solution
and not related to the effects of acetylcholine on heart rate,
myocardial tension development and coronary flow. Hexamethonium
alone did not alter, and excitation of nicotine receptors (by
DMPP) enhanced rather than decreased, the noradrenaline overflow
in response to nerve stimulation (Löffelholz & Muscholl, 1969).
Furthermore, neither acetylcholine nor atropine in the concentrations used altered the uptake of exogenous noradrenaline in the
rabbit heart (Lindmar et al., 1968), excluding the possibility
that changes in overflow were unrelated to changes of the quantity
of transmitter actually being released. Thus, the inhibition of
the stimulation-evoked noradrenaline output could be attributed
to the activation of a muscarine receptor affecting the neuronal
release.

The muscarinic nature of the inhibitory effect of acetylcholine
was confirmed in a subsequent study in which muscarinic agonists
such as oxotremorine, methacholine, carbachol, furtrethonium and
pilocarpine were found to have actions qualitatively similar to
that of acetylcholine, although there were quantitative differences in drug potency (see section VIII); atropine abolished
these inhibitory effects (Fozard & Muscholl, 1972).

Acetylcholine (10 and 100 μM) also caused atropine-sensitive
inhibition of noradrenaline overflow evoked by sympathetic nerve
stimulation at 3 Hz in the chicken heart (Engel & Löffelholz,
1976). Likewise, Langley and Gardier (1977) reported an inhibitory effect of acetylcholine (0.55 μM) on noradrenaline overflow
from the guinea-pig heart when the sympathetic nerves were stimulated at 2.5, 5 and 10 Hz. There was a parallel decrease of the
overflow of dopamine-β-hydroxylase in response to nerve stimulation. This is in line with the other evidence mentioned above
that acetylcholine inhibits the release of transmitter rather
than enhances its inactivation.

A possible physiological role of a muscarinic modulation of
release of the adrenergic transmitter is suggested by the following experiments in which electrical stimulation of the vagus
nerves was employed for releasing endogenous acetylcholine onto

adrenergic nerve fibres. It was thought that the rabbit atrium, for anatomical reasons, might provide a situation favouring the access of released acetylcholine to adrenergic terminals because previous observations had shown that adrenergic and cholinergic terminal axons are juxtaposed in the strands of the autonomic ground plexus innervating the atria of mammalian hearts (Hillarp, 1959; Norberg & Hamberger, 1964; Thoenen & Tranzer, 1968). In order to enhance the small noradrenaline output of the perfused atria (+)-amphetamine was added to the Tyrode solution. Electrical stimulation (10 Hz) of the right postganglionic sympathetic nerves evoked an overflow of noradrenaline that was decreased by 48% when the vagus nerves were stimulated (20 Hz) simultaneously (Löffelholz & Muscholl, 1970). The idea of a presynaptic inhibition, mediated by vagus nerve stimulation, of adrenergic neurotransmission to the heart was strengthened by the recent work of Levy and Blattberg (1976). In this study (using the open chest of the dog) stimulation of the left cardiac sympathetic nerves at 2 and 4 Hz increased ventricular tension development and evoked noradrenaline overflow into the coronary sinus blood. These responses were reduced by 25 and 30%, respectively, when both vagi were stimulated simultaneously at 15 Hz. The vagally induced changes in tension development and noradrenaline overflow were prevented by atropine (1 mg/kg). Since most of the noradrenaline that enters the coronary sinus is derived from the nerve terminals in the ventricular myocardium the muscarinic inhibition must have occurred in this region.

Vascular preparations. Because of the small amount of tissue involved the quantity of endogenous noradrenaline released from perfused vessels is minute (Bevan, Chesher & Su, 1969; Bell & Vogt, 1971). Therefore, the following experiments were rendered feasible only by incorporating labelled noradrenaline into the amine stores and by measuring the stimulation-evoked overflow of radioactivity above resting efflux. In three of the studies quoted below the radioactive compounds were separated by adsorption and ion exchange chromatography. Evidence was obtained that the increase in overflow of tritium produced by electrical stimulation of periarterial nerves reflected an increase of the [^{3}H] noradrenaline fraction, and that acetylcholine inhibited release of [^{3}H]noradrenaline to a larger extent than that of total tritium (Vanhoutte, Lorenz & Tyce, 1973; Vanhoutte & Verbeuren, 1976; Endo, Starke, Bangerter & Taube, 1977).

On the rabbit ear artery, nerve stimulation at 10 Hz enhanced extra- and intraluminal release of tritium that was decreased by 85% when acetylcholine (1.7 μM) was added (Steinsland, Furchgott & Kirpekar, 1973). Acetylcholine, in the range 30 nM - 10 μM, caused a concentration-dependent inhibition of tritium overflow by 5 Hz stimulation that was prevented by atropine (290 nM) but not affected by hexamethonium (10 μM) (Allen, Glover, McCulloch, Rand & Story, 1975). In both investigations there was a parallel suppression by acetylcholine of the vasoconstrictor response to nerve stimulation, and their restoration by atropine.

More extensive work has been carried out on dog saphenous vein
and pulmonary artery and vein (Vanhoutte *et al.*, 1973; Vanhoutte,
1974; Vanhoutte & Verbeuren, 1976). Acetylcholine (275 nM -
2.8 µM) decreased tritium overflow evoked by nerve stimulation at
2 Hz, but not that evoked by infusion of tyramine (12 or 23 µM).
On saphenous vein and pulmonary artery, the constrictor effect of
nerve stimulation was decreased by acetylcholine but on the mesenteric vein it was enhanced (see section VII). The tyramine-
induced tension was not altered by acetylcholine. Isoprenaline
relaxed the saphenous vein previously contracted by nerve stimulation but did not decrease tritium overflow. This result and
the observation, mentioned above, of a specific effect of acetylcholine on [^{3}H]noradrenaline overflow indicate that the changes
in radioactivity of the perfusate were not due to parallel
changes in mechanical expulsion of tritiated compounds. It was
further ascertained that the muscarinic inhibition of noradrenaline release evoked by nerve stimulation at 2 Hz (and that by
50 mM potassium ions) was still obtained on saphenous vein strips
treated with phentolamine (32 µM) or phenoxybenzamine (29 µM).
Thus, complete blockade of the presynaptic α-receptor mediated
negative feedback system did not interfere with the muscarinic
inhibitory mechanism, ruling out the possibility that acetylcholine acts through a facilitation of the presynaptic effect of
noradrenaline.

Starke, Endo, Taube and Borowski (1975) and Endo *et al.* (1977)
investigated agonists and antagonists of various receptor systems,
including acetylcholine and atropine, for their action on stimulation-evoked [^{3}H]noradrenaline release from rabbit pulmonary
strips. They found that the evoked overflow of [^{3}H]noradrenaline,
[^{3}H]dihydroxyphenylethylglycol (DOPEG) and [^{3}H]normetanephrine
was proportionally decreased by acetylcholine (1 µM). This is
further evidence that acetylcholine increases neither the uptake
and subsequent deamination of the released noradrenaline (the
DOPEG fraction should then increase) nor the metabolic inactivation by O-methylation (the normetanephrine fraction should then
increase). Consequently, the inhibitory action of acetylcholine
on tritium overflow was found to be unaltered in the presence of
the neuronal and extraneuronal uptake blockers, cocaine (30 µM)
and corticosterone (40 µM), but was antagonized by atropine
(100 nM).

Various organs. The rather ubiquitous occurrence of presynaptic
muscarine receptors on peripheral noradrenergic nerves is under-
lined by the following observations. Stimulation-evoked noradrenaline overflow (30 Hz) from the perfused cat spleen was
decreased by 58% in the presence of carbachol (55 µM) and this
effect was reversed by atropine (2.9 µM) (Kirpekar, Prat, Puig &
Wakade, 1972). In a subsequent study it was found that the inhibitory action of acetylcholine (5.5 µM) on stimulation-evoked
release of noradrenaline was more pronounced at low than at high
frequencies of sympathetic nerve stimulation (Kirpekar, Prat &
Wakade, 1975). Since this result indicates an analogy between
muscarinic inhibition and calcium deprivation it will be discussed

in section IX.

On the guinea-pig vas deferens (uptake blockers present), exogenous acetylcholine (1 and 5 µM) depressed [^{3}H]noradrenaline secretion in response to field stimulation at 1 Hz, but enhanced the
contractions induced by nerve stimulation. Both effects were
antagonized by atropine (1 µM). Atropine alone increased the
secretion of [^{3}H]noradrenaline, indicating that the release of
noradrenaline induced by field stimulation is normally restricted
by acetylcholine secreted from simultaneously stimulated cholinergic nerves (Stjärne, 1975b). Similar observations were made
on the isolated dog retractor penis muscle preincubated in [^{3}H]
noradrenaline (Klinge & Sjöstrand, 1977). Physostigmine (12 µM)
reduced and scopolamine (520 nM) enhanced tritium efflux evoked
by field stimulation at 2 Hz. A much lower concentration of
scopolamine (26 nM) markedly increased the adrenergic excitatory
response to field stimulation while acetylcholine (55 µM) and
physostigmine (240 nM) decreased it.

Mathé, Tong and Tisher (1977) have recently developed a perfused
rabbit lung preparation with the sympathetic and parasympathetic
innervation intact. They observed a small overflow of noradrenaline during and shortly after stimulation of the sympathetic
nerves at 10 Hz that was inhibited by methacholine (5 or 51 µM)
or by simultaneous stimulation of the vagi at 10 Hz. No anticholinergic drug was tested.

The various findings presented in this section allow the conclusion that in the peripheral adrenergic nervous system the muscarinic inhibitory mechanism is a widespread phenomenon. However,
it should also be mentioned that in the central nervous system
noradrenergic fibres do exist which lack muscarine receptors
(see chapter by K. Starke).

III   MUSCARINIC INHIBITION OF NORADRENALINE RELEASE EVOKED BY
      NICOTINIC DRUGS

The effect of muscarinic drugs on nicotinic noradrenaline release
from peripheral organs seems to have been tested only on isolated
heart preparations. Under these conditions nicotinic agents
activate receptors on the terminal adrenergic fibres and cause a
brief but massive amine release (for review see Muscholl, 1970;
Starke, 1977; chapter by Löffelholz).

For a long time the role of the muscarinic component of the action
of acetylcholine in modifying its nicotinic effect has been
obscured by usually combining acetylcholine with atropine-like
drugs which were believed to block only the end-organ receptors
and, therefore, to "unmask" its nicotinic effect. The identification of muscarine receptors on the terminal adrenergic fibre
was achieved when the effect of acetylcholine on the noradrenaline output of the rabbit heart was investigated and (a) a large
range of atropine concentrations (2.9 nM - 29 µM), and (b) a
similar range of acetylcholine concentrations (55 nM - 2.1 mM) was

tested (Lindmar *et al.*, 1968). Acetylcholine, even at 209 µM, caused only a small noradrenaline output but the latter was enhanced up to ten-fold if atropine (2.9 nM - 2.9 µM) was added to the perfusion medium. Conversely, these concentrations of atropine did not alter the noradrenaline overflow evoked by DMPP (31 µM) which releases the transmitter from rabbit heart by a calcium-dependent nicotinic action. These observations suggested the possibility that the noradrenaline release by acetylcholine which is mediated by nicotine receptors, is at the same time depressed by its muscarinic activity. In agreement with this, the action of acetylcholine was mimicked by that of a combination of DMPP and methacholine with the result that atropine increased the noradrenaline output after this drug combination, just as it increased the output after acetylcholine. Since the muscarine receptors are activated by much lower concentrations of acetyl-choline (550 nM - 55 µM) than the nicotine receptors (100 µM - 2.1 mM), acetylcholine exhibits more pronounced presynaptic inhi-bitory than excitatory effects and its noradrenaline releasing action needs muscarinic blockade in order to be fully developed (Fig. 1).

Facilitation by atropine of the noradrenaline release elicited by acetylcholine was also observed on perfused hearts of guinea-pigs (Lindmar *et al.*, 1968) and cats (Haeusler, Thoenen, Haefely & Huerlimann, 1968). In agreement with the working hypothesis of a muscarinic inhibitory mechanism, it was found that the noradrena-line output of the rabbit heart in response to DMPP was depressed in a concentration-dependent manner when methacholine, pilocarpine (Lindmar *et al.*, 1968), oxotremorine, carbachol, furtrethonium or MH-1 (see Fig. 2) were added and that these effects were antago-nized by atropine (Fozard & Muscholl, 1972). None of the musca-rinic compounds in the maximally inhibitory concentrations caused a significant rise of noradrenaline output above the resting value.

On the rabbit heart, methacholine (10 and 40 µM) also inhibited the noradrenaline output evoked by p-aminophenethyltrimethyl-ammonium (PAPETA) (32 µM) (Muscholl, 1973a), a drug that is more specific than DMPP at nicotine receptors (Barlow & Franks, 1971). Likewise, on the guinea-pig heart previously perfused with [3H] noradrenaline, acetylcholine (10 µM) or methacholine (10 µM) inhibited the tritium efflux evoked by nicotine (10 µM) (Westfall & Hunter, 1974).

IV   MUSCARINIC INHIBITION OF NORADRENALINE RELEASE EVOKED BY
      A HIGH POTASSIUM ION CONCENTRATION

The muscarinic inhibition of transmitter release appeared to affect a process which, in the sequence of events leading to secretion, occurs after excitation of nicotine receptors. Blockade of nico-tine receptors with hexamethonium did not prevent the inhibitory action of acetylcholine on transmitter overflow produced by electrical stimulation of sympathetic nerves (Löffelholz & Muscholl, 1969). Propagation of orthodromic impulses is a prere-quisite for noradrenaline release by electrical nerve stimulation.

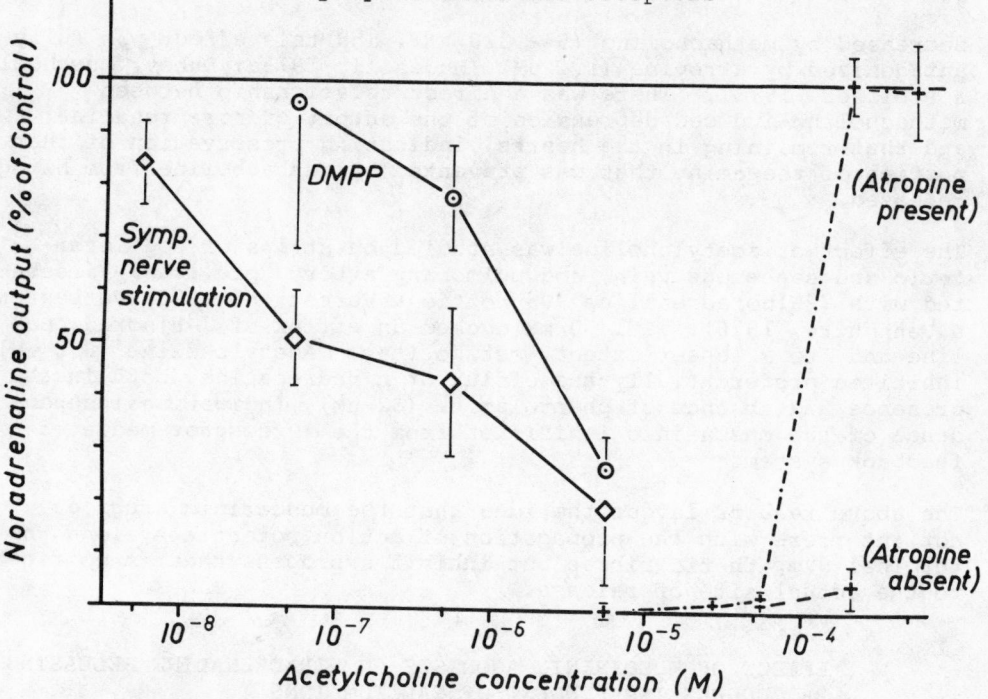

Fig. 1. Muscarinic and nicotinic effects of acetylcholine on the release of noradrenaline from the
perfused rabbit heart. Ordinate, noradrenaline
output as % of control output (sympathetic nerve
stimulation, 600 impulses at 10 Hz; DMPP 31 μM
for 2 min) or as % maximum output (acetylcholine
above 10 μM in the presence or absence of atropine 1.4 μM). Abscissa, molar concentration of
acetylcholine. Given are means ± S.E. of 3 - 8
observations. Note that muscarinic inhibition
occurs at concentrations of acetylcholine which
are below the threshold for a nicotinic release
of noradrenaline. Reproduced from Muscholl
(1970).

Antidromic impulses have been recorded from postganglionic sympathetic nerves after injection of nicotinic drugs into the blood
supply of cat spleen and heart (Ferry, 1963; Cabrera, Torrance &
Viveros, 1966), though they may not be causally involved in
transmitter release (Haeusler et al., 1968). However, the noradrenaline release evoked by a high concentration of potassium is
independent of impulses (Kirpekar & Wakade, 1968; Haeusler et al.,
1968). This stimulation procedure was chosen in order to see
whether muscarinic inhibition is due to blockade of propagation
of impulses travelling along the terminal axons. The noradrenaline output of the rabbit heart in response to 135 mM KCl
(isosmotic replacement of NaCl) was concentration-dependently

decreased by methacholine (5 - 320 μM), and this effect was fully
antagonized by atropine (1.4 μM) (Muscholl, 1973a; Dubey, Muscholl
& Pfeiffer, 1975). There was a direct relationship between
methacholine-induced depression of the output of noradrenaline
and that remaining in the hearts, indicating preservation of that
portion of the amine that was prevented by methacholine from being
released.

The effect of acetylcholine was studied on strips of dog mesenteric and saphenous vein, and pulmonary artery, previously incubated with [³H]noradrenaline (Vanhoutte & Verbeuren, 1976; Verbeuren
& Vanhoutte, 1976). KCl 50 mM evoked an efflux of [³H]noradrena-
line and, to a lesser extent, metabolites. Acetylcholine (0.6 μM)
inhibited preferentially the efflux of noradrenaline, both in the
presence and absence of phentolamine (32 μM), indicating indepen-
dence of the muscarinic inhibition from the α-receptor mediated
feedback system.

The above results favour the idea that the muscarinic drugs do
not interfere with the propagation of action potentials along the
terminal sympathetic fibres but inhibit a process that is confined
to the actual site of release.

V   EFFECT OF MUSCARINIC AGONISTS ON NORADRENALINE RELEASING PROCEDURES INDEPENDENT OF CALCIUM IONS

Löffelholz and Muscholl (1969) found that methacholine (38 μM)
did not alter the noradrenaline overflow evoked by tyramine
(29 μM) although it resulted in the cessation of beating of rabbit
hearts. In view of the evidence obtained with nicotinic drugs
and nerve stimulation, they concluded that mechanisms of release
linked to electrical events on the membrane and to entry of calcium ions are susceptible to muscarinic inhibition, in contrast
to the mechanism involved in release by an indirectly acting
amine. This observation is not restricted to cardiac nerve
fibres. Vanhoutte (1974) administered a vasoconstrictor dose of
tyramine to dog pulmonary artery strips preloaded with [³H]nor-
adrenaline. Acetylcholine (1.1 μM) had no inhibitory action on
the tritium overflow and tension development produced by tyramine.

Another procedure causing amine release independent of external
calcium ions is the perfusion of tissues with solutions having a
low sodium ion content (see Table 1). Methacholine (320 μM) had
no effect on noradrenaline release from the rabbit heart 5 - 10
min after introduction, or 0 - 5 min after cessation, of a low
Na⁺ solution, at times when there was little or no calcium
dependence of release (Dubey et al., 1975). When the heart is
perfused for 30 min with a medium containing a high potassium
and low sodium ion concentration, noradrenaline release occurs
in two phases. Resolution of the two phases by kinetic analysis
showed that the noradrenaline release during the first phase
($t_{1/2}$ = 1.6 min) was calcium-dependent and inhibited by methacholine (40 and 320 μM), but that during the second phase ($t_{1/2}$ =
17 min) was unaffected by omission of calcium ions or presence of

methacholine (Muscholl, Ritzel & Rössler, 1975).

VI   EFFECT OF METHACHOLINE ON THE RELEASE OF AN ADRENERGIC FALSE TRANSMITTER

It is known that adrenergic false transmitters, among them α-methyl-adrenaline, are taken up by the neuronal amine pump, transferred to the storage vesicles and released by nerve impulses or nicotinic drugs in the same proportion to endogenous noradrenaline as they are stored in the tissue (Muscholl, 1972). Hearts from rabbits which had received an infusion of α-methyladrenaline were isolated, the sympathetic nerves were stimulated at 10 Hz and an infusion of the nicotinic drug, PAPETA, or a solution containing 54 mM KCl was given (Fuder, Muscholl & Wegwart, 1976). All these procedures evoked a release of both α-methyladrenaline and noradrenaline that was greatly decreased by methacholine (40 µM) or lowering of the calcium ion concentration. Atropine (1.4 µM) antagonized the effect of methacholine on PAPETA and high K^+ induced amine release. However, tyramine (36 µM) evoked a preferential release of the false transmitter that was not altered by methacholine or calcium deprivation. The results of this study show that the muscarinic inhibition of neuronal noradrenaline release and the requirement of calcium ions for its liberation by depolarizing stimuli can be extended to a false transmitter amine.

VII   INDIRECT EVIDENCE FOR MUSCARINIC MODULATION OF TRANSMITTER RELEASE

After the muscarinic inhibition of noradrenaline release had been established, several reports have appeared in which muscarinic drugs were found to decrease the end-organ responses to electrical stimulation of sympathetic nerves. Although such observations have been regarded as indirect evidence for a presynaptic inhibitory effect of muscarine receptor activation, care must be taken in their interpretation. This is illustrated by the work of Vanhoutte (1974) who showed that on isolated strips of dog saphenous vein or pulmonary, mesenteric and femoral arteries acetylcholine (28 and 55 nM) decreased the rise of isometric tension evoked by electrical stimulation of sympathetic nerves at 2 - 5 Hz, but increased it on strips of pulmonary and mesenteric veins. Yet on both pulmonary artery and mesenteric vein previously incubated in [^{3}H]noradrenaline, the efflux of tritium evoked by nerve stimulation was decreased when acetylcholine (1.1 µM) was added. Apparently, the postsynaptic effect of acetylcholine on the mesenteric vein masks the presynaptic inhibitory effect on the sympathetic nerves, and this might be true also for the pulmonary vein. Without the information obtained by measuring the overflow of tritium, a muscarinic inhibition of transmitter release from mesenteric and pulmonary vein would have to be denied, especially since on both preparations acetylcholine also enhanced the contractions induced by noradrenaline (Vanhoutte 1974).

With these reservations in mind the inhibitory actions of acetylcholine, methacholine, muscarine, arecoline and carbachol on
vasoconstrictor responses elicited by periarterial nerve stimulation of perfused rabbit ear arteries (Rand & Varma, 1970), and
that of acetylcholine on perfused rat mesenteric arteries (Malik
& Ling, 1969) or the rabbit ear artery (Hume, de la Lande &
Waterson, 1972) may be taken as indirect evidence for a muscarinic
modulation of noradrenaline release. However, pilocarpine up to
600 μM did not inhibit the vasoconstrictor responses to nerve
stimulation (at 20 Hz) on the rabbit ear artery (Rand & Varma,
1970) although this concentration corresponded to that causing a
50% inhibition of stimulation-evoked (10 Hz) noradrenaline overflow from the rabbit heart (Fozard & Muscholl, 1972). As later
shown by Steinsland *et al*. (1973), pilocarpine (0.1 - 1 mM)
completely inhibited the response of the ear artery to nerve
stimulation at 1 - 4 Hz but produced only 50% inhibition at frequencies of 8 - 10 Hz.

When the end-organ response to nerve stimulation rather than
transmitter release is taken as a measure of the presynaptic
activity of a drug, the interpretation of results on cardiac
tissues is even more complicated than that on vascular preparations. Most tissues available for such experiments are not only
innervated by adrenergic but also by cholinergic fibres, and the
postsynaptic responses resulting from a combination of acetylcholine and noradrenaline administered are not simply the alge-
braic sum of the effects of each of these compounds. This has
been shown for the dog heart *in situ* (for detailed review of
various papers see Levy, 1971; Higgins, Vatner & Braunwald, 1973),
rabbit atria (Carrier & Bishop, 1972), rat atria (Grodner, Lahrtz,
Pool & Braunwald, 1970), cat papillary and chicken ventricular
muscle (Kissling, Reuter, Sieber, Nguyen-Duong & Jacob, 1972).
The dominant effect of acetylcholine on automaticity and contractility has previously been regarded as a result of mainly postsynaptic interactions (Grodner *et al.*, 1970; Levy, 1971). This
view was based on various observations that cholinergic interven-
tions on adrenergic responses definitely occurred when the latter
were produced by administration of catecholamines, thus excluding
a presynaptic effect. However, the presynaptic inhibitory influence of acetylcholine, in addition to its postsynaptic effects,
is now considered as a functionally important site of action
(Higgins *et al.*, 1973; Levy & Blattberg, 1976).

VIII   THE TYPE OF MUSCARINE RECEPTOR INVOLVED IN THE INHIBITORY
       EFFECT

Pharmacological characteristics of presynaptic muscarine receptors. The evidence for the unequivocal distinction between the
presynaptic muscarinic and nicotinic effects of acetylcholine has
been presented in sections II and III and illustrated by Fig. 1
(see also Fozard & Muscholl, 1974a).

In order to characterize the muscarine receptors of the terminal
adrenergic nerve fibres, nine compounds with differing potencies
on cardiac postsynaptic muscarine receptors were selected, and

their muscarinic affinities as inhibitors of noradrenaline
release determined (Fozard & Muscholl, 1972). In this study on
the perfused rabbit heart, noradrenaline release was evoked by
sympathetic nerve stimulation or infusion of DMPP, and the postsynaptic responses tested were those of atrial tension development
and ventricular rate. If a series of compounds produce their
effects through activation of the same receptors then their order
of potency and relative potencies should be identical on all
tissues containing those receptors. The muscarinic compounds
(except AHR 602, N-benzyl-3-pyrrolidyl acetate methobromide, and
McN-A-343, 4-(m-chlorophenylcarbamoyloxy)-2-butynyltrimethyl-
ammonium chloride) each produced atropine-sensitive inhibition of
noradrenaline release evoked both by nerve stimulation and DMPP.
The order of potency on both parameters and the potencies relative to acetylcholine were in good agreement with those for inhibition of atrial tension (Fig. 2), or ventricular rate (Fozard &

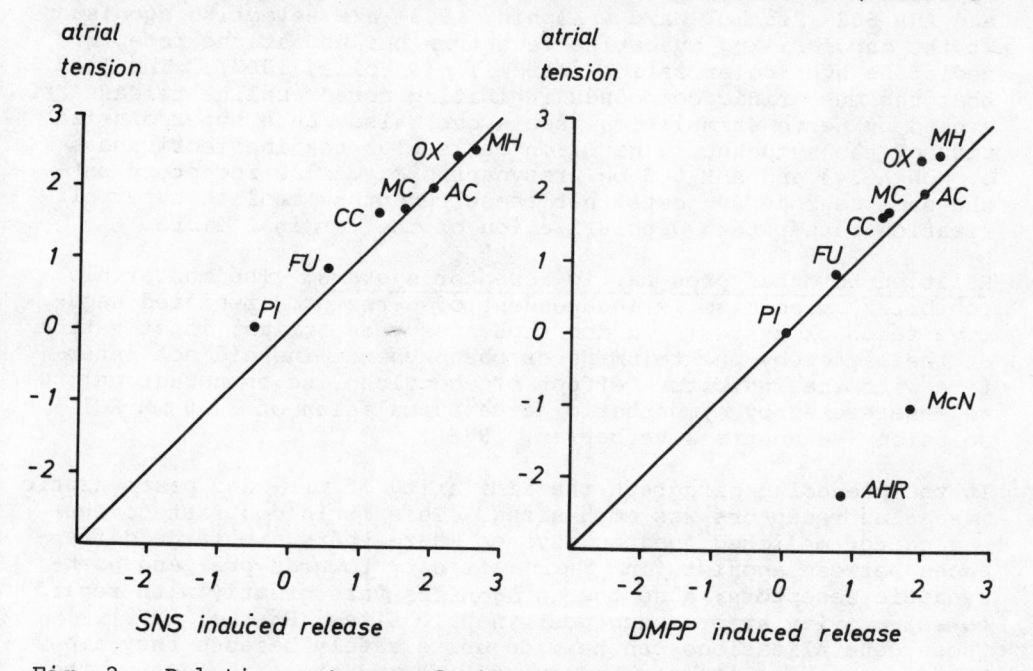

Fig. 2.   Relative potency of nine muscarinic agonists on
          atrial tension development and noradrenaline
          output evoked by sympathetic nerve stimulation
          (SNS) or DMPP on the perfused rabbit heart.
          Relative potencies (log. scale), calculated from
          the negative log. of ED_{50} molar concentrations,
          with that of acetylcholine (AC) expressed as log.
          100. SNS, 600 pulses at 10 Hz; DMPP, 96 µM for
          3 min. MH, N-methyl-1,2,5,6, tetrahydro-nicotinic
          acid prop-2-yne ester (MH-1); OX, oxotremorine;
          MC, methacholine; CC, carbachol; FU, furtretho-
          nium; PI, pilocarpine; McN, McN-A-343; AHR, AHR
          602. Values taken from Fozard and Muscholl
          (1972).

Muscholl, 1972). These results suggest that the muscarine receptors mediating the pre- and postsynaptic inhibitory responses are
similar.

Two compounds (AHR 602 and McN-A-343) were found to increase noradrenaline output evoked by nerve stimulation (therefore they
were omitted from Fig. 2, left panel) and to decrease the noradrenaline output in response to DMPP by a non-muscarinic mechanism, being thereby relatively more potent than the other muscarinic drugs (Fig. 2 right panel). In a subsequent study it was
shown that the facilitated release of noradrenaline after nerve
stimulation and the inhibition of release after DMPP produced by
McN-A-343 and AHR 602 were the result of their combined local
anaesthetic action and inhibition of neuronal amine uptake
(Fozard & Muscholl, 1974b). On the somadendritic membrane of the
superior cervical ganglion cells, McN-A-343 (Roszkowski, 1961)
and AHR 602 (Franko, Ward & Alphin, 1963) are selective agonists
at the depolarizing muscarine receptors but not at the receptors
mediating hyperpolarization (Jaramillo & Volle, 1967). The fact
that the muscarinic compounds inhibiting noradrenaline release
evoked by nerve stimulation (see above) also cause hyperpolarization of the sympathetic ganglion cells plus the ineffectiveness
of McN-A-343 and AHR 602 on presynaptic muscarine receptors on
the same neurone suggests that these receptors mediate hyperpolarization rather than depolarization of the terminal fibre.

Relation to other presynaptic receptor systems. The muscarinic
inhibitory mechanism is independent of α-receptor mediated negative feedback system. On dog saphenous vein strips, inactivation
of the latter by phentolamine or phenoxybenzamine did not interfere with the inhibitory effect of acetylcholine on noradrenaline
release evoked by sympathetic nerve stimulation or a 50 mM KCl
solution (Vanhoutte & Verbeuren, 1976).

In the preceding paragraph the similarity of pre- and postsynaptic
muscarine receptors was emphasized. This is in contrast to the
α-receptor mediated feedback system where there are large differences between agonists in their affinity towards pre- and postsynaptic receptors; also the antagonists vary greatly with regard
to selectivity at pre- and postsynaptic sites (Starke, 1977).
These generalizations can be made quite safely because they are
based on experiments carried out on one and the same tissue, the
rabbit pulmonary artery.

On rabbit heart and pulmonary artery, bradykinin has been demonstrated to inhibit noradrenaline release by an indirect presynaptic effect that is mediated through enhanced formation of prostaglandins of the E series (Starke, Peskar, Schumacher & Taube,
1977). A mechanism of this kind was ruled out for the muscarinic
inhibition of noradrenaline release. Fuder and Muscholl (1974)
perfused rabbit hearts with indomethacin (30 μM). In agreement
with previous work (Chanh, Junstad & Wennmalm, 1972), the noradrenaline output in response to sympathetic nerve stimulation at
3 Hz was increased. Under these conditions the output of prostaglandins of the E series was blocked (Chanh et al., 1972). Both

in the presence and absence of indomethacin, methacholine (40 μM)
decreased the stimulation-evoked output of noradrenaline by a
similar percentage (Fuder & Muscholl, 1974).

Antimuscarinic drugs. In most of the experiments mentioned above,
atropine was used as a muscarine receptor antagonist. Apparently,
no comparative study has been made in which various anticholinergic drugs were tested for their potency to block presynaptic inhibitory muscarine receptors. However, occasionally drugs other
than atropine have been used to antagonize the presynaptic action
of acetylcholine, e.g., scopolamine in the experiments by Klinge
and Sjöstrand (1977), and propantheline or hyoscine-N-methyl
bromide by Hume et al. (1972).

In high concentrations, atropine has effects on neurotransmission
not attributable to blockade of muscarinic sites. For instance,
on the rabbit pulmonary artery presynaptic α-receptors were
blocked by concentrations > 1 μM (Starke et al., 1975; Endo
et al., 1977; Nedergaard & Schrold, 1977), postsynaptic α-receptors
by 10 μM and neuronal noradrenaline uptake by > 60 μM (Nedergaard
& Schrold, 1977). However, 100 nM is a concentration suitable
for muscarinic presynaptic blockade because it did not antagonize
the effect of a low concentration of the α-receptor agonist,
tramazoline, but prevented the inhibitory effect of acetylcholine
(100 nM) on stimulation-evoked noradrenaline overflow (Endo et al.,
1977). Methylatropinium which on the presynaptic muscarine receptors of the rabbit heart is equipotent to atropine (Muscholl,
unpublished observation) is, up to 300 μM, devoid of a postsynaptic α-receptor blocking action on the rabbit pulmonary artery
(Nedergaard & Schrold, 1977) and may therefore be preferred when
administration of a large concentration of an anticholinergic drug
is unavoidable.

Facilitation of adrenergic neurotransmission by muscarine receptor agonists. A possible facilitation of adrenergic transmission
by low concentrations of acetylcholine has aroused some interest,
mainly because such an action is a postulate of the cholinergic
link hypothesis (Burn & Rand, 1962). Malik and Ling (1969)
described 3 experiments in which acetylcholine (275 pM) increased
by 8 ± 4% the response of the rat mesenteric artery preparation
to sympathetic nerve stimulation at 7 Hz. Rand and Varma (1970)
reported a few experiments on the rabbit ear ertery in which very
low concentrations of acetylcholine or muscarine sometimes
enhanced the constrictor effect of periarterial nerve stimulation
at < 10 Hz. There was also no statistical evaluation of the
results.

Trials to obtain facilitation of noradrenaline release with low
doses of acetylcholine have yielded controversial results, depend-
ing on the preparation used and perhaps also on the technical
question as to whether noradrenaline or total radioactivity was
determined. In experiments designed specifically to investigate
the suggested enhancement of transmitter release Muscholl (1973a)
failed to observe any increase in noradrenaline output from the
rabbit heart evoked by nerve stimulation at 10 Hz after acetyl-

choline (55 and 550 pM). Previously it was shown that acetylcholine (5.5 nM) had also no effect while 55 nM - 55 μM produced
inhibition of noradrenaline release (Löffelholz & Muscholl, 1969).
On the rabbit pulmonary artery stimulated at 2 Hz acetylcholine
(10 pM - 10 nM) had no effect, independent of whether the superfusion medium contained cocaine and corticosterone or not (Endo
et al., 1977). However, Allen et al. (1975) found that picomolar
concentrations of acetylcholine enhanced stimulation-evoked (5 Hz)
mechanical responses and tritium overflow from rabbit ear arteries
preincubated with [³H]noradrenaline. It is questionable whether
these facilitatory actions of acetylcholine are due to muscarine
receptor activation because they were neither enhanced by neostig-
mine (Allen et al., 1975) nor antagonized by atropine (Allen
et al., 1975; Malik & Ling, 1969). Furthermore, the facilitatory
effects of picomolar concentrations of acetylcholine persisted
after its withdrawal while the inhibitory actions of nanomolar
concentrations were reversed by perfusion with drug-free medium
(Allen et al., 1975). In this context it should be noted that
Hume et al. (1972) failed to confirm the enhancement by low concentrations of acetylcholine of vasoconstrictor responses to
nerve stimulation although they used the same technique and perfusion medium as Rand and Varma (1970).

IX   THE RELATIONSHIP BETWEEN MUSCARINIC INHIBITION AND DEPENDENCE ON CALCIUM FOR RELEASE

The following evidence which has partially been reviewed above
strongly favours the idea (Löffelholz & Muscholl, 1969; Kirpekar
et al., 1972, 1975; Muscholl, 1973a and b; Dubey et al., 1975)
that activation of muscarine receptors inhibits exocytotic
release: (a) The procedures shown to be affected by muscarinic
inhibition (depolarizing stimuli such as electrical stimulation,
nicotinic drugs, and elevation of the potassium ion concentration
above 50 mM) are all calcium-dependent (Table 1). Moreover,
release of dopamine-β-hydroxylase has been established, although
the proportion to that of noradrenaline is still a matter of
debate (Baldessarini, 1975; Kirpekar, 1975), and acetylcholine
was found to inhibit dopamine-β-hydroxylase release in response
to nerve stimulation (Langley & Gardier, 1977). (b) Lowering of
the calcium ion concentration potentiated the inhibitory effect
of methacholine on potassium-evoked noradrenaline output, indicating that muscarinic inhibition interferes with the availability
of calcium for the secretory process (Dubey et al., 1975), as has
been suggested for the α-receptor mediated negative feedback
system (Stjärne, 1973). (c) Methacholine affected the release
of the false neurotransmitter, α-methyladrenaline, in the same
manner as that of endogenous noradrenaline (Fuder et al., 1976).
This is true with regard to calcium-dependent and independent
releasing procedures. These experiments also show that the
muscarinic inhibition cannot be explained by an alteration of the
biosynthesis of the transmitter, or its metabolism. (d) The
rapid onset of the muscarinic inhibition is consistent with the
hypothesis that a membrane phenomenon is involved. Thus,

independent of the time of preperfusion (0.5 - 15 min) of methacholine the potassium-evoked noradrenaline release was reduced by
the same proportion (Muscholl *et al.*, 1975).

TABLE 1   Relationship between Occurrence of Muscarinic
          Inhibition and Calcium Requirement of Nor-
          adrenaline Release from Peripheral Adrenergic
          Neurons

NA release	Muscarinic Inhibition of NA release	Calcium requirement for NA release
Electrical nerve stimulation	+ see section II	+ Huković & Muscholl (1962) + Kirpekar & Misu (1967)
Nicotinic drugs	+ see section III	+ Lindmar, Löffelholz & Muscholl (1967) + Löffelholz (1967)
Potassium ions	+ see section IV	+ Kirpekar & Wakade (1968) + Sorimachi, Oesch & Thoenen (1973)
Tyramine	- see section V	- Lindmar *et al.* (1967) - Thoenen, Huerlimann & Haefely (1969)
Low Na$^+$ solutions	- see section V	- Bogdanski & Brodie (1969) - Garcia & Kirpekar (1973)

NA, noradrenaline. Action defined in heading has been established
(+) or was not found (-).

Apart from the correlation between calcium dependence of release
and its susceptibility to muscarinic inhibition, no further
details of the processes which finally link the receptor activation to the control mechanisms of neurotransmitter secretion are
known.   Drugs activating presynaptic inhibitory muscarine receptors hyperpolarize the somadendritic portion of the neuron (see
section VIII).   Haeusler *et al.* (1968) observed on cardiac sympathetic nerves that pilocarpine reduced the amplitude of asynchronous discharges evoked by acetylcholine and suggested that muscarinic drugs hyperpolarize the terminals.   It is conceivable that
hyperpolarization counteracts a moderate depolarizing stimulus
triggering release.   It is, however, unlikely that in the presence of 135 mM KCl (cf. Dubey *et al.*, 1975) methacholine could
really lead to a substantial inhibition of the depolarization
caused by the excess of potassium.   An alternative possibility,
suggested by Kirpekar *et al.* (1972), is the opposing influence of

an outward movement of potassium on calcium influx. Enhancement
of potassium permeability by 10 - 20 mM KCl or a muscarinic drug
would then decrease the transmitter release. This is compatible
with observations on dog saphenous vein strips that 10 - 20 mM
KCl (Lorenz & Vanhoutte, 1975) or acetylcholine (0.6 µM)
(Vanhoutte *et al.*, 1973) inhibited [3H]noradrenaline overflow
evoked by nerve stimulation but not that evoked by tyramine. It
is not known whether KCl 10 - 20 mM interferes with the propagation of impulses along the splenic nerves (Kirpekar *et al.*, 1972)
and thereby inhibits transmitter release, although this was less
likely in the experiments of Lorenz and Vanhoutte (1975) who
applied field stimulation.

Since calcium is believed to be rate-limiting for transmitter
release by nervous impulses (Stjärne, 1975) and calcium entry
into the neuron may be frequency-dependent (Kirpekar, 1975),
alterations of the rate of stimulation should also affect the
muscarinic inhibition if the calcium availability hypothesis is
valid. Experiments on vessels and cat spleen agree with this
proposal while confirmatory evidence on hearts is lacking. The
inhibition by acetylcholine of vasoconstrictor responses to nerve
stimulation (10 Hz for 10 - 40 sec) was decreased as the duration
of the stimulation period increased (Hume *et al.*, 1972).
Similarly, frequency -vasoconstrictor response curves also
obtained on the rabbit ear artery showed a much greater inhibitory
effect of acetylcholine (0.14 and 1.4 µM) at 10 Hz than at 35 Hz
(Steinsland *et al.*, 1973). On the perfused cat spleen the inhibition by acetylcholine (5.5 µM) of stimulation-evoked release of
noradrenaline was 98% at 1Hz, 70% at 5 Hz and only 13% at 30 Hz
(Kirpekar *et al.*, 1975). On the rabbit heart there is no comparable evidence based on a similar range of impulse rates. However,
a 3-fold increase in the frequency of nerve stimulation had no
conspicuous effects on the inhibition produced by methacholine
(30 - 40 µM) because the noradrenaline overflow at 3 Hz was
decreased by 84% (Fuder & Muscholl, 1974) and that at 10 Hz by
73% (Fozard & Muscholl, 1972). On the guinea-pig heart the inhibition by acetylcholine (0.6 µM) of stimulation-evoked noradrenaline and dopamine-β-hydroxylase overflow was independent of the
frequency when tested at 2.5, 5 and 10 Hz (Langley & Gardier,
1977).

X   POSSIBLE PHYSIOLOGICAL AND PHARMACOLOGICAL SIGNIFICANCE
       OF THE MUSCARINIC INHIBITORY MECHANISM

Evidence that the muscarinic inhibition might have a physiological
role comes from two kinds of observations: (a) Although most of
the experiments demonstrating a muscarinic inhibition of transmitter release have been carried out on saline-perfused organs or
on isolated tissues under *in vitro* conditions, there are equally
conclusive results which were obtained *in vivo* on the dog heart
(Levy & Blattberg, 1976) or saphenous vein (Vanhoutte, 1976).
(b) On organs innervated by both cholinergic and adrenergic
postganglionic fibres electrical stimulation of the parasympathetic nerve trunks decreased the overflow of noradrenaline elicited

by simultaneous electrical stimulation of the sympathetic supply
(Löffelholz & Muscholl, 1970; Mathé *et al.*, 1977), and this effect
was atropine-sensitive (Levy & Blattberg, 1976).

The recognition of the principle of the presynaptic muscarinic
control of adrenergic nervous activity will not only lead to
re-interpretation of previous findings but also to the design of
new experimental studies to further elucidate the functional role
of reciprocal innervation of organs by the two divisions of the
autonomic nervous system. Which organs will be the most likely
candidates in the search for a physiologically occurring muscarinic inhibitory system? As discussed in section II the morphological basis for this cholinergic-adrenergic interaction is the
autonomic ground plexus (Hillarp, 1959). There is electron microscopic evidence for axo-axonal synapses between neighbouring
adrenergic and cholinergic terminal fibres in rat iris and atrium
(Ehinger, Falck & Sporrong, 1970), and it remains to be seen
whether these synapses permit a particularly efficient interaction. A reciprocal influence has also to be taken into consideration, in view of the evidence for the α-adrenoceptor mediated
inhibition of acetylcholine release (Paton & Vizi, 1969). In
this case it is less clear, however, whether the α-receptors are
located presynaptically or on the somadendritic membrane.
Moreover, cholinergic neurones have also been considered to have
presynaptic muscarine receptors mediating a negative feedback
control. This was first suggested from results on brain tissue
by Polak (1971) but similar evidence has been obtained for peripheral cholinergic neurones (Kilbinger, 1977).

A pharmacological significance of the muscarinic inhibition of
noradrenaline release is rendered likely by the possibility that
atropine-like drugs relieve the restriction by endogenous parasympathetic activity of sympathetic tone, and that muscarinic
drugs inhibit the effect of a sympathetic drive. As far as the
sites of these actions are concerned one is faced with two different systems. Adrenergic nerve fibres endowed with presynaptic
inhibitory muscarine receptors occur not only in organs innervated
by the autonomic ground plexus but also in organs without a func-·
tionally important cholinergic innervation such as veins, abdominal
arteries and spleen. Atropine-like drugs are supposed to exert
relief from parasympathetic influence only in the former tissues
while muscarine receptor agonists might interfere with functions
in all organs receiving an adrenergic supply.

XI   REFERENCES

Allen, G.S., Glover, A.B., McCulloch, M.W., Rand, M.J. & Story,
    D.F. (1975). Modulation by acetylcholine of adrenergic
    transmission in the rabbit ear artery. *Br. J. Pharmacol.* 54,
    49-53.

Bacq, Z.M. (1976). Les contrôles de la libération des médiateurs
    aux terminaisons des nerf adrénergiques. *J. Physiol. (Paris)*
    72, 371-542.

Baldessarini, R.J. (1975). Release of catecholamines. In:
Handbook of Psychopharmacology (eds.) L.L. Iversen, S.D.
Iversen & S.H. Snyder, Vol. 3, pp. 37-137, Plenum Press, New
York.

Barlow, R.B. & Franks, F. (1971). Specificity of some ganglion
stimulants. *Br. J. Pharmacol.* 42, 137-142.

Bell, C. & Vogt, M. (1971). Release of endogenous noradrenaline
from an isolated muscular artery. *J. Physiol. (Lond.)* 215,
509-521.

Bevan, J.A., Chesher, G.B. & Su, C. (1969). Release of adrenergic transmitter from terminal nerve plexus in artery. *Agents
Actions* 1, 20-26,

Bogdanski, D.F. & Brodie, B.B. (1969). The effects of inorganic
ions on the storage and uptake of H^3-norepinephrine by rat
heart slices. *J. Pharmacol. Exp. Ther.* 165, 181-189.

Burn, J.H. & Rand, M.J. (1962). A new interpretation of the
adrenergic nerve fibre. *Adv. Pharmacol.* 1, 1-30.

Cabrera, R., Torrance, R.W. & Viveros, H. (1966). The action of
acetylcholine and other drugs upon the terminal parts of the
postganglionic sympathetic fibre. *Br. J. Pharmacol.* 27, 51-
63.

Carrier, G.O. & Bishop, V.S. (1972). The interaction of acetylcholine and norepinephrine on heart rate. *J. Pharmacol. Exp.
Ther.* 180, 31-37.

Chanh, P.H., Junstad, M. & Wennmalm, A. (1972). Augmented noradrenaline release following nerve stimulation after inhibition of prostaglandin synthesis with indomethacin. *Acta
Physiol. Scand.* 86, 563-567.

Dubey, M.P., Muscholl, E. & Pfeiffer, A. (1975). Muscarinic
inhibition of potassium-induced noradrenaline release and its
dependence on the calcium concentration. *Naunyn Schmiedeberg's
Arch. Pharmacol.* 291, 1-15.

Ehinger, B., Falck, B. & Sporrong, B. (1970). Possible axo-axonal
synapses between peripheral adrenergic and cholinergic nerve
terminals. *Z. Zellforsch.* 107, 508-521.

Endo, T., Starke, K., Bangerter, A. & Taube, H.D. (1977). Presynaptic receptor systems on the noradrenergic neurones of
the rabbit pulmonary artery. *Naunyn Schmiedeberg's Arch.
Pharmacol.* 296, 229-247.

Engel, U. & Löffelholz, K. (1976). Presence of muscarinic inhibitory and absence of nicotinic excitatory receptors at the
terminal sympathetic nerves of chicken hearts. *Naunyn
Schmiedeberg's Arch. Pharmacol.* 295, 225-230.

Ferry, C. (1963). The sympathomimetic effect of acetylcholine in the spleen of the cat. *J. Physiol. (Lond.)* 167, 487-504.

Fozard, J.R. & Muscholl, E. (1972). Effects of several muscarinic agonists on cardiac performance and the release of noradrenaline from sympathetic nerves of the perfused rabbit heart. *Br. J. Pharmacol.* 45, 616-629.

Fozard, J.R. & Muscholl, E. (1974a). Do adrenergic fibres have muscarinic inhibitory receptors? - A reply. *J. Pharm. Pharmacol.* 26, 662-664.

Fozard, J.R. & Muscholl, E. (1974b). Atropine-resistant effects of the muscarinic agonists McN-A-343 and AHR 602 on cardiac performance and the release of noradrenaline from sympathetic nerves of the perfused rabbit heart. *Br. J. Pharmacol.* 50, 531-541.

Franko, B.V., Ward, J.W. & Alphin, R.S. (1963). Pharmacological studies of N-benzyl-3-pyrrolidyl acetate methobromide (AHR-602), a ganglion stimulating agent. *J. Pharmacol. Exp. Ther.* 139, 25-30.

Fuder, H. & Muscholl, E. (1974). The effect of methacholine on noradrenaline release from the rabbit heart perfused with indomethacin. *Naunyn Schmiedeberg's Arch. Pharmacol.* 285, 127-132.

Fuder, H., Muscholl, E. & Wegwart, R. (1976). The effects of methacholine and calcium deprivation on the release of the false transmitter, α-methyladrenaline, from the isolated rabbit heart. *Naunyn Schmiedeberg's Arch. Pharmacol.* 293, 225-234.

Garcia, A.G. & Kirpekar, S.M. (1973). Release of noradrenaline from the cat spleen by sodium deprivation. *Br. J. Pharmacol.* 47, 729-747.

Grodner, A.S., Lahrtz, H., Pool, P.E. & Braunwald, E. (1970). Neurotransmitter control of sinoatrial pacemaker frequency in isolated rat atria and in intact rabbits. *Circ. Res.* 27, 867-873.

Haeusler, G., Thoenen, H., Haefely, W. & Huerlimann, A. (1968). Electrical events in cardiac adrenergic nerves and noradrenaline release from the heart induced by acetylcholine and KCl. *Naunyn Schmiedeberg's Arch. Pharmacol. Exp. Pathol.* 261, 389-411.

Higgins, C.B., Vatner, S.F. & Braunwald, E. (1973). Parasympathetic control of the heart. *Pharmacol. Rev.* 25, 119-155.

Hillarp, N.-A. (1959). The construction and functional organization of the autonomic innervation apparatus. *Acta Physiol. Scand.* 46, 1-68.

Huković, S. & Muscholl, E. (1962). Die Noradrenalin-Abgabe aus dem isolierten Kaninchenherzen bei sympathischer Nervenreizung und ihre pharmakologische Beeinflussung. *Naunyn Schmiedeberg's Arch. Exp. Pathol. Pharmacol.* 244, 81-96.

Hume, W.R., de la Lande, I.S. & Waterson, J.G. (1972). Effect of acetylcholine on the response of the isolated rabbit ear artery to stimulation of the perivascular sympathetic nerves. *Eur. J. Pharmacol.* 17, 227-233.

Jaramillo, J. & Volle, R.L. (1967). Ganglionic blockade by muscarine, oxotremorine and AHR-602. *J. Pharmacol. Exp. Ther.* 158, 80-88.

Kilbinger, H. (1977). Modulation by oxotremorine and atropine of acetylcholine release evoked by electrical stimulation of the myenteric plexus of the guinea-pig ileum. *Naunyn Schmiedeberg's Arch. Pharmacol.* 300, 145-151.

Kirpekar, S.M. (1975). Factors influencing transmission at adrenergic synapses. *Prog. Neurobiol.* 4, 163-212.

Kirpekar, S.M. & Misu, Y. (1967). Release of noradrenaline by splenic nerve stimulation and its dependence on calcium. *J. Physiol. (Lond.)* 188, 219-234.

Kirpekar, S.M., Prat, J.C., Puig, M. & Wakade, A.R. (1972). Modification of the evoked release of noradrenaline from the perfused cat spleen by various ions and agents. *J. Physiol. (Lond.)* 221, 601-615.

Kirpekar, S.M., Prat, J.C. & Wakade, A.R. (1975). Effect of calcium on the relationship between frequency of stimulation and release of noradrenaline from the perfused spleen of the cat. *Naunyn Schmiedeberg's Arch. Pharmacol.* 287, 205-212.

Kirpekar, S.M. & Wakade, A.R. (1968). Release of noradrenaline from the cat spleen by potassium. *J. Physiol. (Lond.)* 194, 595-608.

Kissling, G., Reutter, K., Sieber, G., Nguyen-Duong, H. & Jacob, R. (1972). Negative Inotropie von endogenem Acetylcholin beim Katzen- und Hühnerventrikelmyokard. *Pflügers Arch.* 333, 35-50.

Klinge, E. & Sjöstrand, N.O. (1977). Suppression of the excitatory adrenergic neurotransmission; a possible role of cholinergic nerves in the retractor penis muscle. *Acta Physiol. Scand.* 100, 368-376.

Kosterlitz, H.W. & Lees, G.M. (1972). Interrelationships between adrenergic and cholinergic mechanisms. In: *Catecholamines* (eds.) H. Blaschko & E. Muscholl, *Handbook of Experimental Pharmacology*, Vol. 33, pp. 762-812, Springer, Berlin.

Langley, A.E. & Gardier, R.W. (1977). Effect of atropine and acetylcholine on nerve stimulated output of noradrenaline and dopamine-beta-hydroxylase from isolated rabbit and guinea-pig hearts. *Naunyn Schmiedeberg's Arch. Pharmacol.* 297, 251-256.

Levy, M.N. (1971). Sympathetic-parasympathetic interactions in the heart. *Circ. Res.* 29, 437-445.

Levy, M.N. & Blattberg, B. (1976). Effect of vagal stimulation on the overflow of norepinephrine into the coronary sinus during cardiac sympathetic nerve stimulation in the dog. *Circ. Res.* 38, 81-85.

Lindmar, R., Löffelholz, K. & Muscholl, E. (1967). Unterschiede zwischen Tyramin und Dimethylphenylpiperazin in der Ca^{++}-Abhängigkeit und im zeitlichen Verlauf der Noradrenalin-Freisetzung am isolierten Kaninchenherzen. *Experientia* 23, 933-934.

Lindmar, R., Löffelholz, K. & Muscholl, E. (1968). A muscarinic mechanism inhibiting the release of noradrenaline from peripheral adrenergic nerve fibres by nicotinic agents. *Br. J. Pharmacol.* 32, 280-294.

Löffelholz, K. (1967). Untersuchungen über die Noradrenalin-Freisetzung durch Acetylcholin am perfundierten Kaninchen-herzen. *Naunyn Schmiedeberg's Arch. Pharmacol. Exp. Pathol.* 258, 108-122.

Löffelholz, K., Lindmar, R. & Muscholl, E. (1967). Der Einfluß von Atropin auf die Noradrenalin-Freisetzung durch Acetylcholin. *Naunyn Schmiedeberg's Arch. Pharmacol. Exp. Pathol.* 257, 308.

Löffelholz, K. & Muscholl, E. (1969). A muscarinic inhibition of the noradrenaline release evoked by postganglionic sympathetic nerve stimulation. *Naunyn Schmiedeberg's Arch. Pharmacol.* 265, 1-15.

Löffelholz, K. & Muscholl, E. (1970). Inhibition of parasympathetic nerve stimulation of the release of the adrenergic transmitter. *Naunyn Schmiedeberg's Arch. Pharmacol.* 267, 181-184.

Lorenz, R.R. & Vanhoutte, P.M. (1975). Inhibition of adrenergic neurotransmission in isolated veins of the dog by potassium ions. *J. Physiol. (Lond.)* 246, 479-500.

Malik, K.U. & Ling, G.M. (1969). Modification by acetylcholine of the response of rat mesenteric arteries to sympathetic stimulation. *Circ. Res.* 25, 1-9.

Mathé, A.A., Tong, E.Y. & Tisher, P.W. (1977). Norepinephrine release from the lung by sympathetic nerve stimulation inhibition by vagus and methacholine. *Life Science* 20, 1425-1430.

Muscholl, E. (1970). Cholinomimetic drugs and release of the adrenergic transmitter. In: *New Aspects of Storage and Release Mechanisms of Catecholamines* (eds.) H.J. Schümann & G. Kroneberg, pp. 168-186, Springer, Berlin.

Muscholl, E. (1972). Adrenergic false transmitters. In: *Catecholamines* (eds.) H. Blaschko & E. Muscholl, *Handbook of Experimental Pharmacology*, Vol. 33, pp. 618-660, Springer, Berlin.

Muscholl, E. (1973a). Muscarinic inhibition of the norepinephrine release from peripheral sympathetic fibres. *Proc. 5th Int. Cong. Pharmacol.*, Karger, Basel, 4, 440-457.

Muscholl, E. (1973b). Regulation of catecholamine release. The muscarinic inhibitory mechanism. In: *Frontiers in Catecholamine Research* (eds.) E. Usdin & S.H. Snyder, pp. 537-542, Pergamon Press, Oxford.

Muscholl, E., Ritzel, H. & Rössler, K. (1975). The time course of noradrenaline release caused by high potassium-low sodium solution. Effects of methacholine or decrease of the calcium ion concentration. *Br. J. Pharmacol.* 55, 248P.

Nedergaard, O.A. & Schrold, J. (1977). Effect of atropine on vascular adrenergic neuroeffector transmission. *Blood Vessels,* 14, 325-347.

Norberg, K.-A. & Hamberger, B. (1964). The sympathetic adrenergic neuron. *Acta Physiol. Scand.* 63, Suppl. 238, 1-42.

Paton, W.D.M. & Vizi, E.S. (1969). The inhibitory action of noradrenaline and adrenaline on acetylcholine output by guinea-pig ileum longitudinal muscle strip. *Br. J. Pharmacol.* 35, 10-28.

Polak, R.L. (1971). Stimulating action of atropine on the release of acetylcholine by rat cerebral cortex *in vitro*. *Br. J. Pharmacol.* 41, 600-606.

Rand, M.J. & Varma, B. (1970). The effects of cholinomimetic drugs on responses to sympathetic nerve stimulation and noradrenaline in the rabbit ear artery. *Br. J. Pharmacol.* 38, 758-770.

Roszkowski, A.P. (1961). An unusual type of sympathetic ganglionic stimulant. *J. Pharmacol. Exp. Ther.* 132, 156-170.

Sorimachi, M., Oesch, F. & Thoenen, H. (1973). Effects of colchicine and cytochalasin B on the release of ^{3}H-norepinephrine from guinea-pig atria evoked by high potassium, nicotine and tyramine. *Naunyn Schmiedeberg's Arch Pharmacol.* 276, 1-12.

Starke, K. (1977). Regulation of noradrenaline release by pre-synaptic receptor systems. *Rev. Physiol. Biochem. Pharmacol.* 77, 1-124.

Starke, K., Endo, T., Taube, D.H. & Borowski, E. (1975). Pre-synaptic receptor systems on noradrenergic nerves. In: *Chemical Tools in Catecholamine Research* (eds.) O. Almgren, A. Carlsson & J. Engel, pp. 193-200, North-Holland, Amsterdam.

Starke, K., Peskar, B.A., Schumacher, K.A. & Taube, H.D. (1977). Bradykinin and postganglionic sympathetic transmission. *Naunyn Schmiedeberg's Arch. Pharmacol.* 299, 23-32.

Steinsland, O.S., Furchgott, R.F. & Kirpekar, S.M. (1973). Inhi-bition of adrenergic neurotransmission by parasympathomimetics in the rabbit ear artery. *J. Pharmacol. Exp. Ther.* 184, 346-356.

Stjärne, L. (1973). Michaelis-Menten kinetics of secretion of sympathetic neurotransmitter as a function of external calcium: Effect of graded alpha-adrenoceptor blockade. *Naunyn Schmiedeberg's Arch. Pharmacol.* 278, 323-327.

Stjärne, L. (1975a). Basic mechanisms and local feedback control of secretion of adrenergic and cholinergic neurotransmitters. In: *Handbook of Psychopharmacology* (eds.) L.L. Iversen, S. Iversen & S.H. Snyder, pp. 179-233, Plenum Press, New York.

Stjärne, L. (1975b). Pre- and post-junctional receptor-mediated cholinergic interactions with adrenergic transmission in guinea-pig vas deferens. *Naunyn Schmiedeberg's Arch Pharmacol.* 288, 305-310.

Thoenen, H., Huerlimann, A. & Haefely, W. (1969). Cation depen-dence of the noradrenaline-releasing action of tyramine. *Eur. J. Pharmacol.* 6, 29-37.

Thoenen, H. & Tranzer, J.P. (1968). Chemical sympathectomy by selective destruction of adrenergic nerve endings with 6-hydroxydopamine. *Naunyn Schmiedeberg's Arch. Pharmacol.* 261, 271-288.

Vanhoutte, P.M. (1974). Inhibition by acetylcholine of adrenergic neurotransmission in vascular smooth muscle. *Circ. Res.* 34, 317-326.

Vanhoutte, P.M. (1976). Inhibition of acetylcholine of adrenergic neurotransmission in vascular smooth muscle. In: *Physiology of Smooth Muscle* (eds.) E. Bülbring & M.F. Shuba, pp. 369-377, Raven Press, New York.

Vanhoutte, P.M., Lorenz, R.R. & Tyce, G.M. (1973). Inhibition of norepinephrine-^{3}H release from sympathetic nerve endings in veins by acetylcholine. *J. Pharmacol. Exp. Ther.* 185, 386-394.

Vanhoutte, P.M. & Verbeuren, T.J. (1976).   Inhibition by acetyl-
    choline of ^{3}H-norepinephrine release in cutaneous veins after
    alpha-adrenergic blockade. *Arch. Int. Pharmacodyn.* 221, 344-
    346.

Verbeuren, T.J. & Vanhoutte, P.M. (1976).   Acetylcholine inhibits
    potassium evoked release of ^{3}H-norepinephrine in different
    blood vessels of the dog. *Arch. Int. Pharmacodyn.* 221, 347-
    350.

Westfall, T.C. & Hunter, P.E. (1974).   Effect of muscarinic
    agonists on the release of [^{3}H]noradrenaline from the guinea-
    pig perfused heart. *J. Pharm. Pharmacol.* 26, 458-460.

ROLE OF PROSTAGLANDINS AND CYCLIC ADENOSINE MONOPHATE IN RELEASE

L. Stjärne

I   INTRODUCTION

Release of noradrenaline from (nor-)adrenergic nerves may be
caused by different processes. Under resting conditions there is
a spontaneous 'leakage' of noradrenaline. Accelerated release
may be induced either by indirectly acting sympathomimetic amines
(or other drugs), or by the depolarization which is normally
caused by the arrival of propagated nerve impulses to the nerve
terminals. The latter process is subject to complex local feedback control (see Chapter 5, this Volume).

It has been proposed that the secretory mechanism as such, in
nerves as well as in other secretory cells, may be dependent on
the generation of cyclic adenosine monophate (cAMP) (Rasmussen,
1970), and that the released noradrenaline triggers negative
feed-back control of further noradrenaline release, by initiating
the (synthesis and) release of E-type prostaglandins (PGE)
(Hedqvist, 1969a). Since many of the actions of PGE seem to be
expressed via cAMP (Kuehl, 1974), it seems a priori possible that
the two control mechanisms may be interconnected.

These two types of influence on noradrenaline release form the
subject of this review. Its scope is essentially limited to such
control in peripheral adrenergic nerves. After discussing effects
and mechanisms of action of exogenous prostaglandins (PG:s) on
noradrenaline release, an attempt is made to evaluate the evidence
in the literature for and against the concepts that the release
mechanism in these nerves is normally dependent on, or regulated
by, generation of endogenous PG:s and/or cAMP.

II   PROSTAGLANDINS AND RELEASE OF NORADRENALINE

The powerful hypotensive action of human seminal plasma, or of
crude extracts of sheep vesicular gland, one of the characteristic
effects leading to the discovery of the PG:s (Goldblatt, 1933;
Euler, 1934, 1935), is to a large extent due to the mixed effects
of PG:s of the E-series (PGE:s) contained in the preparations
tested. The hypotensive effect is mainly due to vasodilatation,
caused both by direct relaxation of the smooth muscle in different
segments of the vascular system (Bergström, Dunér, Euler, Pernow
& Sjövall, 1959), and by inhibition of adrenergic vasomotor tone,
due to depression of noradrenaline release from adrenergic nerves
(Hedqvist, 1969a, 1970a).

This latter effect was discovered in experiments prompted by the finding that PGE$_1$ depressed the vasoconstrictor response both to nerve stimulation and to exogenous noradrenaline in cat spleen (Hedqvist, 1968), and inhibited the luminal occlusion induced by nerve stimulation in rabbit oviduct (Brundin, 1968). That these effects were at least in part due to inhibition of noradrenaline release was later directly shown for PGE$_1$ (though its effects in cat spleen were not consistent, Hedqvist & Brundin, 1969) and for its close congener PGE$_2$ (Hedqvist, 1969a). Since it was known that sympathetic nerve stimulation may cause release of PGE:s (Davies, Horton & Withrington, 1967, 1968; Gilmore, Vane & Wyllie, 1968), Hedqvist (1969a) proposed that endogenous PGE$_2$, "locally mobilized by sympathetic nerve stimulation, may counteract further release of noradrenaline by a negative feed-back mechanism, thus exerting a braking effect on the sympathetic neuro-effector system". If this hypothesis is correct (and if the PGE:s are not metabolized), the effluent from tissues exposed to sympathetic nerve stimulation should inhibit the release of noradrenaline evoked by renewed nerve stimulation, and inhibition of PGE synthesis should cause an increase in noradrenaline release per nerve impulse. The fulfillment of both criteria was first reported for the perfused rabbit heart (Wennmalm & Stjärne, 1971; Samuelsson & Wennmalm, 1971), and has been confirmed in other tissues.

That exogenous PGE:s are potent inhibitors of noradrenaline release in most adrenergic nerves is by now generally accepted. Opinions concerning a physiological role for endogenous PGE:s as mediators of a feed-back control of noradrenaline release in peripheral adrenergic nerves, are more divided (for recent reviews see Hedqvist, 1976a, 1977; Stjärne, 1975; Starke, 1977). Some workers have failed to reproduce the key experimental results on which this concept is based (see Dubocovich & Langer, 1975; Langer, Enero, Adler-Graschinsky, Dubocovich & Celuchi, 1975), and therefore remain in doubt. The extreme position is that "prostaglandins, in spite of their remarkable potency (may be) metabolites with no special function" (Horton, 1976).

A.   Effects of Exogenous PG:s on Release of Noradrenaline

Most results concerning the effects of PG:s on noradrenaline release are based on work with isolated, saline-perfused or -superfused tissues. Two different approaches have been used to estimate noradrenaline release: Either recording of the electrical and/or mechanical responses to nerve stimulation, or measurement of the overflow of total and/or labelled noradrenaline and its metabolites, and of the enzyme dopamine β-hydroxylase, into the effluent from stimulated tissues (for a discussion of the fallacies of each of these methods, see Starke, 1977). Since PG:s often affect both the release of noradrenaline from nerves and the responsiveness of the effector organ to the transmitter released, judgement of their effect on noradrenaline release based exclusively on recording of the effector response to nerve stimulation may be misleading (see for example Stjärne, 1973a).

1.   Comparison between different PG:s and related compounds

a)   PGE:s: The findings that PGE_1 and/or PGE_2 are capable of
inhibiting noradrenaline release from the adrenergic nerves of
cat spleen (Hedqvist & Brundin, 1969; Hedqvist, 1969a) have been
confirmed and found to apply both to central and to most peripheral adrenergic nerves in the different species tested (for
experimental conditions and references, see Table 4 in Starke,
1977; the Table lists 14 different tissues from 6 species). PGE_2
has been found to be equipotent with (Hedqvist, 1974a), or more
potent than PGE_1 (Hedqvist, 1970a), inhibiting noradrenaline
release evoked by nerve stimulation at concentrations from 3 x
$10^{-10}M$ (at low external calcium, in guinea-pig vas deferens;
Stjärne, 1973b).

While adrenergic nerves are generally sensitive to the inhibitory
effect of PGE:s on transmitter release, exceptions have been
reported. The adrenergic nerves of dog spleen (Davies &
Withrington, 1969), cat nictitating membrane (Brody & Kadowitz,
1974; Illés, Vizi & Knoll, 1974; Langer *et al.*, 1975), and rat
vas deferens (Ambache, Dunk, Verney & Zar, 1972; Hedqvist &
Euler, 1972; Illés, Hadházy, Torma, Vizi & Knoll, 1973) have been
found to be highly resistant to the inhibitory effect of PGE:s.
In dog subcutaneous adipose tissue, PGE_2 depressed the release of
[^{3}H]noradrenaline, but only after treatment with phenoxybenzamine
(Fredholm & Hedqvist, 1973a).

There are, however, also a few reports that PGE:s may enhance
noradrenaline release. This was found to be the case in rat
brain synaptosomes (Roberts & Hillier, 1976). The report that
PGE_1 increased the overflow of noradrenaline on nerve stimulation
in cat spleen perfused with whole blood *in vitro* (but not in the
spleen *in situ*, Blakeley, Brown, Dearnaley & Woods, 1969) need
not imply that PGE_1 enhanced the release of noradrenaline. As
pointed out by Hedqvist (1970a, 1977) very high concentrations of
PGE_1 were used in this study. The rise in overflow of noradrenaline might thus well be due to inhibition of platelet aggregation,
and to the resulting improvement in microcirculation, leading to
more complete washout of the noradrenaline released from the nerves.

b)   Other PG:s or related compounds: Figure 1 provides a simplified diagram of the biosynthetic pathways for PGE_2 and related
compounds. The effects of the parent compounds, the various intermediaries, or PG:s other than PGE_2, on the release of noradrenaline
have not been extensively examined. One reason for this is the
extreme lability of several of the intermediaries; the endoperoxides, PGG_2 and PGH_2, are non-enzymatically degraded in saline
into various metabolites, mainly PGE_2 (their $t_{1/2}$ in salinic media
is approximately 5 min, at 37°C; Hamberg, Svensson, Wakabayashi &
Samuelsson, 1974).

The endoperoxides, PGG_2 and PGH_2 (and therefore probably also
their derivatives TxA_2 and PGI_2) have been reported to be less
than half as potent as PGE_2, as inhibitors of the release of
[^{3}H]noradrenaline from guinea-pig isolated vas deferens (Hedqvist,

114   L. Stjärne

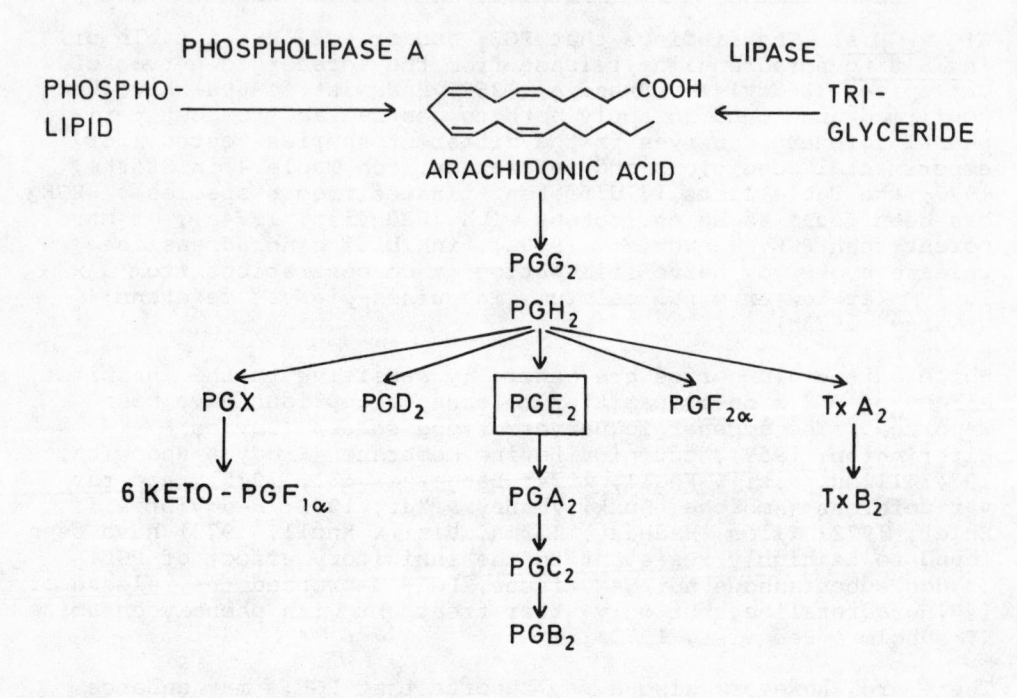

Fig. 1.   Simplified presentation of the synthesis of, and interrelationships between, the different members of the branch of the
PG family to which PGE_2 belongs.   It should be noted that the
drugs commonly used to inhibit the synthesis of PGE_2, i.e., ETA,
indomethacin or meclofenamate, inhibit the enzyme(s) responsible
for the first step (Flower, 1974) in the synthesis of both PGE_1
and PGE_2 (in the latter case, the conversion of arachidonic acid
into the endoperoxides PGG_2 and/or PGH_2), and therefore prevent
the formation of all PG:s, including the recently discovered TxA_2
and PGI_2.   For references see Samuelsson, Granström, Green,
Hamberg & Hammarström (1975); Pace-Asciak (1977); Johnson, Morton,
Kinner, Gorman, McGuire & Sun (1976); Prostaglandins 13, 375
(1977).

1976a).   Their true potency may be even lower, since part of the
effect observed could be due to conversion to PGE_2.   Of the other
PG:s, PGD_2 has been found to be practically inactive (potency
less than 1/100 of PGE_2), and PGA_2 and PGB_2 were also either without effect or very weakly active as inhibitors of noradrenaline
release (see Hedqvist, 1976a, 1977; Frame, 1976).

$PGF_{2\alpha}$, one of the PG:s released from tissues as the result of
nerve stimulation (together with PGE_2 and/or PGE_1, Gilmore et al.,
1968; for other references see Hedqvist, 1977), potentiates the
mechanical response to sympathetic nerve stimulation, without increasing the response to exogenous noradrenaline, in a number of

preparations (Ducharme, Weeks & Montgomery, 1968; Kadowitz, Sweet
& Brody, 1971; Malik & McGiff, 1975), suggesting that this PG may
increase noradrenaline release per nerve impulse. However, direct
evidence for such presynaptic facilitation is lacking. In isolated rabbit heart $PGF_{2\alpha}$ was without effect on noradrenaline
release at concentrations up to $10^{-6}M$ (Hedqvist & Wennmalm, 1971),
and in rabbit pulmonary artery high concentrations of this PG
depressed noradrenaline release (Taube et al., 1976). The potentiating effect of this and other PG:s on the effector response to
sympathetic nerve stimulation is thus probably due to induced
changes in the responsiveness of the effector organ (Hedqvist,
1977).

2. Level and mechanism of action of exogenous PGE:s
   on noradrenaline release

Although there exist tissue and/or species differences with
respect to the sensitivity to PGE:s, nerve stimulation induced
overflow of noradrenaline is depressed by very low concentrations
of PGE_1 and/or PGE_2, in most adrenergic nerves. The following
different levels and mechanisms of action have been considered:

a) PGE:s and the spread of excitation in nerve terminals: PGE_1
has been shown to block invasion of nerve terminals in the rat
phrenic nerve-diaphragm preparation (Gripenberg, Jansson,
Heinänen, Heinonen, Hyvärinen & Tolppanen, 1976), at concentrations not affecting conduction in the nerve trunk (Jansson,
Hyvärinen, Tolppanen & Gripenberg, 1974), but only on stimulation
at more than 10 Hz and at 37°C. Even though PGE_2 did not block
impulse conduction in an adrenergic (bovine splenic) nerve trunk
(Hedqvist, 1970a), the possibility thus exists that it may block
invasion of terminal ramifications of adrenergic nerves. However,
exogenous PGE_2 depresses the tetrodotoxin-resistant release of
noradrenaline evoked by direct depolarization of nerve terminals
with high K^+ (Stjärne, 1973c; Westfall & Brasted, 1974). This
shows that at least a major part of the inhibitory effect of PGE:s
is directed towards the noradrenaline release mechanism in individual varicosities.

b) PGE:s depress the release of noradrenaline: The inhibitory
effect of PGE:s on nerve stimulation induced noradrenaline overflow is due to depression of noradrenaline release as such, and
not to interference with the synthesis, storage/leakage, enzymatic
degradation or rebinding of noradrenaline. PGE:s depress the
stimulation induced overflow of endogenous and exogenous
(labelled) noradrenaline to about the same extent; therefore
their effect is not due to interference with synthesis and/or
preferential secretion of newly synthesized noradrenaline
(Hedqvist, 1970a). Furthermore, they do not affect the efflux of
noradrenaline from isolated ('large dense core') storage vesicles
from bovine splenic nerve trunk (Hedqvist, 1970a), the degradation
of noradrenaline by monoamine oxidase or catechol-O-methyl transferase (Bhagat, Dhalla, Montagne & Montier, 1972), or the neuronal
(Blakely et al., 1969; Hedqvist, 1970a; Ciofalo, 1973) or extraneuronal (Salt, 1972) uptake of noradrenaline. These facts taken
together show that PGE:s inhibit noradrenaline release induced by

nerve stimulation. This conclusion gains further strength from
the demonstration that both PGE_1 and PGE_2 depressed the overflow
of dopamine-β-hydroxylase as well as that of noradrenaline, in
guinea-pig vas deferens (Johnson, Thoa, Weinshilboum, Axelrod &
Kopin, 1971).

Concerning the effects of PGE:s on other kinds of noradrenaline
'release' the evidence is unclear. They do not affect the resting
'leakage' of noradrenaline (Hedqvist, 1970b; Hedqvist, Stjärne &
Wennmalm, 1970; George, 1975). There are reports of variable
effects on the noradrenaline release produced by sympathomimetic
amines. In cat spleen, the release of noradrenaline by tyramine
was not affected by PGE_2 at concentrations depressing noradrenaline release by nerve stimulation (Hedqvist, 1970b). On the
other hand PGE_2 (but not PGE_1) was reported to enhance the tyramine-induced release of [^{3}H]noradrenaline in guinea-pig perfused
heart (Westfall & Brasted, 1974), while both PGE_1 and PGE_2
depressed the release of [^{3}H]noradrenaline induced by sympathomimetic amines in rat mesenteric artery (George, 1975).

c) Inhibitory effect of PGE_2 independent of cyclic AMP: Since
cAMP has been proposed to be critically involved in excitation-
secretion coupling (Rasmussen, 1970), and since PGE:s are known
to increase the content of cAMP in nervous tissue (Sattin & Rall,
1970; Kuehl, 1974), alterations in tissue cAMP might be expected
to alter the inhibitory potency of PGE:s on noradrenaline release.
However, addition of dibutyryl cAMP or of theophylline did not
alter the inhibitory effect of PGE_2 on the release of [^{3}H]nor-
adrenaline by nerve stimulation, in guinea-pig vas deferens
(Stjärne, 1976).

d) Relation between external calcium and inhibitory effect of
PGE:s: On the grounds that the depression of noradrenaline release induced by PGE_2, in cat spleen, was in part reversed by
raising the calcium level of the medium it has been proposed that
PGE:s inhibit noradrenaline release by restricting the availability of external calcium for the secretory mechanism (Hedqvist,
1970b). In view of the pivotal role of calcium in excitation-
secretion coupling (Douglas, 1968; Rubin, 1970), this may be correct. PGE:s and other agents that markedly affect neurotransmitter release in adrenergic nerves, may do so by regulating
access of external calcium ions to some 'trigger site' in the
nerves. Direct proof for this is still lacking. In favour of
the hypothesis are the findings that the inhibitory potency of
PGE:s on the release of [^{3}H]noradrenaline in guinea-pig isolated
vas deferens varied inversely with the calcium level in the medium
(Hedqvist, 1973a,b, 1974b; Stjärne, 1973b; Stjärne & Alberts,
(1979). During nerve stimulation with trains of 300 impulses at
5 Hz, the ID_{50} for PGE_2 increased 10-fold (from 3×10^{-10}M to
3×10^{-9}M) as the external calcium level was raised from 0.3 -
0.5 to 1.8 mM (Stjärne, 1973b). However, conflicting results
have been obtained by other workers. Also in guinea-pig vas deferens, Johnson et al. (1971) found that the inhibitory effect of
PGE:s on the overflow of noradrenaline and dopamine-β-hydroxylase
induced by prolonged and intense nerve stimulation actually
increased with the calcium level in the medium. In cat spleen

Dubocovich and Langer (1975) did not observe any marked change in the inhibitory potency of PGE$_2$ related to changes in the calcium level.

By an unconventional application of methods commonly used in enzyme kinetic studies, an attempt has been made to more quantitatively define the calcium dependence of the inhibitory effect of PGE$_2$ on the secretion of [^{3}H]noradrenaline in guinea-pig vas deferens. The conclusion, based on Lineweaver-Burk and Eadie and Hofstee plots, that PGE$_2$ may inhibit noradrenaline release by depressing the 'apparent affinity' of the release mechanism for external calcium (Stjärne, 1973d) has not been supported by later work with the same preparation, which suggests rather that PGE$_2$ depressed the 'maximal secretory velocity' (V$_{max}$) essentially without altering the apparent K$_m$ (the calcium concentration required for half maximal secretory velocity; Stjärne & Alberts, 1979).

Additional circumstantial evidence indicating that the inhibitory action of PGE:s may be related to control of calcium-mediated activation of the release mechanism will be discussed in the following sections.

e) Inhibitory potency of PGE:s as a function of stimulation parameters: The inhibitory effect of PGE:s on the release of noradrenaline has been reported to be inversely related to the duration of impulses (Hedqvist, 1976b; Stjärne, 1978a), to the number of impulses in each stimulus train (Illés *et al.*, 1973; Knoll, Illés & Torma, 1975; Stjärne, 1977, 1978b) and to the frequency of nerve stimulation (Hedqvist, 1973a; Illés *et al.*, 1973; Junstad & Wennmalm, 1973; Stjärne, 1973e, 1978a; Dubocovich & Langer, 1975; Frame & Hedqvist, 1975; Stjärne & Brundin, 1977a). Since both increased pulse duration (Katz & Miledi, 1967) and repetitive pulses (Katz & Miledi, 1968) may enhance transmitter secretion by promoting the formation of a calcium-dependent trigger complex in the nerves, these findings are compatible with a calcium-related mechanism for the inhibitory effect of PGE:s on noradrenaline secretion (see section II.A.2.d).

f) Effects of tetraethylammonium or rubidium on inhibitory potency of PGE:s: Both tetraethylammonium (TEA) and rubidium, agents believed to prolong the duration of nerve action potentials (Koketsu, 1958; Baker, Hodgkin & Shaw, 1962) by inactivating K$^+$ channels (Katz & Miledi, 1969), thereby promoting calcium influx during nerve stimulation, have been reported to reduce the inhibitory effect of PGE$_2$ on [^{3}H]noradrenaline release in field stimulated guinea-pig vas deferens (Hedqvist, 1976b; Stjärne, 1978a). Apparently agents (such as TEA, Stjärne, 1973f) that cause 'flooding' of intraneuronal trigger sites with calcium, during nerve stimulation, may thereby counteract, and possibly ultimately abolish the inhibitory effect of PGE:s on noradrenaline release. The conclusion, that PGE only inhibits noradrenaline release during conditions when calcium influx is rate limiting for the secretory mechanism, is again in support of the calcium hypothesis for PGE action (see section II.A.2.d).

g)   Antagonism between PGE:s and α-adrenoceptor blocking drugs:
PGE:s prevent and/or abolish the enhancing effect of α-blockers
on noradrenaline release (Hedqvist, 1969b, 1974a; Stjärne, 1972a;
1973c,d).   In dog subcutaneous adipose tissue PGE_2 in fact
inhibited the release of [^{3}H]noradrenaline by nerve stimulation
only after release had been enhanced by treatment with phenoxybenzamine (Fredholm & Hedqvist, 1973a).

That the release of noradrenaline under normal conditions, when
it is 'auto-inhibited' by previously released noradrenaline remaining in the 'junctional space' (see Chapter 5, this volume),
is less susceptible to further inhibition by PGE:s than is release after removal of α-adrenoceptor-mediated feedback inhibition
of the release mechanism, has also been directly demonstrated in
guinea-pig vas deferens (Hedqvist, 1974a, 1976b; Stjärne, 1978a).

There is thus an interesting contrast between the effects of TEA
and α-blocking agents on the inhibitory potency of PGE_2.   Both enhance noradrenaline release per nerve impulse, but while the inhibitory effect of PGE_2 on noradrenaline release increased with
the degree of disinhibition of the secretory mechanism, by increasing concentrations of phentolamine, the inhibitory effect of PGE_2
declined with the increase in secretion caused by increasing concentrations of TEA.   Direct kinetic comparison of the calcium dependence of the TEA- and phentolamine-mediated increase in [^{3}H]nor-
adrenaline release in guinea-pig vas deferens (Stjärne, 1973f) has
shown that the maximum secretory velocity obtained with the two
drugs is essentially identical.   In the presence of phentolamine
the secretory rate remained a strict function of external calcium
or less in the presence of 6 mM TEA.   From this one may conclude
that TEA saturates the secretory mechanism with calcium at relatively low external calcium levels, whereas with phentolamine saturation is attained only at 'infinite' levels of calcium in the
medium.

The finding that the inhibitory effect of PGE:s on noradrenaline
release is normally inversely related to external calcium (see
II.A.2.d), but ceases to be so under treatment with agents (such
as TEA) which cause intraneuronal calcium 'flooding', indicates
that PGE:s oppose secretion only as long as they manage to depress
the free intraneuronal Ca^{+2} level.   In view of the report that
PGE_1 may act as a 'calcium ionophore' (Kirtland & Baum, 1972) one
may speculate that PGE:s probably lower the free intraneuronal Ca^{2+}
by promoting its sequestration into a 'calcium store' (Fig. 2)
rather than by opposing Ca^{2+} entry during depolarization.   In
that case it seems likely that the PGE-independent α-adrenoceptor
mediated control of the release mechanism triggered by noradrenaline in the junctional cleft operates at the next step in
'electro-secretory coupling' by restricting the 'utilization' of
free intraneuronal Ca^{2+}, for example by depressing the calcium
'affinity' of the hypothetical binding site 'K', thus counter-
acting formation of the fully charged complex Ca_nx, which triggers
transmitter release (Del Castillo & Katz, 1954).   This may explain why the inhibitory potency of PGE:s increased with the degree
of phentolamine-mediated disinhibition of the release mechanism
from α-adrenoceptor mediated control, since under such conditions
the rate of release should, to an increasing extent, become a

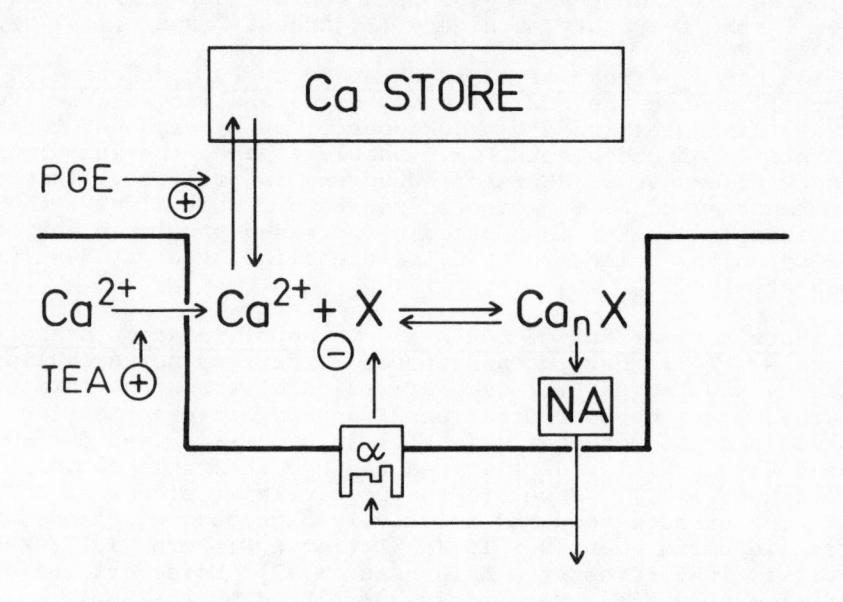

Fig. 2. Model of adrenergic nerve secretory varicosity to illustrate the proposed level and mechanism of action of PGE$_2$ (and of
α-adrenoceptor mediated feedback) on depolarization-secretion
coupling. For details see the text.

simple function of the level of free intraneuronal Ca^{2+}, which
(as suggested above), may be under the control of PGE:s (for a
somewhat different, earlier model for these interactions, see
Stjärne, 1975a).

While the inhibitory potency of PGE:s on noradrenaline release
depends on the functional state of the α-adrenoceptor control system, it should be pointed out that the antagonism between PGE:s
and the drug phentolamine as such is not a competitive one. An
increase in phentolamine concentration from 7.5×10^{-9}M to $7.5 \times$
10^{-6}M did not materially alter the ED$_{50}$ for PGE$_2$ in guinea-pig vas
deferens (Stjärne, 1973g). More recent experiments in the same
preparation show that an increase in phentolamine concentration,
from 10^{-9}M to 10^{-6}M increased the inhibitory effect of (5×10^{-8}M)
PGE$_2$ to a very small, but significant, extent from 48% to 72%
(Stjärne, 1978a).

h) Inhibitory potency of PGE:s unaffected by β-adrenoceptor
stimulation: While PGE:s depress noradrenaline release, β-adreno-
ceptor stimulation causes the opposite effect in many tissues
(see Chapter 5, this volume for references). The finding that
the inhibitory effect of PGE$_2$ on the release of [^{3}H]noradrenaline
evoked by field stimulation of human isolated blood vessels was
unchanged in the presence of the β-agonist isoprenaline at a concentration causing a 90% increase in release per nerve impulse,

indicates that PGE:s and β-agonists do not compete for the same sites in the secretory machinery (Stjärne & Brundin, 1977b).

i) Inhibitory effect of PGE:s enhanced by PG synthetase inhibitor: If endogenous PGE restricts noradrenaline release (Hedqvist, 1969a), disinhibition from such control by blockade of formation and release of endogenous PGE:s should enhance the inhibitory potency of exogenous PGE:s on noradrenaline release. This has been reported to be the case in perfused rabbit kidney; the PG synthetase inhibitor indomethacin increased the inhibitory effect of PGE_2 on the release of $[^3H]$noradrenaline by about 50% (Frame & Hedqvist, 1975).

j) Inhibitory effect of PGE:s due to depolarization of nerve membrane: PGE:s have been proposed to depress noradrenaline release by causing partial depolarization of the nerve terminals, since PGE_1 at the concentrations found to depress the size of evoked junction potentials (EJP:s) in guinea-pig vas deferens frequently partially depolarized the smooth muscle cells (Sjöstrand, 1972). However, the depolarizing effect of PGE:s in different tissues required relatively high concentrations, the threshold being about $3 \times 10^{-7}M$ (Taylor & Einhorn, 1972; Kuriyama & Suzuki, 1976; Grosset & Mironneau, 1977). Moreover, the depression of evoked EJP:s was poorly correlated to the amplitude of depolarization of muscle cells caused by PGE_1 (Sjöstrand, 1972; Taylor & Einhorn, 1972). This raises doubt that depolarization of the nerve terminals is the cause of the inhibitory effect of PGE:s on noradrenaline release. Final evaluation of this possibility requires direct evidence concerning the depolarizing effect of PGE:s on nerve terminals, and about the possible correlation between this and the depression of noradrenaline release.

B.   Do Endogenous PGE:s Play a Role in the
      Control of Noradrenaline Release

The concept that endogenous PGE:s serve as chemical mediators of one type of negative feedback control of noradrenaline release from adrenergic nerves, (Hedqvist, 1969a), has received considerable experimental support. However, conflicting evidence has also appeared and has led to doubts about its physiological importance (see for example Dubocovich & Langer, 1975). This section presents the key arguments on which the hypothesis rests, and also discusses the experimental evidence for each of them.

1. Adrenergic nerves possess inhibitory receptors for PGE:s

The finding that extremely small amounts of PGE:s depress the release of noradrenaline from adrenergic nerves in most tissues and species is in favour of a physiological role for PGE:s in the control of noradrenaline release, since it indicates that most adrenergic nerves possess specific receptor functions for these compounds (for references see section II.A.1.a., and also Table 4 in Starke, 1977). On the other hand, some adrenergic nerves are highly resistant, or completely insensitive, to the inhibitory effect of PGE:s (for references see section II.A.1.a). This indicates that such PGE-mediated control is not generalized, but may be completely lacking in some nerves.

2. Sympathetic nerve stimulation causes release of PGE:s

The reports that sympathetic nerve stimulation causes (*de novo* synthesis and) release of PGE:s (mainly PGE_2 and/or PGE_1, together with $PGF_{2\alpha}$; for references see Hedqvist, 1977), in amounts sufficient to depress noradrenaline release, is in favour of a role for PGE:s in the control of noradrenaline release. Direct evidence for this has been obtained by stimulation during reperfusion with 'stimulated effluent' in rabbit heart (Wennmalm & Stjärne, 1971).

However, some findings weaken this argument for a role for endogenous PGE:s in the control of noradrenaline release. Firstly, sympathetic nerve stimulation is not specific as trigger of PGE synthesis and release, nor is the infusion of catecholamines (Davies *et al.*, 1967, 1968; Gilmore *et al.*, 1968). PGE:s are also released by infusion of acetylcholine (Junstad & Wennmalm, 1974), bradykinin (McGiff, Terragno, Malik & Lonigro, 1972), angiotensin (McGiff, Crowshaw, Terragno & Lonigro, 1970a) and adenosine tri- or diphosphate (Minkes, Douglas & Needleman, 1973). Moreover, PGE synthesis and release is initiated by many non-specific stimuli involving some degree of tissue damage, such as mechanical stirring and/or vibration (Piper & Vane, 1971; Gryglewski & Vane, 1972), ischemia (McGiff, Crowshaw, Terragno, Lonigro, Strand, Williamson, Lee & Ng, 1970b), hypoxia (Wennmalm, 1975) etc. Secondly, sympathetic nerve stimulation causes much greater PGE output from tissues such as dog spleen, in which the adrenergic nerves are relatively resistant to their inhibitory effect (Davies & Withrington, 1969), than in cat spleen in which the nerves are highly sensitive (Gilmore *et al.*, 1968; Ferreira, Moncada & Vane, 1973). Thirdly, both the resting and the nerve stimulation induced output of PGE:s in saline perfused tissues such as cat spleen or rabbit heart were initially quite low, in well-preserved preparations, but tended to increase with the duration of the experiments and thus probably with the degree of non-specific tissue damage (Ferreira *et al.*, 1973; Peskar & Hertting, 1973; Junstad & Wennmalm, 1974; Hoszkowska & Paczenko, 1974; Bedwani & Millar, 1975; Dubocovich & Langer, 1975). On these grounds it has been questioned whether sympathetic nerve activity under physiological conditions *in vivo* is accompanied by release of PGE:s, and whether therefore PGE:s contribute at all to the physiological control of noradrenaline secretion (Dubocovich & Langer, 1975; Langer *et al.*, 1975).

3. Inhibitors of PGE synthesis enhance noradrenaline release

If endogenous PGE:s restrict noradrenaline release, blockade of PG synthesis and release, or of its effects on specific receptors, ought to enhance noradrenaline release. Specific receptor blocking agents for PG:s are still lacking (Samuelsson & Wennmalm). That blockade of PGE synthesis (with 5,8,11,14-eicosa tetrayonic acid, ETA; Downing, Ahern & Bachta, 1970) augments the release of

noradrenaline by nerve stimulation was first shown by Samuelsson
and Wennmalm (1971), in perfused rabbit heart. Similar observations have been made with ETA, indomethacin or meclofenamate as
inhibitors of PGE synthesis (Flower, 1974), in many isolated
tissues from several species, in central (Starke,& Montel,
1973a) or peripheral adrenergic nerves (Hedqvist, Stjärne &
Wennmalm, 1971; Wennmalm, 1971; Chanh, Junstad & Wennmalm, 1972;
Stjärne, 1972a; Fredholm & Hedqvist, 1973b; Hedqvist, 1973c,
1974c; Starke & Montel, 1973b; Stjärne & Gripe, 1973; Fuder &
Muscholl, 1974; Frame & Hedqvist, 1975; Hedqvist & Moawad, 1975;
Taube *et al.*, 1976). Furthermore, administration of indomethacin
to rats *in vivo*, at dose levels that markedly inhibit PGE synthesis, has been reported to cause a rise in the urinary excretion
of noradrenaline, under resting conditions or during cold exposure
(Stjärne, 1971, 1972b; Junstad & Wennmalm, 1972), and also a
marked and apparently selective increase in noradrenaline turnover in certain tissues without marked effects on the metabolism
of noradrenaline by monoamine oxidase or catechol-O-methyl transferase (Fredholm & Hedqvist, 1975a).

This evidence, obtained with three chemically different inhibitors
of PGE synthesis (Flower, 1974), and with many tissues from several species, is strongly in favour of a role for endogenous PGE:s
in the control of noradrenaline release. However, other results
are at variance with those described above. Inhibition of PGE
synthesis with meclofenamate or indomethacin did not enhance the
release of noradrenaline by nerve stimulation at 5-10 Hz, in cat
spleen (Hoszowska & Panczenko, 1974; Dubocovich & Langer, 1975;
Langer *et al.*, 1975). Similarly, indomethacin, at concentrations
blocking the formation and release of PGE:s, did not enhance the
release of [^{3}H]noradrenaline by nerve stimulation at 4 Hz, in dog
subcutaneous adipose tissue (Fredholm & Hedqvist, 1975b). In this
case it should be noted that the secretion of [^{3}H]noradrenaline
was also resistant to exogenous PGE$_2$, except after treatment with
phenoxybenzamine (Fredholm & Hedqvist, 1973a).

It is at present difficult to explain the discrepancy between
these experimental results, since many of them were obtained in
the same type of tissue and species, with the use of closely similar techniques. However, the concept that endogenous PGE:s play
a role in the control of noradrenaline release would be more
severely shaken if treatment with inhibitors of PG synthesis
failed to enhance noradrenaline release on stimulation at even
lower frequencies (1 Hz), since the efficiency of the postulated
PGE-mediated feedback control of noradrenaline release has been
reported to be inversely related to the stimulation frequency
(Junstad & Wennmalm, 1973; Stjärne, 1973e; Stjärne & Brundin,
1977a).

4. Enhanced synthesis of PGE depresses noradrenaline release

If noradrenaline release is restricted by PGE:s, enhanced synthesis of PGE:s ought to further depress noradrenaline output.
This has been reported to be the case. Administration of arachidonic acid, the precursor of PGE$_2$, reversibly depressed the

release of [3H]noradrenaline by nerve stimulation, in rabbit kidney; this effect was abolished by indomethacin (Frame & Hedqvist, 1975).

5. Effector response to sympathetic nerve activity influenced by PGE synthesis

If endogenous PGE:s restrict neurotransmission in adrenergic neuro-effector junctions, the effector response to sympathetic nerve stimulation ought to vary inversely with PGE synthesis and release. This has been reported to be the case in many tissues *in vitro* (for references see Hedqvist, 1977). Since PGE:s act both pre- and postjunctionally (Hedqvist, 1970a), this can only be regarded as circumstantial evidence. Moreover, some workers report that inhibition of PGE formation did not alter the effector response to sympathetic nerve stimulation (Dubocovich & Langer, 1975).

C. Characteristics of the Postulated PGE-Mediated Control of Noradrenaline Release

The results in favour of a role for endogenous PGE:s in the control of noradrenaline release indicate that this type of negative feedback control of sympathetic neurotransmitter secretion has the following characteristics:

1. The increased noradrenaline release is a result of inhibition of PGE synthesis

It seems likely that the enhanced nerve stimulation induced over-flow of noradrenaline produced by ETA, indomethacin or meclofenamate, is due to increased release, resulting from inhibition of PGE synthesis: Firstly, the three inhibitors are chemically widely different, and should therefore not have many side effects in common. Since ETA is an irreversible inhibitor (Downing et al., 1970), it can be washed out of the tissue; this should minimize the risk for non-specific effects. Secondly, neither ETA nor indomethacin inhibit noradrenaline binding or uptake in tissues (Hedqvist et al., 1971; Samuelsson & Wennmalm, 1971; Chanh et al., 1972; Zimmerman, Ryan, Gomer & Kraft, 1973c). Furthermore, although ETA, indomethacin and meclofenamate may at higher concentrations interfere with the functions of other enzymes, they seem to act, at the concentrations required to enhance noradrenaline release, mainly by blocking PGE synthetase (Flower, 1974; however, see also Jobke, Peskar & Hertting, 1976, for a discussion of possible side effects of these drugs.

2. Trigger and source of PGE involved in control of noradrenaline release

Since the release of PGE:s caused by sympathetic nerve stimulation, and/or by the infusion of catecholamines can be blocked by α-adrenoceptor antagonists, (Davies et al., 1967; 1968; Gilmore et al., 1968), or by a combination of α- and β-adrenoceptor antagonists (Wennmalm, 1975), it seems likely that the synthesis and release of PGE involved in control of noradrenaline release is

triggered by the noradrenaline released from the nerves, and is
mediated via adrenoceptors.

The source of the PGE:s shown to be capable of interfering with
noradrenaline release is not known. Most of the PGE:s released
as the result of sympathetic nerve stimulation must be derived
from extraneuronal sources, since   essentially 'normal' PGE
release may· be induced by infusion of catecholamines, even after
complete degeneration of the adrenergic nerves (Gilmore *et al.*,
1968). On these grounds it has been assumed that the trigger for
PGE release is the contractile response to the noradrenaline released from the nerves. The source of PGE would in that case
probably be muscle, and PGE would serve as a chemical link in
'trans-synaptic' negative feedback control of noradrenaline release. However, as pointed out by Hedqvist (1969a), it is possible that the PGE fraction mediating control of noradrenaline
release may be derived from the nerves. In support of this,
treatment with ETA to block PGE synthesis enhanced noradrenaline
release by nerve stimulation even in the absence of a contractile
response (i.e., stimulation of guinea-pig vas deferens at 5 Hz
and low external calcium, Stjärne, 1972a). The PGE-mediated control thus may not be mechanically, but chemically triggered, by
stimulation of (neural?) α-adrenoceptors, causing release of
(neural?) PGE (Stjärne, 1973i).

3. Frequency dependence of PGE mediated
    control of noradrenaline release

The increase in noradrenaline release induced by inhibitors of PGE
synthesis was apparent only on stimulation at low frequencies
(Junstad & Wennmalm, 1973; Stjärne, 1973e; Stjärne & Brundin
(1977a). Clearly this type of feedback control of noradrenaline
release was overcome by the facilitation caused by repetitive
·stimulation (Stjärne, 1978). Part of the reason could be that the
output of endogenous PGE$_2$ does not increase very steeply with the
frequency of nerve stimulation (Dunham & Zimmerman, 1970; Junstad
& Wennmalm, 1973). With respect to frequency dependence blockers
of PGE synthesis were similar to exogenous PGE$_2$, the inhibitory
effect of which was also inversely related to the frequency of
nerve stimulation (for references see section II.A.2.e), or to the
number of impulses applied per stimulus train (Stjärne, 1978).

4. Does endogenous PGE restrict invasion of nerve terminals?

While exogenous PGE$_2$ depressed both the tetrodotoxin-sensitive
[^{3}H]noradrenaline release evoked by electrical field stimulation,
and the tetrodotoxin-resistant release produced by direct depolarization of the nerve terminals with high K$^+$, treatment with ETA
enhanced only the release by electrical nerve stimulation (Stjärne,
1973c). If both types of stimulation released PGE, the results
suggest a difference between the actions of endogenous and exogenous PGE$_2$. While exogenous PGE$_2$ inhibited noradrenaline release
(at least) at the level of depolarization-secretion coupling,
endogenous PGE did not appear to be 'in the position' to do so,

but only depressed the release of noradrenaline which depended on
impulse conduction, and therefore seemed to act by restricting
invasion of nerve terminals by propagated impulses. This interpretation receives some support from the finding that PGE$_1$ may
induce terminal conduction block in cholinergic nerves, at least
at high frequency stimulation at 37°C (Jansson et al., 1974;
Gripenberg et al., 1976).

However, before such a concept is accepted, other possible explanations for the differential effect of exogenous and endogenous PGE
must be ruled out. It is possible that the K$^+$-induced depolarization in the above mentioned study (Stjärne, 1973c) was too
'massive' (Dismukes & Mulder, 1976). In that case the failure of
ETA to potentiate K$^+$-induced secretion would be analogous to its
failure to potentiate the release of noradrenaline evoked by high
frequency nerve stimulation (Junstad & Wennmalm, 1973; Stjärne,
1973e; Stjärne & Brundin, 1977a).

In conclusion, it is not known if each nerve impulse normally in-
vades all terminal ramifications of the neuron, and the evidence
is as yet insufficient to allow conclusions whether or not feedback control of noradrenaline release is exerted at this level.

D.   PGE-Dependent and -Independent α-Adrenoceptor
      Mediated Control of Noradrenaline Release

The postulated PGE-dependent control of noradrenaline release may
be triggered via (possibly neural) α-adrenoceptors (Stjärne,
1973i). However, both the inhibitory effect of α-agonists (Starke
& Montel, 1973b; Stjärne, 1973j), and the enhancing effect of
α-antagonists(Stjärne, 1972a, 1973c,h; Hedqvist, 1973c; Starke &
Montel, 1973b; Dubocovich & Langer, 1975), on the release of noradrenaline by nerve stimulation, are essentially unaffected by
treatment with PGE synthesis inhibitors. It can thus be concluded
that, although the postulated feedback control of noradrenaline
release mediated by release of endogenous PGE:s may be triggered
via α-adrenoceptors, the release mechanism is in addition controlled by a different and much more 'powerful' α-adrenoceptor mediated
feedback system (see Chapter 5, this volume), which is independent
of the local release of PGE.

In contrast to the PGE synthesis inhibitor ETA (see above under
II.C.4), phentolamine (even in the presence of ETA) enhanced the
release of noradrenaline both when caused by nerve stimulation
and by high K$^+$ (Stjärne, 1973c). It follows therefore that the
PGE-independent, α-adrenoceptor mediated control operated at least
to a major extent by depressing depolarization-secretion coupling.
This opens the possibility that the postulated dual PGE-dependent
and -independent control of noradrenaline release (Stjärne, 1973i)
may be complementary, the two components exerting their actions at
different levels in the neuron, possibly triggered via different
sets of (neural?) α-adrenoceptors (Stjärne, 1973j).

E.   Interactions Between PGE- and Adrenoceptor
      Mediated Controls of Noradrenaline Release

In many adrenergic nerves the release of noradrenaline can be influenced by three different sets of receptors: PGE- and α-adrenoceptors, mediating inhibition, and β-adrenoceptors mediating
enhancement, of noradrenaline release (see Chapter 5, this volume).

While treatment with PGE synthesis inhibitors alone does not
appreciably alter the effects of α-agonists or -antagonists (see
section II.D), it has been shown to greatly increase the sensitivity of certain preparations (i.e., human omental vein) to the
effects of β-agonists such as isoprenaline, both with respect to
the increase in [3H]noradrenaline release and to the contractile
response, caused by electrical field stimulation (Stjärne &
Brundin, 1976, 1977a,b). Combined pretreatment with a PGE synthesis inhibitor (ETA) and a β-agonist (isoprenaline) also strongly potentiated the enhancing effect of the α-antagonist phentolamine on the release of [3H]noradrenaline evoked by nerve stimulation, in human omental blood vessels (Stjärne & Brundin, 1977a).

Although the details of the mechanism of interaction between these
different receptor-mediated controls of noradrenaline release are
not yet known, these additive and/or potentiating effects indicate
that the three control systems are directed towards different
links in the chain of events starting with the generation of propagated nerve impulses and ending with the discharge of noradrenaline into the junctional cleft.

III   CYCLIC ADENOSINE MONOPHATE AND NORADRENALINE SECRETION

Rasmussen proposed in 1970 that the process of secretion in general, including that of hormones and neurotransmitters, may, in
addition to being critically dependent on extracellular calcium,
also require the generation of cyclic adenosine monophosphate
(cAMP) in secretory cells. This proposal has stimulated much work
to clarify the relative roles of calcium and cAMP for excitation-
secretion coupling in many secretory systems. However, firm evidence whether or not cAMP plays a critical role for the release of
the adrenergic neurotransmitter is still lacking.

A.   cAMP and Release of Transmitter from
      Central Catecholaminergic Neurons

There is a lack of agreement concerning the role of cAMP in the
release of neurotransmitter from catecholaminergic neurons in the
brain. In rat striatal slices various treatments intended to enhance intraneuronal cAMP (i.e., addition of dibutyryl cAMP alone,
or of cAMP in the presence of inhibitors of phosphodiesterase,
PDE) potentiated the release of [3H]dopamine induced by electrical
field stimulation (6000 shocks at 50 Hz), but not the resting release (Westfall, Kitay & Wahl, 1976). On the other hand, the release of [3H]noradrenaline from rat neocortical slices, induced by
submaximal stimulation with K^+, was reported to be dose-dependently
depressed by three structurally different inhibitors of PDE, but

not by 0.5 mM monobutyryl cAMP (Dismukes & Mulder, 1976).

In both papers the possibility was discussed that the observed effects of treatments designed to alter the cAMP content in catecholaminergic nerve terminals were indirect, and mediated via local neuronal loops. This possibility is excluded in studies of isolated synaptosomes where the addition of dibutyryl cAMP to synaptosomes prepared from rat striatum, doubled the rate of dopamine synthesis, but did not alter either the spontaneous or the veratridine-induced calcium-dependent and tetrodotoxin-sensitive release of endogenous dopamine (Patrick & Barchas, 1976a,b). This opens the possibility that intraneuronal cAMP, while controlling processes such as neurotransmitter synthesis (Harris, Baldessarini, Morgenroth III & Roth, 1975), may not be critically involved in excitation-secretion coupling in these nerves. The drastic but opposite effects of manipulation of intracellular cAMP in the two studies of rat brain slices quoted above (Westfall *et al.*, 1976; Dismukes & Mulder, 1976) could thus be expressions of altered postsynaptic responsiveness to nerve stimulation in neurons belonging to local neuronal loops and perhaps containing an adenylate cyclase specifically sensitive to the transmitter by which they are normally controlled (Westfall *et al.*, 1976).

B.   cAMP and Release of Noradrenaline in
      Peripheral (Nor-) Adrenergic Nerves

While some experimental findings are compatible with a critical role for cAMP in excitation-secretion coupling in these nerves, other results do not support such a concept. This applied to results obtained in the two tissues (guinea-pig vas deferens and cat spleen) in which this problem has been studied directly, by determining the effects on the overflow of noradrenaline, and its metabolites, and of dopamine-β-hydroxylase, evoked by electrical nerve stimulation, of agents that alter the intracellular content of cAMP.

1.   cAMP and noradrenaline release in guinea-pig vas deferens

In this tissue, Wooten, Thoa, Kopin and Axelrod (1973) found that dibutyryl cAMP (0.1 mM), but not theophylline (1 mM), enhanced the resting overflow both of noradrenaline and of dopamine-β-hydroxylase, in the presence or absence of calcium in the medium. Both agents enhanced the overflow of noradrenaline and of dopamine-β-hydroxylase, evoked by preganglionic nerve stimulation (45000 impulses at 25 Hz during 1 hr) in the presence of 50 μM phenoxybenzamine, both in the presence and absence of calcium. The authors concluded that the cAMP formed intraterminally following depolarization of the nerve membrane acted "in series" with calcium entering from the external medium, and in addition acted "directly in parallel with calcium to activate the presumed neurotubule-neurofilament-vesicle complex, resulting in exocytosis".

There are a number of reasons to regard these conclusions with some reservation, however. The methods used in the study are in part technically difficult. While it is useful to monitor the overflow of dopamine-β-hydroxylase as well as that of noradrenaline

as a measure of release in adrenergic nerves, this applies particularly to tissues where the outflow of dopamine-β-hydroxylase
can be accurately measured; the extremely small amounts of dopamine-β-hydroxylase released into the medium from guinea-pig vas
deferens must be very difficult to assay. This may account in
part for the large variations in the noradrenaline/dopamine-β-
hydroxylase ratios in the medium under the different experimental
conditions tested, which raises some doubt about the reliability
of the results reported. The high frequency (25 Hz) and long
duration (1 h) of the preganglionic nerve stimulation, and the
high concentration of phenoxybenzamine used (50 μM), also make it
questionable whether the results apply to release evoked by more
physiological, short-term postganglionic nerve stimulation. In
particular the finding that in the presence of dibutyryl cAMP or
theophylline, the secretory mechanism was in part independent of
external calcium is surprising, and has not been confirmed in
other studies.

In contrast, studies of the release of [3H]noradrenaline evoked
by mild, short-term postganglionic nerve stimulation in the same
preparation (field stimulation with trains of 300 impulses at
5 Hz) indicate that the release mechanism remains completely dependent on external calcium even in the presence of dibutyryl,
cAMP or theophylline at the concentrations used by Wooten *et al.*
(Stjärne, 1976b). Neither compound materially altered the fractional release of [3H]noradrenaline, either at zero, or at 0.5 or
1.8 mM calcium, during stimulation with trains of 300 impulses at
5 Hz, or with trains of 1500 impulses at 25 Hz, in the presence
or absence of 50 μM phenoxybenzamine. The results were thus at
variance with those of Wooten *et al.*, and the conclusion drawn was
that the release mechanism has an absolute requirement for external calcium, but is not critically dependent on generation of
cAMP.

2. cAMP and noradrenaline release in cat spleen

In perfused cat spleen several analogues of cAMP (but not cAMP
itself, which penetrates poorly into cells), as well as drugs
shown to be capable of inhibiting cat spleen PDE, were found to
markedly enhance the overflow of [3H]noradrenaline and of total
noradrenaline, as well as of dopamine-β- hydroxylase, evoked by
postganglionic nerve stimulation with trains of 300 impulses at
5 Hz (Cubeddu, Barnes & Weiner, 1974; 1975). This in itself indicates that cAMP is probably involved in electro-secretory
coupling in these nerves. However, papaverine (Cubeddu *et al.*,
1974), and phentolamine (Cubeddu *et al.*, 1975), the two agents
that most strongly enhanced the secretory response to nerve stimulation, were not, or were not specific as, inhibitors of cat
spleen PDE, at the concentrations used. It was therefore concluded that "cyclic nucleotides are not directly responsible for the
release of the adrenergic neurotransmitter, but may facilitate
the normal process of release by nerve stimulation" (Cubeddu
et al., 1975).

Even this rather conservative conclusion may not be entirely justified by the results presented, however. As pointed out above,
a cGMP analogue was at least as potent as the cAMP analogues tested. Theoretically the effect of 8-Br cGMP might be explained as
a result of inhibition of PDE, leading to a rise in endogenous
cAMP. However, calculations based on the data of Cubeddu *et al*.
(1974, 1975) show absolutely no correlation between the reported
degree of inhibition of PDE (in whole spleen) and the enhancement
in the secretory response obtained with the PDE inhibitors 'MIX'
or Ro-20-1724, or with monobutyryl cAMP or 8-Br cGMP. The inhibition of PDE at the highest concentrations of these drugs was
about 93, 67, 63 and 20%, while the enhancement of overflow of
dopamine-β-hydroxylase was about 10, 67-94, 31 and 91%, respectively. The possibility that neural PDE differed from the average
splenic PDE with respect to sensitivity to these agents must be
kept in mind, but at the present time remains mere speculation.
The authors were fully aware that there data did not conclusively
prove that cAMP in adrenergic nerves controls the secretory mechanism. They pointed out that the enhanced secretion during treatment with the various drugs could represent an indirect effect,
and be due to an increase in cAMP in non-neural cells, which (by
some unknown mechanism) might be able to influence the secretory
responsiveness of the adrenergic nerves (Cubeddu *et al*., 1975).

The finding in perfused cat spleen that papaverine shifted the
concentration - effect curve of (-)-isoprenaline on neurotransmitter release to the left, and that this effect of papaverine
was reduced by propranolol, has been taken as circumstantial evidence in favour of a role for cAMP in the control of noradrenaline
release, since it appeared a priori likely that the β-adrenoceptor
mediated enhancement of noradrenaline release would operate via
stimulation of adenylate cyclase (Langer, 1976). However,
papaverine has been shown to enhance noradrenaline release by
mechanisms other than inhibition of PDE, such as by a 'reserpine-
like' effect on the storage vesicles (Cubeddu *et al*., 1974).
Since this drug has in addition been reported to exert a number
of other effects, such as stimulation of the (Na-K)-adenosine
triphosphatase in nerve tissue (Woods & Lieberman, 1976), blocking
of oxidative phosphorylation (Santi, Ferrari & Contessa, 1964) and
direct alteration of excitation-contraction coupling in smooth
muscle by binding to calcium sites in the plasma membrane
(Tashiro & Tomita, 1970), observations based on the use of papaverine cannot be used as evidence either for or against the role
of cAMP in electro-secretory coupling.

While much of the available evidence is compatible with the possibility that cAMP does play a modulatory role in the control of
noradrenaline release in the adrenergic nerves of cat spleen, as
suggested by Cubeddu *et al*. (1975), more direct demonstration is
required before the concept can be finally accepted.

IV   SUMMARY AND CONCLUSIONS

A.   Role of PG:s in Noradrenaline Secretion

There is general agreement that PGE$_1$ and/or PGE$_2$ belong to the
most potent known biologically occurring inhibitors of noradrenaline release in adrenergic nerves from most tissues and species
tested. Opinion is still divided, however, concerning the physiological importance of endogenous PGE:s in the control of the release of sympathetic neurotransmitter.

In favour of such a role is the finding that sympathetic nerve
stimulation, in many saline perfused tissues, initiates selective
synthesis and release of PGE$_1$ and/or PGE$_2$, which are capable of
depressing noradrenaline release. The only additional PG thus
released in any quantity, from most tissues, is PGF$_{2\alpha}$. Although
this PG does not alter noradrenaline release, it may still contribute to modulation of sympathetic neuro-effector transmission
by altering the responsiveness of the postjunctional effector
cells to the transmitter. The selection of PG:s released thus
corresponds with the specificity of receptor functions control-
ing transmission in sympathetic neuro-effector junctions.

In addition, it has been demonstrated that treatment with PGE
synthesis inhibitors enhances the release of noradrenaline produced by nerve stimulation, in many isolated tissues from several
species, and also enhances the urinary excretion and the turnover
of noradrenaline (in rats) *in vivo*. There thus can be little
question that endogenous PGE:s <u>may</u> play a role in the control of
noradrenaline release.

On the other hand, a number of factors argue against the
<u>importance</u> of such a role for endogenous PGE:s. Firstly, such
control is apparently not generalized, since PGE:s do not inhibit
noradrenaline release from some adrenergic nerves (e.g., rat vas
deferens and cat nictitating membrane). Secondly, PGE release
by sympathetic nerve stimulation has been mainly studied in isolated saline perfused tissues. In these both the resting and
nerve stimulation induced output of PGE:s generally increases
with time and (probably) tissue deterioration. This has generated
doubt that sympathetic nerve activity under more physiological
conditions causes the release of enough PGE to affect noradrenaline release. Thirdly, even in tissues in which PGE-mediated
control of noradrenaline release has been demonstrated, it is
quantitatively far less marked than the PGE-independent α-adrenoceptor mediated negative feedback system. It is evident that
more work is needed to clarify the physiological role of PG:s
in the control of noradrenaline release.

B.   Role of cAMP in Noradrenaline Release

While there is evidence that cAMP in adrenergic nerves may be
critically involved in the control of short-term acceleration of
noradrenaline biosynthesis, the evidence that cAMP plays an equally central role in the control of excitation-secretion coupling

is not yet convincing, for either adrenergic, or dopaminergic
nerves. This unsatisfactory situation is probably due to the
lack of technical means to selectively and specifically manipulate
the functional cAMP compartment which may possibly be concerned
with such control. Some of the drugs used to enhance endogenous
intraneuronal cAMP levels by blocking PDE, have not turned out to
be specific inhibitors of this enzyme. Elevation of the overall
intracellular cAMP may be meaningless, if different intraneuronal
pools of cAMP mediate different, and possibly, antagonistic processes. It is thus not surprising that there is a lack of agreement concerning the role of cAMP for essentially all secretory
processes so far examined.

One example of such nonspecific inhibitors of PDE is the group of
methylxanthines, e.g., theophylline, which besides inhibiting PDE
also block the formation of cAMP in brain tissue induced by nerve
stimulation, probably mainly by blocking neural adenosine receptors (Sattin & Rall, 1970). This is particularly relevant to a
discussion concerning the role of cAMP for the mechanism of neurotransmitter release, since adenosine, which is known to enhance
neural cAMP levels, has in fact been observed to depress the release of neurotransmitter in adrenergic nerves (see chapter by
Clanachan). In view of these considerations it appears that the
question of the role of cAMP in excitation-secretion coupling is
still not settled.

V   REFERENCES

Ambache, N., Dunk, L.P., Verney, J. & Zar, M.A. (1972). Inhibi-
    tion of postganglionic motor transmission in the vas deferens
    by indirectly acting sympathomimetic drugs. *J. Physiol.*
    [Lond.] 246, 433-456.

Baker, P.F., Hodgkin, A.L. & Shaw, T.I. (1962). The effect of
    changes in internal ionic concentrations on the electrical pro-
    perties of perfused giant axons. *J. Physiol. [Lond.]* 164, 335-
    374.

Bedwani, J.R. & Millar, G.C. (1975). Prostaglandin release from
    cat and dog spleen. *Br. J. Pharmacol.* 54, 499-505.

Bergström, S., Dunér, H., Euler, U.S. v., Pernow, B. & Sjövall, J.
    (1959). Observations on the effects of prostaglandin E in man.
    Acta Physiol. Scand. 45, 145-151.

Bergström, S., Farnebo, L.O. & Fuxe, K. (1973). Effect of prosta-
    glandin E$_2$ on central and peripheral catecholamine neurons.
    Eur. J. Pharmacol. 21, 362-368.

Berkowitz, B.A. & Spector, S. (1971). Effect of caffeine and
    theophylline on peripheral catecholamines. *Eur. J. Pharmacol.*
    13, 193-196.

Bhagat, B., Dhalla, N.S., Ginn, D.m Montagne, A.E. & Montier, A.D. (1972). Modification by prostaglandin E_2 (PGE2) of the response of guinea-pig isolated vasa deferentia and atria to adrenergic stimuli. *Br. J. Pharmacol.* 44, 689-698.

Blakeley, A.G.H., Brown, L., Dearnaley, D.P. & Woods, R.I. (1969). Perfusion of the spleen with blood containing prostaglandin E_1: transmitter liberation and uptake. *Proc. Roy. Soc. B.* 174, 281-292.

Brundin, J. (1968). The effect of prostaglandin E_1 on the response of the rabbit oviduct to hypogastric nerve stimulation. *Acta Physiol. Scand.* 73, 54-57.

Ciofalo, F.R. (1973). Prostaglandins and synaptosomal transport of ^3H-norepinephrine and ^3H-5-hydroxytryptamine. *Res. Commun. Chem. Pathol. Pharmacol.* 5, 551-554.

Cubeddu, L.X., Barnes, E. & Weiner, N. (1974). Release of norepinephrine and dopamine-β-hydroxylase by nerve stimulation. II. Effect of papaverine. *J. Pharmacol. Exp. Ther.* 191, 444-457.

Cubeddu, L.X., Barnes, E. & Weiner, N. (1975). Release of norepinephrine and dopamine-β-hydroxylase by nerve stimulation. IV. An evaluation of a role for cyclic adenosine monophosphate. *J. Pharmacol. Exp. Ther.* 193, 105-127.

Davies, B.N., Horton, E.W. & Withrington, P.G. (1967). The occurrence of prostaglandin E_2 in splenic venous blood of the dog following splenic nerve stimulation. *J. Physiol. [Lond.]* 188, 38P-39P.

Davies, B.N., Horton, E.W. & Withrington, P.G. (1968). The occurrence of prostaglandin E_2 in splenic venous blood of the dog following splenic nerve stimulation. *Br. J. Pharmacol.* 32, 127-135.

Davies, B.N. & Withrington, P.G. (1969). Actions of prostaglandins A_1, A_2, E_1, E_2, $F_{1\alpha}$, and $F_{2\alpha}$ on splenic vascular and capsular smooth muscle and their interactions with sympathetic nerve stimulation, catecholamines and angiotensin. In: *Prostaglandins, Peptides and Amines* (eds.) P. Mantegazza & E.W. Horton, pp. 53-56, Academic Press, London-New York.

Del Castillo, J. & Katz, B. (1954). Quantal components of the end-plate potential. *J. Physiol. [Lond.]* 124, 560-573.

Dismukes, R.K. & Mulder, A.H. (1976). Cyclic AMP and α-receptor-mediated modulation of noradrenaline release from rat brain slices. *Eur. J. Pharmacol.* 39, 383-388.

Douglas, W.W. (1968). Stimulus-secretion coupling: the concept and clued from chromaffin and other cells. *Br. J. Pharmacol.* 34, 451-474.

Downing, D.T., Ahern, D.G. & Bachta, M. (1970). Enzyme inhibition by acetylenic compounds. *Biochem. Biophys. Res. Commun.* 40, 218-223.

Dubocovich, M.L. & Langer, S.Z. (1975). Evidence against a physiological role of prostaglandins in the regulation of noradrenaline release in the cat spleen. *J. Physiol.* [*Lond.*] 251, 737-762.

Ducharme, D.W., Weeks, J.R. & Montgomery, R.G. (1968). Studies on the mechanism of the hypertensive effect of prostaglandin F$_{2\alpha}$. *J. Pharmacol. Exp. Ther.* 160, 1-10.

Dunham, E.W. & Zimmermann, B.G. (1970). Release of prostaglandin-like material from dog kidney during renal nerve stimulation. *Am. J. Physiol.* 219, 1279-1285.

Euler, U.S. von (1934). Zur Kenntnis der pharmakologischen Wirkungen von Nativsekreten und Extrakten männlicher accessorischer Geschlechtsdrüsen. *Naunyn-Schmiedeberg's Arch. Exp. Pathol. Pharmacol.* 175, 78-84.

Euler, U.S. von (1935). Uber die spezifische blutdrucksenkende Substanz des menschlichen Prostata- und Samenblasensekretes. *Klin. Wochenschr.* 14, 1183-1184.

Ferreira, S.H., Moncada, S. & Vane, J.R. (1973). Some effects of inhibiting endogenous prostaglandin formation on the responses of the cat spleen. *Br. J. Pharmacol.* 47, 48-58.

Flower, R.J. (1974). Drugs which inhibit prostaglandin biosynthesis. *Pharmacol. Rev.* 26, 33-67.

Frame, M.H. (1976). A comparison of the effects of prostaglandins A$_2$, E$_2$ and F$_{2\alpha}$ on the sympathetic neuroeffector system of the isolated rabbit kidney. In: *Advances in Prostaglandin and Thromboxane Research* (eds.) B. Samuelsson & R. Paoletti, pp. 369-373, Raven Press, New York.

Frame, M.H. & Hedqvist, P. (1975). Evidence for prostaglandin mediated prejunctional control of renal sympathetic transmitter release and vascular tone. *Br. J. Pharmacol.* 54, 189-196.

Fredholm, B. & Hedqvist, P. (1973a). Role of pre- and postjunctional inhibition by prostaglandin E$_2$ of lipolysis induced by sympathetic nerve stimulation in dog subcutaneous adipose tissue *in situ*. *Br. J. Pharmacol.* 47, 711-718.

Fredholm, B. & Hedqvist, P. (1973b). Increased release of noradrenaline from stimulated guinea-pig vas deferens after indomethacin treatment. *Acta Physiol. Scand.* 87, 570-572.

Fredholm, B. & Hedqvist, P. (1975a). Indomethacin-induced increase in noradrenaline turnover in some rat organs. *Br. J. Pharmacol.* 54, 295-300.

134   L. Stjärne

Fredholm, B. & Hedqvist, P. (1975b). Indomethacin and the role
    of prostaglandins in adipose tissue. *Biochem. Pharmacol.* **24**,
    61-66.

George, A.J. (1975). The effect of prostaglandin E_1 and E_2 on
    drug-induced release of (^3H)-noradrenaline from rat mesenteric
    arteries. *Br. J. Pharmacol.* **55**, 243P.

Gilmore, N., Vane, J.R. & Wyllie, M.G. (1968). Prostaglandins
    released by the spleen. *Nature [Lond.]* **218**, 1135-1140.

Goldblatt, M.W. (1933). A depressor substance in seminal fluid.
    J. Soc. Chem. Ind. Lond. **52**, 1056-1057.

Gripenberg, J., Jansson, S.-E., Heinänen, V., Heinonen, E.,
    Hyvärinen & Tolppanen (1976). Effect of prostaglandin E_1 on
    neuromuscular transmission in the rat. *Br. J. Pharmacol.* **57**,
    387-393.

Grosset, A. & Mironneau (1977). An analysis of the actions of
    prostaglandin E_1 on membrane currents and contraction in
    uterine smooth muscle. *J. Physiol. [Lond.]* **270**, 765-784.

Gryglewski, R. & Vane, J.R. (1972). The release of prostaglandins
    and rabbit aorta contracting substance (RCS) from rabbit spleen
    and its antagonism by antiinflammatory drugs. *Br. J. Pharmacol.*
    45, 37-47.

Hamberg, M., Svensson, J., Wakabayashi, T. & Samuelsson, B. (1974).
    Isolation and structure of two prostaglandin endoperoxides
    that cause platelet aggregation. *Proc. Nat. Acad. Sci. [USA]*
    71, 345-349.

Harris, J.E., Baldessarini, R.J., Morgenroth III, V.H. & Roth,
    R.H. (1975). Activation by cyclic 3':5'-adenosine monophos-
    phate of tyrosine hydroxylase in the rat brain. *Proc. Nat.
    Acad. Sci. [Wash.]* **72**, 789-793.

Hedqvist, P. (1968). Reduced effector response to nerve stimu-
    lation in the cat spleen after administration of prostaglandin
    E_1. *Acta Physiol. Scand.* **74**, 7A.

Hedqvist, P. (1969a). Modulating effect of prostaglandin E_2 on
    noradrenaline release from the isolated cat spleen. *Acta
    Physiol. Scand.* **75**, 511-512.

Hedqvist, P. (1969b). Antagonism between prostaglandin E_2 and
    phenoxybenzamine on noradrenaline release from the cat spleen.
    Acta Physiol. Scand. **76**, 383-384.

Hedqvist, P. (1970a). Studies on the effect of prostaglandins
    E_1 and E_2 on the sympathetic neuromuscular transmission in
    some animal tissues. *Acta Physiol. Scand. Suppl.* **345**.

Hedqvist, P. (1970b). Antagonism by calcium of the inhibitory
    action of prostaglandin E$_2$ on sympathetic neurotransmission
    in the cat spleen. *Acta Physiol. Scand.* 80, 269-275.

Hedqvist, P. (1973a). Aspects on prostaglandin and α-receptor
    mediated control of transmitter release from adrenergic nerves.
    In: *Frontiers in Catecholamine Research* (eds.) E. Usdin &
    S.H. Snyder, pp. 583-587, Pergamon Press, New York.

Hedqvist, P. (1973b). Prostaglandin as a tool for local control
    of transmitter release from sympathetic nerves. *Brain Res.*
    62, 483-488.

Hedqvist, P. (1973c). Dissociation of prostaglandin and α-recep-
    tor mediated control of adrenergic transmitter release. *Acta
    Physiol. Scand.* 87, 42-43A.

Hedqvist, P. (1974a). Prostaglandin action on noradrenaline re-
    lease and mechanical responses in the stimulated guinea pig
    vas deferens. *Acta Physiol. Scand.* 90, 86-93.

Hedqvist, P. (1974b). Interactions between prostaglandins and
    calcium ions on noradrenaline release from the stimulated
    guinea pig vas deferens. *Acta Physiol. Scand.* 90, 153-157.

Hedqvist, P. (1974c). Effect of prostaglandins and prostaglandin
    synthesis inhibitors on norepinephrine release from vascular
    tissue. In: *Prostaglandin Synthetase Inhibitors* (eds.)
    H.J. Robinson & J.R. Vane, pp. 303-309, Raven Press, New York.

Hedqvist, P. (1976a). Prostaglandin action on transmitter re-
    lease at adrenergic neuroeffector junctions. In: *Advances in
    Prostaglandin and Thromboxane Research* (eds.) B. Samuelsson &
    R. Paoletti, pp. 357-363, Raven Press, New York.

Hedqvist, P. (1976b). Further evidence that prostaglandins in-
    hibit the release of noradrenaline from adrenergic nerve ter-
    minals by restriction of availability of calcium. *Br. J.
    Pharmacol.* 58, 599-603.

Hedqvist, P. (1977). Basic mechanisms of prostaglandin action on
    autonomic neurotransmission. *Ann. Rev. Pharmacol. Toxicol.* 17,
    259-279.

Hedqvist, P. & Brundin, J. (1969). Inhibition by prostaglandin
    E$_1$ of noradrenaline release and of effector response to nerve
    stimulation in the cat spleen. *Life Sci.* 8, 389-395.

Hedqvist, P. & Euler, U.S. von (1972). Prostaglandin-induced
    neurotransmission failure in the field stimulated, isolated
    vas deferens. *Neuropharmacol.* 11, 177-187.

Hedqvist, P. & Fredholm, B. (1976). Effects of adenosine on ad-
    renergic neurotransmission: Prejunctional inhibition and post-
    junctional enhancement. *Naunyn-Schmiedeberg's Arch. Pharmacol.*
    293, 217-223.

Hedqvist, P., Stjärne, L. & Wennmalm, Å. (1970). Inhibition by
    prostaglandin E_2 of sympathetic neurotransmission in the rab-
    bit heart. *Acta Physiol. Scand.* 79, 139-141.

Hedqvist, P., Stjärne, L. & Wennmalm, Å. (1971). Facilitation of
    sympathetic neurotransmission in the cat spleen after inhibi-
    tion of prostaglandin synthesis. *Acta Physiol. Scand.* 83,
    156-162.

Hedqvist, P. & Wennmalm, Å. (1971). Comparison of the effects of
    prostaglandins E_1, E_2 and $F_{2\alpha}$ on the sympathetically stimulated
    rabbit heart. *Acta Physiol. Scand.* 83, 156-162.

Horton, E.W. (1976). Prostaglandins - mediators, modulators or
    metabolites? *J. Pharm. Pharmacol.* 28, 389-392.

Hoszowska, A. & Panczenko, B. (1974). Effects of inhibition of
    prostaglandin biosynthesis on noradrenaline release from iso-
    lated perfused spleen of the cat. *Pol. J. Pharmacol. Pharm.*
    26, 137-142.

Illés, P., Hadházy, P., Torma, Z., Vizi, E.S. & Knoll, J. (1973).
    The effect of number of stimuli and rate of stimulation on the
    inhibition by PGE_1 of adrenergic transmission. *Eur. J. Pharma-
    col.* 24, 29-36.

Illés, P., Rónai, A. & Knoll, J. (1974). Adrenergic neuroeffector
    junctions sensitive and insensitive to the effect of PGE_1.
    Pol. J. Pharmacol. Pharm. 26, 127-136.

Jansson, S.-E., Hyvärinen, J., Tolppanen, E.-M. & Gripenberg, J.
    (1974). Prostaglandin E_1 on neuromuscular transmission. *Acta
    Physiol. Scand.* 91, 26A.

Jobke, A., Peskar, B.A. & Hertting, G. (1976). On the relation
    between release of prostaglandins and contractility of rabbit
    splenic capsular strips. *Naunyn-Schmiedeberg's Arch. Pharmacol.*
    292, 35-42.

Johnson, D.G., Thoa, N.B., Weinshilboum, R., Axelrod, J. & Kopin,
    I.J. (1971). Enhanced release of dopamine- - hydroxylase from
    sympathetic nerves by calcium and its reversal by prostagland-
    ins. *Proc. Nat. Acad. Sci.* [*Wash.*] 68, 2227-2230.

Johnson, R.A., Morton, D.R., Kinner, J.H., Gorman, R.R., Mcguire,
    J.C. & Sun, F. (1976). The chemical structure of prostaglandin
    X (prostacyclin). *Prostaglandins* 12, 915-928.

Junstad, M. & Wennmalm, Å. (1972). Increased renal excretion of
    noradrenaline in rats after treatment with prostaglandin syn-
    thesis inhibitor indomethacin. *Acta Physiol. Scand.* 85, 573-
    576.

Junstad, M. & Wennmalm, Å. (1974). Release of prostaglandin from
    the rabbit isolated heart following vagal nerve stimulation or
    acetylcholine infusion. *Br. J. Pharmacol.* 52, 375-379.

Kadowitz, P.J., Sweet, C.S. & Brody, M.J. (1971). Differential effects of prostaglandins E_1, E_2, $F_{1\alpha}$ and $F_{2\alpha}$ on adrenergic vasoconstriction in the dog hindpaw. *J. Pharmacol. Exp. Ther.* 177, 641-649.

Katz, B. & Miledi, R. (1967). The release of acetylcholine from nerve endings by graded electric pulses. *Proc. Roy. Soc. B.* 167, 23-28.

Katz, B. & Miledi, R. (1968). The role of calcium in neuromuscular facilitation. *J. Physiol.* [*Lond.*] 195, 481-492.

Katz, B. & Miledi, R. (1969). Tetrodotoxin resistant electric activity in presynaptic terminals. *J. Physiol.* [*Lond.*] 203, 459-487.

Knoll, J., Illés, P. & Torma, Z. (1975). The effect of PGE_2 on contraction delay and velocity of the field stimulated guinea-pig vas deferens. *Neuropharmacol.* 14, 314-324.

Koketsu, K. (1958). Action of tetraethylammonium chloride on neuromuscular transmission in frogs. *Am. J. Physiol.* 193, 213-215.

Kuehl, F.A. (1974). Prostaglandins, cyclic nucleotide and cell function. *Prostaglandins* 5, 325-340.

Kuriyama, H. & Suzuki, H. (1976). Effects of prostaglandin E_2 on and oxytocin on the electrical activity of hormone-treated and pregnant myometria. *J. Physiol.* [*Lond.*] 260, 335-349.

Kirtland, S.J. & Baum, H. (1972). Prostaglandin E_1 may act as a "calcium ionophore". *Nature New Biol.* 236, 47-49.

Langer, S.Z. (1976). The role of α- and β-presynaptic receptors in the regulation of noradrenaline release elicited by nerve stimulation. *Clin. Sci. Mol. Med.* 51, 423-426.

Langer, S.Z., Enero, M., Adler-Graschinsky, E., Dubocovich, M.L. & Celuchi, S.M. (1975). Presynaptic regulatory mechanisms for noradrenaline release by nerve stimulation. In: *Central Action of Drugs in Blood Pressure Regulation* (eds.) D.S. Davies & J.L. Reid, pp. 133-150, Pitman, Tunbridge Wells.

Malik, K.U. & McGiff, J.C. (1975). Modulation by prostaglandins of adrenergic transmission in the isolated perfused rabbit and rat kidney. *Circ. Res.* 36, 599-609.

McGiff, J.C., Crowshaw, K., Terragno, N.A. & Lonigro, A.J. (1970a). Release of prostaglandin-like substance into renal venous blood in response to angiotensin II. *Circ. Res.* 26-27, I-121-I-130.

McGiff, J.C., Crowshaw, K., Terragno, N.A., Lonigro, A.J., Strand, J.C., Williamson, M.A., Lee, J.B. & Ng, K.K.F. (1970b). Prostaglandin-like substances appearing in canine renal venous blood during renal ischemia. *Circ. Res.* 27, 765-782.

McGiff, J.C., Terragno, N.A., Malik, K.U. & Lonigro, A.J. (1972). Differential effect of noradrenaline and renal nerve stimulation on vascular resistance in the dog kidney and the release of a prostaglandin E-like substance. *Clin. Sci.* 42, 223-233.

Minkes, M.S., Douglas, J.R. & Needleman, P. (1973). Prostaglandin release by the isolated perfused rabbit heart. *Prostaglandins* 3, 439-445.

Pace-Asciak, C.R. (1977). Minireview: Oxidative biotransformations of arachidonic acid. *Prostaglandins* 13, 811-817.

Patrick, R.L. & Barchas, J.D. (1976a). Dopamine synthesis in rat brain striatal synaptosomes. I. Correlation between veratridininduced synthesis stimulation and endogenous dopamine release. *J. Pharmacol. Exp. Ther.* 197, 89-96.

Patrick, R.L. & Barchas, J.D. (1976b). Dopamine synthesis in rat brain striatal synaptosomes. II. Dibutyrl cyclic adenosine 3':5'-monophosphoric acid and 6-methyltetrahydropteridineinduced synthesis increases without an increase in endogenous dopamine release. *J. Pharmacol. Exp. Ther.* 197, 97-104.

Peskar, B. & Hertting, G. (1973). Release of prostaglandins from isolated cat spleen by angiotensin and vasopressin. *Naunyn-Schmiedeberg's Arch. Pharmacol.* 279, 227-234.

Piper, P. & Vane, J.R. (1971). The release of prostaglandins from lung and other tissues. *Ann. N.Y. Acad. Sci.* 180, 363-385.

Rasmussen, H. (1970). Cell communication, calcium ion, and cyclic adenosine monophosphate. *Science* 170, 404-412.

Roberts, P.J. & Hillier, K. (1976). Facilitation of noradrenaline release from rat brain synaptosomes by prostaglandin E_2. *Brain Res.* 112, 425-428.

Rubin, R.P. (1970). The role of calcium in the release of transmitter substances and hormones. *Pharmacol. Rev.* 22, 389-428.

Salt, P.J. (1972). Inhibition of noradrenaline uptake$_2$ in the isolated rat heart by steroids, clonidine and methoxylated phenylethylamines. *Eur. J. Pharmacol.* 20, 329-340.

Samuelsson, B. & Wennmalm, Å. (1971). Increased nerve stimulation induces release of noradrenaline from the rabbit heart after inhibition of prostaglandin synthesis. *Acta Physiol. Scand.* 83, 163-168.

Samuelsson, B., Granström, E., Green, K., Hamberg, M. & Hammarström, S. (1975). Prostaglandins. *Ann. Rev. Biochem.* 44, 669-695.

Santi, R., Ferrari, M. & Contessa, A.R. (1964). On the mechanism of spasmolytic effect of papaverine and certain derivatives. *Biochem. Pharmacol.* 13, 153-158.

Sattin, A. & Rall, T.W. (1970). The effect of adenosine and adenineenucleotides on the cyclic adenosine 3',5'-phosphate content of guinea-pig cerebral cortex slices. *Mol. Pharmacol.* 6, 13-23.

Sjöstrand, N.O. (1972). A note on the dual effect of prostaglandin E_1 on the responses of the guinea-pig vas deferens to nerve stimulation. *Experientia* 28, 431-432.

Starke, K. (1977). Regulation of noradrenaline release by presynaptic receptor systems. *Rev. Physiol. Biochem. Pharmacol.* 77, 1-116.

Starke, K. & Montel, H. (1973a). Interaction between indomethacin, oxymetazoline and phentolamine on the release of (^3H)-noradrenaline from brain slices. *J. Pharm. Pharmacol.* 25, 758-759.

Starke, K. & Montel, H. (1973b). Sympathomimetic inhibition of noradrenaline release: Mediated by prostaglandins? *Naunyn-Schmiedeberg's Arch. Pharmacol.* 278, 111-116.

Stjärne, L. (1971). Hyperexcretion of catecholamines induced by indomethacin. *Acta Physiol. Scand.* 83, 574-576.

Stjärne, L. (1972a). Prostaglandin E restricting noradrenaline secretion - neural in origin? *Acta Physiol. Scand.* 86, 574-576.

Stjärne, L. (1972b). Enhancement by indomethacin of cold-induced hypersecretion of noradrenaline in the rat *in vivo* - by suppression of PGE mediated feedback control? *Acta Physiol. Scand.* 86, 3880397.

Stjärne, L. (1973a). Lack of correlation between profiles of transmitter efflux and of muscular contraction in response to nerve stimulation in isolated guinea-pig vas deferens. *Acta Physiol. Scand.* 88, 137-144.

Stjärne, L. (1973b). Inhibitory effect of prostaglandin E_2 on noradrenaline secretion from sympathetic nerves as a function of external calcium. *Prostaglandins* 3, 105-109.

Stjärne, L. (1973c). Comparison of secretion of sympathetic neurotransmitter induced by nerve stimulation with that evoked by high potassium, as triggers of dual alpha-adrenoceptor mediated negative feedback control of noradrenaline secretion. *Prostaglandins* 3, 421-426.

Stjärne, L. (1973d). Kinetics of secretion of sympathetic neurotransmitter as a function of external calcium: Mechanism of inhibitory effect of prostaglandin E. *Acta Physiol. Scand.* 87, 428-430.

Stjärne, L. (1973e). Frequency dependence of dual negative feed-
    back control of secretion of sympathetic neurotransmitter in
    guinea-pig vas deferens. *Br. J. Pharmacol.* 49, 358-360.

Stjärne, L. (1973f). Michaelis-Menten kinetics of calcium depen-
    dence of sympathetic neurotransmitter secretion in guinea-pig
    vas deferens: Comparison between the effects of phentolamine
    and of tetraethylammonium. *Acta Physiol. Scand.* 89, 142-144.

Stjärne, L. (1973g). Uncompetitive character of inhibition by
    prostaglandin E_2 of the enhancing effect of α-adrenoceptor
    blocking drugs on noradrenaline secretion in isolated guinea-
    pig vas deferens. *Acta Physiol. Scand.* 89, 278-282.

Stjärne, L. (1973h). Prostaglandin- versus α-adrenoceptor med-
    iated control of sympathetic neurotransmitter secretion in
    isolated guinea-pig vas deferens. *Eur. J. Pharmacol.* 22, 233-
    238.

Stjärne, L. (1973i). Dual alpha-adrenoceptor mediated control of
    secretion of sympathetic neurotransmitter: one mechanism de-
    pendent and one independent of prostaglandin E. *Prostaglandins*
    3, 111-116.

Stjärne, L. (1973j). Role of alpha-adrenoceptors in prostaglandin
    E mediated negative feedback control of the secretion of nor-
    adrenaline from the sympathetic nerves of guinea-pig vas de-
    ferens. *Prostaglandins* 4, 845-851.

Stjärne, L. (1975). Basic mechanisms and local feedback control
    of secretion of adrenergic and cholinergic transmitters. In:
    Handbook of Psychopharmacology (eds.) L.L. Iverson,
    S.D. Iversen & S.H. Snyder, pp. 179-233, Plenum Publishing Co.,
    New York.

Stjärne, L. (1976). Relative importance of calcium and cyclic
    AMP for noradrenaline secretion from sympathetic nerves of
    guinea-pig vas deferens and for prostaglandin E-induced de-
    pression of noradrenaline secretion. *Neuroscience* 1, 19-22.

Stjärne, L. (1977). Inhibitory effects of noradrenaline and
    prostaglandin E_2 on neurotransmitter secretion evoked by single
    shocks or by short trains of nerve stimuli. *Acta Physiol.
    Scand.*, in press.

Stjärne, L. & Alberts, P. (1978). Factors influencing neurotrans-
    mitter secretion in guinea-pig isolated vas deferens: III.
    Roles of calcium and frequency. *Acta Physiol. Scand*, in press.

Stjärne, L. & Brundin, J. (1976). Additive stimulating effects
    of inhibitor of prostaglandin synthesis and of β-adrenoceptor
    agonist on sympathetic neuroeffector function in human omental
    blood vessels. *Acta Physiol. Scand.*, 97, 267-269.

Stjärne, L. & Brundin, J. (1977a). Frequency dependence of ^{3}H-noradrenaline secretion from human vasoconstrictor nerves: Modification by factors interfering with α- and β-adrenoceptor or prostaglandin E$_2$ mediated control. *Acta Physiol. Scand.* in press.

Stjärne, L. & Brundin, J. (1977b). Prostaglandin E$_2$- and α- or β-adrenoceptor mediated interferences with ^{3}B-noradrenaline secretion from human vasoconstrictor nerves: Comparison between effects on omental arteries and veins. *Acta Physiol. Scand.*, 100, 267-269.

Stjärne, L. & Gripe, K. (1973). Prostaglandin-dependent andα-independent feedback control of noradrenaline secretion in vasoconstrictor nerves of normotensive human subjects: A preliminary report. *Naunyn-Schmiedeberg's Arch. Pharmacol.* 280, 441-446.

Taube, H.D., Endo, T., Bangerter, A. & Starke, K. (1976). Presynaptic receptor systems on the noradrenergic nerves of the rabbit pulmonary artery. *Naunyn-Schmiedeberg's Arch. Pharmacol.* 293, R2.

Taylor, G.S. & Einhorn, V.F. (1972). The effect of prostaglandins on junction potentials in the mouse vas deferens. *Eur. J. Pharmacol.* 20, 40-45.

Wennmalm, Å. (1971). Studies on mechanisms controlling the secretion of neurotransmitters in the rabbit heart. *Acta Physiol. Scand.* 82, Suppl. 365.

Wennmalm, Å. (1975). Prostaglandin release and mechanical performance in the isolated rabbit heart during induced changes in the internal environment. *Acta Physiol. Scand.* 93, 15-24.

Wennmalm, Å. & Hedqvist, P. (1971). Inhibition by prostaglandin E$_1$ of parasympathetic neurotransmission in the rabbit heart. *Life Sci.* 10, 465-470.

Wennmalm, Å. & Stjärne, L. (1971). Inhibition of the release of adrenergic transmitter by a fatty acid in the perfusate from sympathetically stimulated rabbit heart. *Life Sci.* 10, 471-479.

Westfall, T.C. & Brasted, M. (1974). Specificity of blockade of the nicotine-induced release of ^{3}H-norepinephrine from adrenergic neurons of the guinea-pig heart by various pharmacological agents. *J. Pharmacol. Exp. Ther.* 189, 659-664.

Westfall, T.C., Kitay, D. & Wahl, G. (1976). The effect of cyclic nucleotides on the release of ^{3}H-dopamine from rat striatal slices. *J. Pharmacol. Exp. Ther.* 199, 149-157.

Vizi, E.Z. & Knoll, J. (1976). The inhibitory effect of adenosine and related nucleotides on the release of acetylcholine. *Neuroscience* 1, 391-398.

Woods, W.T. & Lieberman, E.M. (1976). The effect of papaverine
    on sodium-potassium adenosine triphosphatase and the ouabain
    sensitive electrical properties of crayfish nerve. *Neuro-
    science* 1, 383-390.

Wooten, G.F., Thoa, N.B., Kopin, I.J. & Axelrod, J. (1973). En-
    hanced release of dopamine β-hydroxylase and norepinephrine
    from sympathetic nerves by dibutyryl cyclic adenosine 3',5'-
    monophosphate and theophylline. *Molec. Pharmacol.* 9, 178-183.

Zimmerman, B.G., Ryan, M.J., Gomer, S. & Kraft, E. (1973).
    Effect of the prostaglandin synthesis inhibitors indomethacin
    and eicosa-5,8,11,14-tetraynoic acid on adrenergic responses
    in dog cutaneous vasculature. *J. Pharmacol. Exp. Ther.* 187,
    315-323.

PRESYNAPTIC REGULATION OF RELEASE IN THE CENTRAL NERVOUS SYSTEM

K. Starke

I INTRODUCTION, DEFINITIONS AND SCOPE

Nerve cells are endowed with receptor sites through which they recognize chemical messages from their environment. Postganglionic sympathetic noradrenergic neurons possess two topographically as well as functionally different groups of receptors. Soma-dendritic receptors are located on the cell bodies and dendrites and regulate the generation of action potentials. Presynaptic receptors are probably located on the axon terminals where, upon interaction with appropriate agonists, they initiate (e.g., nicotine receptors) or modify (e.g., α-adrenoceptors) calcium-dependent release processes (reviews by Langer, 1974; Baldessarini, 1975; Stjärne, 1975; Bacq, 1976; Starke, 1977).

This article deals with mechanisms in the central nervous system (CNS) that are strikingly similar to the presynaptic modulation of transmitter release from peripheral noradrenergic fibres. Relevant observations were first published about 1970. Besson, Cheramy, Feltz and Glowinski (1969) found that acetylcholine releases dopamine in the corpus striatum. The effect is partly analogous to the nicotinic effect of acetylcholine on postganglionic sympathetic nerve endings. Farnebo and Hamberger (1970, 1971) showed that drugs with affinity for α-adrenoceptors modify the release of noradrenaline from cortical nerve endings much like noradrenaline release in the periphery. They also reported similar results with dopaminergic and serotonergic neurons. However, whereas in the periphery a direct action of presynaptic modulators on the nerve endings is widely accepted, such an action is much less certain for the CNS. Central catecholamine-containing varicosites are within reach of numerous other neurotransmitter substances. These may be secreted from nerve endings that impinge upon the varicosites, forming axo-axonic synapses; they may also diffuse from more distant nerve endings that do not make typical synaptic contacts (Beaudet & Descarries, 1976); or they may be released from dendrites (Groves, Wilson, Young & Rebec, 1975). Instead of acting directly on the catecholaminergic varicosities, a drug may primarily act on neighbouring terminals or dendrites, or on the cell bodies from which they project, or even on glial cells, and may influence catecholamine release by way of these structures and their secretion products.

Therefore, throughout this review the term "presynaptic receptor" is used cautiously for sites that (1) are distinct from soma-dendritic receptors and do not control the generation of action

143

potentials in the perikarya; (2) initiate or modify calcium-dependent release processes in the nerve terminals; and (3) are possibly located on the catecholaminergic nerve terminals themselves; however, this location is by no means certain.

"Release" is the passage of a transmitter across the neuronal membrane into the extracellular space. Unless defined further, the term denotes secretion evoked by normal orthodromic action potentials, triggered for instance by electrical stimulation. "Overflow" or "outflow" describes the diffusion of catecholamines or their metabolites from the tissue into the surrounding fluid.

The article reviews the presynaptic regulation of transmitter release from noradrenergic and dopaminergic neurons. Although the CNS contains adrenaline neurons (Hökfelt, Fuxe, Goldstein & Johansson, 1974), nothing is known about presynaptic modulation of their activity. *In vitro* studies are the basis of each section. Since the very location of the receptors is doubtful, little can be said about the steps that lead from receptor activation to changes in release, and this question will rarely be considered. It seemed reasonable to discuss soma-dendritic receptors briefly together with the corresponding presynaptic sites. Both may participate in the physiological regulation as well as in pharmacological modifications of a neuron's activity; these potential *in vivo* functions will be critically analyzed.

II   DETERMINATION OF CATECHOLAMINE RELEASE

The best way to study catecholamine release is to determine the overflow of the transmitter and its metabolites from the tissue into perfusion, superfusion or incubation fluids. Experimental strategies that allow the extrapolation of drug effects on overflow to effects on release have been recently reviewed (Starke, 1977). Only some special points relevant to CNS studies will be discussed here. Most investigations on central presynaptic mechanisms have been carried out on slices or similar dissected parts of the brain. Comparatively few authors have used synaptosomes or *in vivo* preparations.

Brain Slices
When presynaptic drug effects are examined, the possibility that the drug changes the firing rate of the neurons under study, must be excluded. One approach is to use slices that contain axon terminals, but not cell bodies, with the respective transmitter. For instance, the corpus striatum is innervated by dopaminergic neurons that have their cell bodies in the pars compacta of the substantia nigra. The noradrenergic nerve terminals in cerebellum, hypothalamus, hippocampus and cerebral cortex arise from perikarya in the lower brain stem, most notably the locus coeruleus. Slices of corpus striatum and cerebral cortex can thus be employed to study dopamine and noradrenaline release without the interference of the respective soma-dendritic receptors.

In all published studies of presynaptic regulation, the transmitter stores have been labelled either by preincubation with

radioactive noradrenaline or dopamine (which are incorporated by
the neuronal uptake systems) or, in the case of dopamine, by incubation with radioactive tyrosine (which is converted into dopamine).

A possible source of error in experiments with radioactive catecholamines previously taken up is that the labelled compound may
enter into cells other than those containing the endogenous transmitter, and may subsequently be released from the "wrong" structure. For instance, in some areas of the cerebral cortex [^{3}H]-
noradrenaline may be incorporated into dopaminergic nerve endings.
However, this difficulty can be avoided by the choice of areas
without dopaminergic innervation such as the occipital cortex.
Moreover, low preincubation concentrations of the labelled transmitter ensure a high degree of specificity.

In the case of dopamine, specific labelling has been obtained by
incubation of striatal slices with [^{3}H]tyrosine (Besson *et al.*,
1969). Since only catecholamine neurons contain tyrosine hydroxylase, and since the corpus striatum is practically devoid of noradrenergic and adrenergic fibres, the incubation leads to selective formation of [^{3}H]dopamine in dopaminergic nerve terminals.
A refined biochemical procedure allows the effective separation
of [^{3}H]dopamine from other tritiated compounds so that even during
continuous superfusion with [^{3}H]tyrosine the outflow of [^{3}H]dop-
amine is several times greater than the [^{3}H] background
(Giorguieff, Le Floc'h, Westfall, Glowinski & Besson, 1976).

How representative is the release of the label for the secretion
of endogenous transmitter? Nerve endings probably contain at
least two pools of catecholamines with different dynamic properties (Glowinski, 1975). A transmitter molecule that has recently
been taken up or synthesized first enters a "functional" pool
which is normally the major source for release. As time goes on,
the probability that the molecule is released declines; it is
stored in a "reserve" pool which contributes to release mainly
when the neuronal activity is high. According to this view, the
overflow of labelled catecholamines predominantly originates from
the reserve pool if some time (perhaps 30 min) has elapsed since
the labelling procedure; this has been the case in most studies
on presynaptic mechanisms. On the other hand, the outflow mainly
originates from the functional pool, e.g., during continuous superfusion with [^{3}H]tyrosine. There is an indication that the two
pools may respond differently to presynaptic agonists: acetylcholine releases [^{3}H]dopamine that has been formed from [^{3}H]tyro-
sine in the preceding 20 min (and is thus presumably in the functional pool), but fails to release [^{3}H]dopamine that has been
taken up some time previously (and is thus presumably in the reserve pool; Giorguieff *et al.*, 1976). However, this is an excep-
tional situation since acetylcholine initiates *de novo* release.
Such a phenomenon will be most prominent when the labelled compound is readily releasable. Most presynaptic agonists do not
trigger *de novo* release but rather modulate ongoing release processes, in particular release evoked by nerve impulses. It seems
very likely that they exert at least qualitatively the same effect,
whether the ongoing release is fuelled from the functional or the

reserve pool, i.e., whether the effect is tested early or late
after labelling. In fact, in the periphery presynaptic modulators
always change the release of radioactive noradrenaline previously
taken up, and that of endogenous noradrenaline, in a closely
parallel manner (Starke, 1977).

The characteristics of the outflow of labelled monoamines from
brain slices have been described in detail (reviews by Katz &
Chase, 1970; Baldessarini, 1975). In the case of noradrenaline,
there is a basal outflow that is not changed by tetrodotoxin and
not changed or even slightly enhanced (Taube, Starke & Borowski,
1977) by the omission of calcium. When the slices are stimulated
by an electrical field, the outflow increases. Provided the
stimulus strength is sufficiently low, the evoked overflow is completely abolished by tetrodotoxin and lack of calcium. Obviously,
the response requires membrane depolarization by the rapid sodium
inward current as well as calcium-dependent electro-secretory
coupling and thus closely resembles physiological release (cf.,
Orrego & Miranda, 1977). Pulses of alternating polarity, with
the negative pulse immediately following on the positive pulse,
have theoretical advantages (Bradford, 1975). In practice, however, similar results were obtained, whether pulses of constant
or alternating polarity were used (Montel & Starke, unpublished).
Depolarization by high extracellular potassium concentrations or
veratrum alkaloids also elicits calcium-dependent release.

Surprisingly, the outflow of dopamine differs in some respects
from that of noradrenaline. Whether striatal nerve endings are
labelled by uptake of [^{3}H]dopamine or by synthesis from [^{3}H]tyro-
sine, the basal outflow is markedly reduced during superfusion
with tetrodotoxin or calcium-free medium (Dismukes & Mulder, 1977;
Giorguieff, Le Floc'h, Glowinski & Besson, 1977). The reason for
this apparently impulse-induced release in the absence of external
stimuli is not clear. Possibly the irritation caused by the dis-
section can, under certain conditions, lead to the generation of
action potentials in the cut axons. Electrical pulses increase
the outflow of [^{3}H]dopamine. At identical stimulus parameters,
the evoked overflow of [^{3}H]dopamine from striatal slices is smaller than that of [^{3}H]noradrenaline from cortical slices and declines more slowly after the end of stimulation (Farnebo, 1971;
Dismukes & Mulder, 1977). With mild stimuli, the evoked overflow is completely calcium-dependent and blocked by tetrodotoxin,
and is thus similar to physiological release. Farnebo (1971) has
pointed out that striatal, in contrast to cortical, slices undergo rapid changes in their microscopic appearance during incubation.
Thus, some anomalies suggest particular caution when studies on
striatal slices are evaluated.

Synaptosomes
Techniques for the preparation of synaptosomes and for the investigation of their secretory activity have recently been reviewed (Bradford, 1975; Jones, 1975). Both the outflow of endogenous and that of previously stored labelled catecholamines can
be measured. Calcium-dependent release can be elicited by electrical stimulation, high potassium or veratrum alkaloids.

Synaptosomes offer one distinct advantage over slices in studies
on presynaptic receptors. Brain slices still consist of an intri-
cate network of fibres with many short interneurons probably intact. In synaptosome preparations all non-terminal axons are disrupted. Therefore, when a drug similarly modifies the release of
a catecholamine in slice and synaptosome preparations, then a
primary action on the cell bodies or dendrites of interneurons
can definitely be ruled out. However, this experiment is by no
means unequivocal evidence for a direct action of the drug on
catecholaminergic nerve endings. Synaptosomes are not pure presynaptic terminals since many have the postsynaptic membrane still
attached (see Jones, 1975, pp. 83 and 98), and the site of action
may be there. Moreover, presently available synaptosome preparations are always heterogeneous. The primary target of the drug
may well be a non-catecholaminergic synaptosome, and changes in
catecholamine release may be secondary to changes in the release
of the second neurotransmitter. This is particularly prone to
occur in synaptosome beds, i.e., deposits with short intersynapto-
somal distances.

Experiments *In Vivo*
The significance of presynaptic regulation must ultimately be
proven by *in vivo* studies. Progress has been made in recent
years in the measurement of the outflow of catecholamines from
small brain areas *in situ*, in particular with the help of the
push-pull cannula (Philippu, Przuntek & Roensberg, 1973a;
Philippu, Roensberg & Przuntek, 1973b; Bartholini, Stadler,
Gadea Ciria & Lloyd, 1976; Nieoullon, Cheramy & Glowinski, 1977).
Drug-induced changes of outflow have been observed repeatedly.
However, their interpretation is even more difficult than in slice
or synaptosome experiments.

In order to illustrate these difficulties, one example will be
discussed in some detail. Systemic injection of bicuculline and
picrotoxin increases the outflow of endogenous dopamine and newly
synthesized [^{3}H]dopamine into push-pull cannula superfusates of
the caudate nucleus of the cat (Bartholini & Stadler, 1975;
Cheramy, Nieoullon & Glowinski, 1977). The action is central.
Since both drugs block receptors for γ-aminobutyric acid (GABA),
one may safely assume that they interrupt a GABAergic inhibition
of dopamine neurons. Where does this inhibition take place?

In an elegant series of experiments, Bartholini and Stadler (1975)
and Cheramy *et al*. (1977) have pinpointed two sites of action
(Fig. 1). Firstly, the antagonists also enhance the outflow of
dopamine from the caudate nucleus when they are locally infused
into the substantia nigra. The substantia nigra contains high
levels of GABA, a large proportion of which is in the terminals
of a striato-nigral GABA pathway. GABA decreases the firing rate
of units in the substantia nigra, and its effect is blocked by
iontophoretically applied picrotoxin (Crossman, Walker & Woodruff,
1973). It seems likely, therefore, that bicuculline and picrotoxin enhance the release of dopamine because they antagonize a
tonic soma-dendritic inhibition of the nigral dopamine cells by
GABAergic fibres. The target may be GABA receptors on the dopaminergic somata and dendrites themselves (Fig. 1), although an inter-

K. Starke

calation of other small neurons cannot be ruled out.

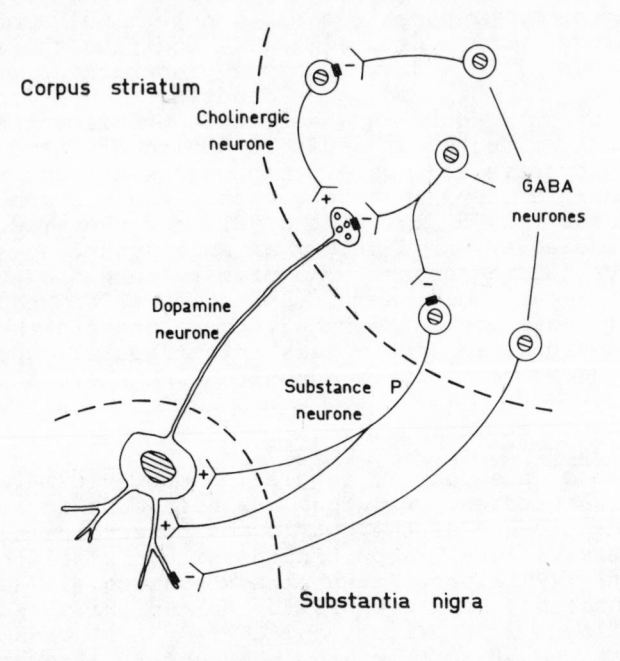

Fig. 1.   The nigro-striatal dopaminergic pathway, and possible
mechanisms for the inhibitory effect of GABA and the facilitatory
effect of GABA antagonists on the release of dopamine *in vivo*.
GABA receptors are represented by rectangles.   The dopaminergic
cell bodies and dendrites in the substantia nigra are innervated
by inhibitory (-) GABA and excitatory (+) substance P neurons.
Within the corpus striatum, the dopaminergic nerve endings receive an inhibitory GABAergic and an excitatory cholinergic input; furthermore, GABA interneurons inhibit cholinergic and substance P-containing cells.   It is emphasized that this survey of
potential sites of action of GABA and its antagonists is not
meant to be exhaustive, and that details of the neuronal connections as shown in the figure are hypothetical.

In a second stage Bartholini and Stadler (1975) and Cheramy
et al. (1977) showed that bicuculline and picrotoxin augment the
outflow of dopamine even when they are added to the medium superfusing the caudate nucleus itself.   Local infusion of GABA
counteracts the facilitation and, given alone, reduces dopamine
outflow.   What is the mechanism of this second, intrastriatal
effect?   One possibility is that the drugs act directly on the
dopaminergic nerve endings which, in this case, would be inhibited by GABA.   Just as possibly they may act on interneurons (in
Fig. 1 a cholinergic cell) which impinge upon the dopaminergic
nerve endings.   Either mode of action would be "presynaptic",
i.e., the drugs would change the release of dopamine per impulse,

with no change in the rate of nigro-striatal impulse flow. However, there is an entirely different alternative. Fibres containing substance P appear to descend from the corpus striatum
to the substantia nigra (Kanazawa, Emson & Cuello, 1977), and
substance P excites nigral cells (Dray & Straughan, 1976; Walker,
Kemp, Yajima, Kitagawa & Woodruff, 1976). Intrastriatally administered GABA may reduce the release of dopamine because it
inhibits these substance P neurons and thereby removes an excitatory input to the dopaminergic cell bodies; the reverse may hold
good for the antagonists. If so, the effect would not be "presynaptic" at all, but would be mediated by a neuronal loop, soma-
dendritic receptors of the dopamine neurons, and a change in
their rate of firing. The potential relevance of this alternative has been underscored by recent studies with rat striatal
slices. In this preparation, in which the dopaminergic terminals
are severed from their perikarya, GABA tends to facilitate rather
than inhibit the release of dopamine (Stoof & Mulder, in press).
In conclusion, the example shows that even direct measurement of
the outflow of catecholamines from brain nuclei and sophisticated
techniques of drug application may fall short of a definite
identification of the location of receptor sites.

Nuclei containing catecholaminergic cell bodies can be electrically stimulated *in vivo*, and the evoked release of transmitter
from the nerve endings can be estimated (e.g., Nieoullon *et al.*,
1977). When a drug affects this release, a presynaptic action
seems plausible. On the other hand, the external pulses are
superimposed on an ongoing endogenous activity, and a change of
the latter cannot be ruled out. Axotomy of the pathway under
study and stimulation of the peripheral stump may be a means to
keep the rate of impulse traffic constant and to make sure that
effects on release are indeed mediated by presynaptic receptors.

III   REGULATION OF NORADRENALINE RELEASE

α-Adrenoceptors
α-Adrenergic agonists reduce, whereas α-adrenoceptor blocking
drugs enhance, the electrically and potassium-evoked overflow of
tritium from brain slices preincubated with [3H]noradrenaline
(Table 1; the facilitatory effect of clonidine in the guinea-pig
hypothalamus may be due to the partial agonist character of this
agent). The decrease of total tritium overflow caused by tramazoline, and the increase caused by phentolamine, reflect propor-
tionate decreases and increases, respectively, of [3H]noradren-
aline and its major metabolite, [3H]3,4-dihydroxyphenylglycol
([3H]DOPEG; Taube *et al.*, 1977). Formation of DOPEG from released noradrenaline largely takes place intraneuronally after re-
uptake. Therefore, drugs like cocaine which block the uptake
mechanism markedly decrease the evoked overflow of DOPEG (Farah,
Adler-Graschinsky & Langer, 1977; Taube *et al.*, 1977). The fact
that phentolamine causes an increase rules out any inhibition of
re-uptake. It confirms previous evidence (see references in
Table 1) showing that drugs with α-adrenoceptor affinity at least
at low concentrations selectively modulate the release of noradrenaline; DOPEG is secondarily decreased by agonists or

Table 1. EFFECT OF DRUGS ON THE ELECTRICALLY AND POTASSIUM-EVOKED RELEASE OF NORADRENALINE IN BRAIN SLICES.

Species & Brain Region	Drug & Concentration (μM)	Stimulation Frequency; Potassium Concentration	Effect	References
Rat cerebral cortex	Noradrenaline 0.01-1	3 Hz; 20 mM	−	Farnebo & Hamberger, 1970, 1971, 1973; Starke & Montel, 1973a,b,c; Starke et al., 1975b; Dismukes & Mulder, 1976; Dismukes et al., 1977; Taube et al., 1977; Baumann & Maître, in press
	Clonidine 0.1-10	5-10 Hz	−	
	Oxymetazoline 0.05-10	5-10 Hz; 13-26 mM	−	
	Tramazoline 0.1	3 Hz	−	
	Phenoxybenzamine 0.1-10	5-10 Hz; 26 mM	+	
	Phentolamine 0.01-10	2-10 Hz; 20-26 mM	+	
	Yohimbine 0.1-1	3 Hz	+	
	Chlorpromazine 1-10	10 Hz	+	
	Dopamine 0.01-1	3 Hz	0	Starke et al., 1975b; Taube et al., 1977
	Isoprenaline 0.01-1	1-10 Hz	0	Farnebo & Hamberger, 1973; Starke et al., 1975b; Taube et al., 1977
	Propranolol 0.1-1	1-10 Hz	0	
	Prostaglandin E1 0.01-1	3 Hz; 20 mM	−	Bergström et al., 1973; Farnebo & Hamberger, 1973; Starke & Montel, 1973c; Taube et al., 1977
	Prostaglandin E2 3	10 Hz	−	
	Indomethacin 30 (plus pretreatment)	5 Hz	+	
	Acetylcholine 0.01-10	3 Hz	0	Starke et al., 1975b; Taube et al., 1977
	Oxotremorine 1-10	3 Hz	0	
	Atropine 0.1-3	3 Hz	0	

....................cont'd.

K. Starke

Species & Brain Region	Drug & Concentration (μM)	Stimulation Frequency; Potassium Concentration	Effect	References
Rat cerebral cortex	Morphine 0.1-10	0.3-3 Hz; 20 mM	–	Montel et al., 1974a,b, 1975a,b; Taube et al., 1976, 1977; Baumann, personal communication; Mulder, personal communication
	Fentanyl 0.01-1	3 Hz; 20 mM	–	
	Pethidine 3	0.3-3 Hz	–	
	Levorphanol 0.1-1	3 Hz	–	
	Dextrorphan 1	3 Hz	0	
	Methionine-enkephalin 0.1-10	1-3 Hz; 20 mM	–	
	Naloxone 1-100	1-3 Hz; 20 mM	0 or +	
	Angiotensin I 0.001-1	3 Hz	0	Starke et al., 1975b; Taube et al., 1977
	Angiotensin II 0.0001-10	3 Hz	0	
	Saralasin 0.01	3 Hz	0	
	Serotonin 0.01-10	3 Hz	0	Taube et al., 1977
	Histamine 1-10	3 Hz	0	
	GABA 100-1000	3 Hz	+	
	Substance P 0.001-1	3 Hz	–	
Rat cerebellum	Acetylcholine 1-10	50 mM	–	Westfall, 1974b
	Morphine 1-10	3 Hz	–	Montel et al., 1975b; Taube et al., 1977
	Methionine-enkephalin 1-10	3 Hz; 20 mM	–	
	Naloxone 1-10	3 Hz	0	
Rat hypo-thalamus	Acetylcholine 1-10	3 Hz; 20 mM	0	Taube et al., 1977
	Morphine 1-10	3 Hz; 20 mM	–	
	Methionine-enkephalin 0.1-10	3 Hz; 20 mM	–	

.............................cont'd.

Species & Brain Region	Drug & Concentration (μM)	Stimulation Frequency; Potassium Concentration	Effect	References
Guinea-pig hypo-thalamus	Noradrenaline 2-50	10 Hz	−	Bryant et al., 1975; Rand et al., 1975
	Adrenaline 5	10 Hz	−	
	Clonidine 0.00005-0.5	10 Hz	+	
	Phenoxybenzamine 10	10 Hz	0	
	Phentolamine 0.05-5	10 Hz	+	
	Piperoxan 10	10 Hz	+	
	Dopamine 10	10 Hz	−	
	Isoprenaline up to 50	10 Hz	0	

Brain slices were preincubated with [³H]noradrenaline and then superfused with fresh medium. They were stimulated electrically or by high potassium concentrations as indicated. The evoked overflow of tritium was taken to represent noradrenaline release. Effects on the evoked overflow: + increase, − decrease, 0 no change. For many drugs with affinity to α-adrenoceptors, for isoprenaline, prostaglandin E1, acetylcholine, opiates, the angiotensins and substance P it was shown that at the concentrations indicated they did not change the basal outflow of tritium. Noradrenaline, dopamine, serotonin and histamine accelerated basal tritium outflow, but this could be prevented by cocaine.

increased by antagonists because of an altered supply of recap-
tured noradrenaline to intraneuronal monoamine oxidase.

A common site of action of agonists and antagonists was borne out
by the finding that clonidine and oxymetazoline at supramaximal
concentrations prevent the facilitatory effect of low concentrations of phentolamine and phenoxybenzamine (Starke & Montel,
1973a,b; cf. Baumann & Maître, in press). Conversely, a high
dose of phentolamine antagonizes the inhibition produced by low
doses of oxymetazoline and noradrenaline (Dismukes & Mulder,
1976; Taube *et al.*, 1977).   The receptors involved can be dif-
ferentiated from other presynaptic receptors. Phentolamine
counteracts the effect of clonidine, but fails to interfere with
the inhibitory effects on release of morphine, methionine-enkephalin and prostaglandin E_1; conversely, naloxone leaves the inhibitory effect of tramazoline unchanged (Taube *et al.*, 1977).

All these findings mirror observations on postganglionic sympathetic neurons. As in the periphery, secretion of transmitter from
central noradrenergic axon terminals appears to be subject to a
presynaptic α-adrenoceptor-mediated feedback control, in which
released noradrenaline activates the α-adrenoceptors and inhibits
its own further release. Antagonists interrupt the feedback
loop. Their facilitatory effect demonstrates that the negative
feedback operates at least *in vitro*.

Drugs with affinity for α-adrenoceptors influence central noradrenergic neurons not only in the presynaptic, but also in the
soma-dendritic region. In 1975, Svensson, Bunney and Aghajanian
showed that intravenously injected clonidine inhibits the firing
of locus coeruleus neurons, presumably the noradrenergic ones.
The rate of firing is also reduced when clonidine, noradrenaline,
adrenaline or dopamine are directly applied in the vicinity of
the locus coeruleus perikarya by microintophoresis. Iontophoretically administered piperoxan attenuates the inhibition and, given
alone, causes slight acceleration. No evidence for β-adrenoceptors and dopamine receptors was found (Svensson *et al.*, 1975;
Cedarbaum & Aghajanian, 1977).

Thus, biochemical combined with electrophysiological studies show
that inhibitory α-adrenoceptors exist near central noradrenergic
nerve endings as well as cell bodies. Although it is presently
not possible to exclude a location outside the noradrenaline
cells, the alternative that the receptors in fact are on or in
these cells has the attractiveness of simplicity and is in accord
with current thinking about peripheral presynaptic α-adrenoceptors. Dismukes, de Boer and Mulder (1977) have recently shown
that the effect of oxymetazoline on the potassium-evoked release
of noradrenaline in brain slices is not changed by tetrodotoxin,
which prevents any action potential-dependent interneuronal communication. Moreover, oxymetalozine and clonidine also depress
potassium-evoked noradrenaline release from synaptosomes (Mulder,
de Langen & Dismukes, personal communication). These findings
clearly indicate that the "presynaptic" α-adrenoceptors are not
located on the cell bodies or dendrites of interneurons, although
location on non-noradrenergic nerve terminals cannot be ruled out

(see p.146).

If the noradrenaline neurons themselves carry α-adrenoceptors, destruction of these neurons, e.g., by 6-hydroxydopamine might be expected to reduce the total number of α-adrenoceptors. The number of receptors can be estimated by the amount of binding of labelled agonists or antagonists to particles in brain homogenates. When rats were pretreated with 6-hydroxydopamine, whole brain levels of noradrenaline decreased by 79%. Contrary to the prediction, the specific binding of [^{3}H]clonidine was not reduced, but even slightly increased (U'Prichard, Greenberg & Snyder, 1977). However, although the outcome is negative, the experiment does not disprove receptor location on noradrenergic somata, dendrites and terminals. These receptors may be a quantitatively minor, yet functionally significant group. Moreover, treatment with 6-hydroxydopamine may lead to a proliferation of postsynaptic α-adrenoceptors that exceeds the loss of receptors on noradrenergic neurons (cf. Taube *et al.*, 1977; U'Prichard *et al.*, 1977).

In some peripheral tissues, presynaptic α-adrenoceptors differ from the postsynaptic ones in their affinity for drugs (see Starke, 1972, 1977; Borowski, Starke, Ehrl & Endo, 1977). Langer (1974) proposed that the presynaptic sites, because of their distinct pharmacological properties, should generally be classified as α_2, and the postsynaptic ones as α_1. Interestingly, the soma-dendritic α-adrenoceptor in the locus coeruleus is more similar to the presynaptic than to the postsynaptic α-adrenoceptor in the pulmonary artery of the rabbit. For instance, clonidine acts on the former two as a particularly potent agonist, and phenylephrine as a particularly weak agonist (Starke, Endo & Taube, 1975a; Cedarbaum & Aghajanian, 1977). Both the peripheral presynaptic and the central soma-dendritic receptors are (probably) located on the noradrenaline fibres themselves. Do such receptors, apart from their common location, generally share common molecular properties? Several considerations leave some doubt. The soma-dendritic receptors in the locus coeruleus are equally sensitive to noradrenaline and dopamine which here act on α- rather than specific dopamine receptors (Cedarbaum & Aghajanian, 1977). On the other hand, the presynaptic sites in the rabbit pulmonary artery are 100 times less sensitive to dopamine than to noradrenaline (Endo, Starke, Bangerter & Taube, 1977). Moreover, there is growing evidence that peripheral postsynaptic α-adrenoceptors are not all of a single type (e.g., Barker, Harper & Hughes, 1977). The same may hold good for soma-dendritic and presynaptic α-adrenoceptors, and similarities between the locus coeruleus cells and peripheral sympathetic nerve endings may be fortuitous. Notwithstanding such cautionary reflections, however, the view that inhibitory α-adrenoceptors of noradrenergic neurons are a distinct pharmacological group remains intriguing.

Do presynaptic and soma-dendritic α-adrenoceptors play a physiological role? There is little doubt that α-adrenoceptors within the CNS physiologically help to control the activity of central noradrenergic neurons. This has been borne out by many demonstrations that α-adrenoceptor antagonists accelerate the synthesis,

utilization, turnover (e.g., Andén, Corrodi, Fuxe & Hökfelt,
1967a; Andén, Grabowska & Strömbom, 1976) and.probably release
(Lloyd & Bartholini, 1975) of noradrenaline in various parts of
the CNS *in vivo*, because they remove a normal α-adrenergic inhibition. Moreover, intravenously injected piperoxan markedly
accelerates locus coeruleus units (see Aghajanian, Cedarbaum &
Wang, in press). Much less is known about where this regulation
takes place. Important possibilities are illustrated in Fig. 2.

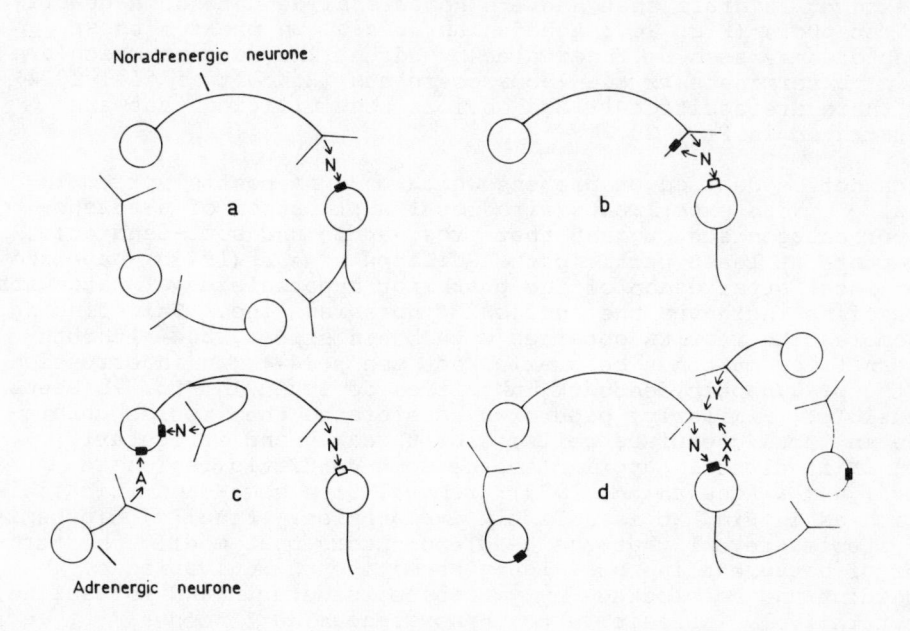

Fig. 2. Models for a physiological α-adrenergic inhibition of
central noradrenaline neurones. Released noradrenaline (N) or
adrenaline (A) act on receptors symbolized by rectangles; filled
rectangles indicate the receptors involved in α-adrenergic inhibition. (a) Shows inhibition of the firing frequency of the
noradrenergic cell via postsynaptic α-adrenoceptors and a neuronal loop. (b) Shows inhibition of the release of noradrenaline
per impulse via presynaptic α-adrenoceptors on the nerve endings.
(c) Shows inhibition of the firing frequency via soma-dendritic
α-adrenoceptors; they are shown to receive a noradrenaline input
from a recurrent axon collateral and an adrenaline input. (d)
Shows less evident possibilities that at present cannot be ruled
out. Activation of postsynaptic α-adrenoceptors may trigger
liberation of a compound X from the postsynaptic cell, and X may
reduce the release of noradrenaline. Or activation of postsynaptic α-adrenoceptors may change impulse traffic in a loop of interneurons that ultimately depress noradrenaline release by an inhibitory transmitter Y. Panel (d) also shows that there may be
inhibitory α-adrenoceptors that receive no endogenous input at
all, but may be reached by exogenous agonists.

The original hypothesis was that activation of postsynaptic
α-adrenoceptors is communicated to the noradrenaline cells
through a neuronal loop, and that the cells compensatorily slow
their firing (Fig. 2a). This model functions without any presynaptic or soma-dendritic α-adrenoceptors. The discovery of
these receptors, however, opens up alternatives. The physiological inhibition may operate presynaptically via receptors on the
nerve endings, and α-adrenolytic drugs may act there (Fig. 2b).
Or noradrenergic neurons may inhibit their own impulse generation
by axon collaterals that secrete noradrenaline onto soma-dendritic receptors (Fig. 2c ; Aghajanian et al., in press); these
receptors may also be innervated by adrenaline neurons which are
known to terminate in the locus coeruleus (Hökfelt et al., 1974).
And there are additional less obvious possibilities that are
illustrated in Fig. 2d.

It cannot be decided at present which mode of control predominates. In vivo experiments with local application of α-adrenoceptor antagonists suggest that presynaptic and soma-dendritic
receptors at least participate. Philippu et al., (1973b) have shown
that local superfusion of the posterior hypothalamus of cats with
tolazoline increases the outflow of noradrenaline. This finding
resembles the results obtained with brain slices, and although
alternatives must not be overlooked (see p.147). an interruption
of the presynaptic feedback inhibition depicted in Fig. 2b seems
plausible. Similarly, piperoxan accelerates the impulse generation in locus coeruleus cells, albeit weakly and irregularly,
when it is directly applied to the soma-dendritic region
(Cedarbaum & Aghajanian, 1977); removal of a soma-dendritic inhibition as in Fig. 2c is a likely explanation. Finally, biochemical studies reveal that the α-adrenoceptors that modify the turnover of noradrenaline are highly sensitive to activation by
clonidine and to blockade by yohimbine, piperoxan and tolazoline,
but relatively insensitive to phenoxybenzamine (Andén et al.,
1976). These properties are reminiscent of peripheral presynaptic α-adrenoceptors (Starke et al., 1975a; Borowski et al., 1977)
and soma-dendritic α-adrenoceptors in the locus coeruleus (Cedarbaum & Aghajanian, 1977). It is tempting to speculate, therefore,
that the main targets of clonidine, yohimbine, piperoxan and tolazoline, and the crucial sites of the physiological α-adrenergic
control, are receptors on the noradrenergic neurons (Fig. 2b and
c). However, it is emphasized again that pharmacological classes
of receptors (sharing common drug sensitivities) are not necessarily identical with topographical classes (on versus outside
noradrenergic cells).

Prostaglandin Receptors
Prostaglandins E_1 and E_2 inhibit the electrically and potassium-
evoked overflow of tritium from rat brain cortex slices preincubated with [^{3}H]noradrenaline, probably by inhibition of
release (Table 1). The evoked overflow of [^{3}H]noradrenaline and
[^{3}H]DOPEG is proportionately decreased (Taube et al., 1977). The
prostaglandins presumably interact with a distinct receptor system, since their effect is not antagonized by phentolamine and
naloxone (Taube et al., 1977).

Indomethacin, which blocks the biosynthesis of prostaglandins,
slightly increases the evoked overflow of tritium (Table 1).
The finding may indicate that in the brain, as in the periphery
(see Hedqvist, 1977), prostaglandins, locally formed upon stimulation, inhibit the release of noradrenaline. However, at the
high concentration used indomethacin may have exerted other
effects (e.g., blockade of noradrenaline re-uptake; Clarenbach,
Raffel, Meyer & Hertting, 1976), so that the evidence is not
conclusive.

Morphine Receptors

Morphine-like analgesics as well as the endogenous agonist
methionine-enkephalin reduce the electrically and potassium-
evoked overflow of tritium from rat brain slices preincubated
with [^{3}H]noradrenaline, in all probability by inhibition of noradrenaline release (Table 1). The evoked overflow of [^{3}H]nor-
adrenaline and [^{3}H]DOPEG is proportionately decreased (Taube *et
al.*, 1977). The inhibition is mediated by specific opiate receptors, for the following reasons: (1) The rank order of the inhibitory potency of various opiates agrees with their analgesic
order of potency (Montel, Starke & Weber, 1974a, b); (2) The
antagonist naloxone causes no change or a slight increase when
given alone, but prevents the effect of the agonists (see references in Table 1); (3) In contrast to levorphanol, its analgesi-
cally inactive enantiomer dextrorphan has no effect (Taube *et al.*,
1977); and (4) As discussed above, the receptors can be differen-
tiated from other presynaptic receptors.

Some recent findings invite conjecture about the mechanism of
opiate-induced inhibition. One indirect mode of action has been
ruled out. Morphine was reported to promote the formation of prostaglandins including prostaglandin E$_2$ in homogenates of rabbit
brain (Collier, McDonald-Gibson & Saeed, 1974). However, the presynaptic inhibition is not mediated by prostaglandins, since it
persists after pretreatment with indomethacin (Taube *et al.*,
1977).

Narcotic analgesics do not affect the calcium-independent basal
outflow of tritium from preincubated brain slices (see references
in Table 1). Moreover, the release of noradrenaline by tyramine
is not changed; as in the periphery, tyramine-evoked release in
brain slices does not require calcium (Taube & Starke, unpublished results). Thus, these drugs appear to inhibit selectively calcium-dependent release processes such as release by nerve impulses
and high potassium, perhaps because they reduce the amount of calcium available for stimulus-secretion coupling. It has been mentioned briefly that morphine does not change the potassium-evoked
loss of noradrenaline from rat hypothalamic synaptosomes (Clouet
& Williams, 1974); for want of details, the finding is difficult
to evaluate. In agreement with a role of calcium, the inhibitory
effect of opiates is inversely related to the frequency of stimulation (Montel *et al.*, 1974a). At high frequencies, large amounts
of calcium probably accumulate intraneuronally which saturate the
calcium-receptive sites (see Bennett & Florin, 1975), so that effects of drugs that reduce the availability of calcium are mini-
mized. Acute injection of morphine to rats decreases the calcium

content of synaptosomes prepared from their brain cortex by no
less than 73% with no change in sodium, potassium and magnesium
(Cardenas & Ross, 1976; cf. Harris, Yamamoto, Loh & Way, 1977).
It is tempting to assume a connection between this decrease of
calcium and the inhibition of noradrenaline release.

The release of noradrenaline has also been examined in cerebral
cortex slices from rats chronically implanted with morphine pel-
lets (Montel, Starke & Taube, 1975a). Tissues were preincubated
with [³H]noradrenaline. After slices from dependent animals had
been washed free of morphine, the electrically evoked overflow
of tritium was higher than in controls. Surprisingly, when morphine or levorphanol were then added to the superfusion medium,
they reduced the evoked overflow at the same threshold concentrations as in slices from control animals. Since, however, the
original overflow in the dependent group had been elevated, low
concentrations of morphine or levorphanol brought it back to
normal values, and higher doses were required for a decrease to
subnormal values.

The results can be interpreted in terms of withdrawal, tolerance
and dependence (Fig. 3). In slices from untreated animals, morphine reduces the release of noradrenaline (Fig. 3b). Tolerance
to this impairment of transmission does not result from subsensitivity of the presynaptic opiate receptors, as shown by the unchanged threshold concentrations. Instead, the basic efficiency

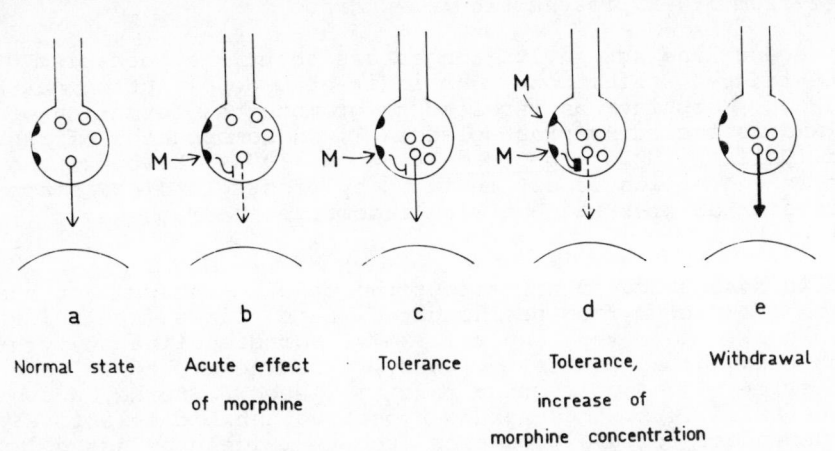

Fig. 3 Acute and chronic effects of morphine on noradrenergic
and dopaminergic nerve endings. Morphine (M) inhibits the release of transmitter from the nerve endings of unpretreated
animals (b). Tolerance develops because, in an unknown manner,
the secretion process becomes more efficient, as arbitrarily indicated by a closer approach of the vesicles to the site of secretion (c). Higher concentrations of morphine are now necessary
to reduce release to subnormal values (d). When morphine is withdrawn, the increased secretory efficiency becomes manifest by an
overshoot of release (e).

of the release mechanism appears to increase, leading to the ex-
aggerated tritium overflow observed during withdrawal (Fig. 3e).
The system is now morphine-dependent, requiring low opiate concentrations to normalize transmission (Fig. 3c), and is tolerant,
since increased concentrations are required to depress transmission (Fig. 3d). Interestingly, dopaminergic nerve endings appear
to develop similar adaptional changes (p.166, Kuschinsky, 1977).

Again, these findings have a striking parallel in the effect of
morphine on brain calcium. Whereas the acute effect is a decrease (see above), chronic administration produces an increase
in synaptosomal calcium in mice (Harris *et al.*, 1977). As discussed by the authors, this increase may be the basis for enhanced neurotransmitter release during withdrawal.

Morphine receptors have also been detected in the soma-dendritic
region of central noradrenergic neurons. Intravenous injection
of morphine depresses the firing of presumably noradrenergic locus coeruleus cells of conscious or anaesthetized rats (Korf,
Bunney & Aghajanian, 1974). More direct evidence is the inhibitory effect of morphine, levorphanol and methionine-enkephalin
when they are applied to the locus coeruleus by iontophoresis
(Bird & Kuhar, 1977; Young, Bird & Kuhar, 1977). The inhibition
can be reversed by naloxone which, given alone, causes no change.

Thus, as in the case of α-adrenoceptors, biochemical combined
with electrophysiological studies suggest that central noradrenergic neurons can be modulated via inhibitory morphine receptors
both in their receptive and in their transmissive part. Again,
the view that the receptors are structural parts of the noradrenaline-containing cells is attractive. Opiates also inhibit transmitter release from some postganglionic sympathetic fibres; the
analogy between the periphery and the CNS makes receptor location
on the one neural element common to the tissues, namely the noradrenergic nerve endings themselves, quite plausible. On the
other hand, in studies of the binding of opiates to brain homogenates no indication of such a location was found. Electrolytic
lesions of the locus coeruleus of the rat reduced the ability of
the ipsilateral cerebral cortex to take up noradrenaline by 58%,
but did not diminish the amount of $[^3H]$dihydromorphine binding
(Kuhar, Pert & Snyder, 1973); in other words, the number of receptors was unchanged despite severe degeneration of noradrenergic
fibres. However, this experiment does not rule out opiate receptors on noradrenergic nerve endings. The noradrenaline-containing
nerve endings are a minute fraction of the total cortical nerve
endings (Lapierre, Beaudet, Demianczuk & Descarries, 1973). Since
many terminals, plus perikarya and dendrites, probably are equipped with opiate receptors (Snyder & Simantov, 1977), disappearance
of only this fraction is unlikely to diminish the overall receptor
density. Interestingly morphine also inhibits the release of noradrenaline in the cerebellum (Montel, Starke & Taube, 1975b) in
spite of the fact that no or almost no receptors can be detected
there in binding studies (Kuhar *et al.*, 1973; Höllt, Haarmann &
Herz, 1976).

Opiate receptors appear to exist for the recently discovered
endorphin peptides such as methionine-enkephalin. Are presynaptic and soma-dendritic opiate receptors of noradrenergic neurons
physiological targets of endorphins? If so, naloxone should
exert effects of its own on noradrenaline economics. However,
iontophoretically applied naloxone does not change the firing of
locus coeruleus units (Bird & Kuhar, 1977; Young *et al.*, 1977);
nor has a change been noticed after systemic administration,
although both conscious and anaesthetized animals were used
(Korf *et al.*, 1974). In brain slices, naloxone failed to modify
the release of noradrenaline except in one series where it caused
a small increase (Taube, Borowski, Endo & Starke, 1976; cf.
Table 1). Finally, naloxone has no effect *in vivo* whatsoever on
the rate of turnover of noradrenaline in the CNS (Gunne, Jonsson
& Fuxe, 1969; Smith, Sheldon, Bednarczyk & Villareal, 1972;
Sugrue, 1974; Paalzow & Paalzow, 1975). The results to date are
largely negative, but do not rule out that under other conditions
the soma-dendritic or presynaptic receptors indeed receive an
endorphin input.

Do exogenous opiates *in vivo* influence noradrenaline neurons
through presynaptic or soma-dendritic receptors? Since both receptor groups are inhibitory, one might expect that narcotic
analgesics would markedly diminish the utilization and turnover
of noradrenaline. It is puzzling, therefore, that such a decrease has been obtained in anaesthetized (Gomes, Svensson &
Trolin, 1976), but never in conscious rats, in which the rate of
turnover is unchanged or even increased (Gunne *et al.*, 1969;
Sugrue, 1974; Paalzow & Paalzow, 1975; Papeschi, Theiss & Herz,
1975; Gomes *et al.*, 1976). In most *in vivo* situations, indirect
excitatory effects apparently balance or even supersede the presynaptic and soma-dendritic inhibition. *In vitro* and *in vivo*
studies on morphine withdrawal agree better. *In vitro*, noradrenaline release is increased (see above). This facilitation may
contribute to the increased turnover of brain noradrenaline during withdrawal *in vivo* (Gunne *et al.*, 1969; Gramsch & Bläsig,
1976).

Cholinoceptors
With few exceptions, postganglionic sympathetic neurons are endowed with two presynaptic receptor systems for cholinergic drugs.
Nicotinic agonists depolarize the nerve endings and evoke a calcium-dependent release of noradrenaline, whereas muscarinic agonists inhibit calcium-dependent release processes such as release
evoked by electrical pulses, high potassium concentrations and
nicotinic drugs (Lindmar, Löffelholz & Muscholl, 1968; see
Starke, 1977).

Nicotine increases the outflow of radioactive material from rat
brain preparations preincubated with labelled noradrenaline (Hall
& Turner, 1972; Balfour, 1973; Goodman, 1974; Westfall, 1974a;
Taube *et al.*, 1977). However, for several reasons it seems likely
that the nature of this phenomenon differs entirely from the releasing effect in the periphery: (1) The concentrations required
are relatively high. Only in one report was less than $10^{-4}M$
nicotine effective (Balfour, 1973). Acetylcholine, in the

presence of atropine, fails to accelerate the outflow of radioactivity at concentrations of up to 10^{-3}M (Taube et al., 1977).
Postganglionic sympathetic nerve endings respond to much lower
concentrations. For instance, nicotine causes half-maximal release in the rabbit heart at 2 x 10^{-5}M, and acetylcholine (in the
presence of atropine) does at 10^{-4}M (Löffelholz, 1970). (2) The
nicotine-evoked release of noradrenaline in the periphery is
short-lasting, whereas the effect in brain is maintained
(Goodman, 1974; Westfall, 1974a; Taube et al., 1977). (3) It has
been reported that the effect of nicotine (10^{-3}M) on hypothalamic
slices is calcium-dependent and strongly reduced by hexamethonium
and acetylcholine, presumably through the latter's muscarinic
action (Westfall, 1974a). However, other investigators did not
observe any dependence on calcium nor an antagonist effect of
hexamethonium (Goodman, 1974; Taube et al., 1977). Gulati and
Shah (1977) recently used [^{3}H]metaraminol to label noradrenergic
nerve endings in hypothalamic slices. 8 x 10^{-4}M Nicotine was
required to increase the outflow of tritium, and neither hexamethonium nor omission of calcium blocked the increase. (4) In
neocortical slices preincubated with [^{3}H]noradrenaline, high
potassium concentrations as well as electrical stimulation mainly
cause an overflow of [^{3}H]noradrenaline with only a minor increase
in [^{3}H]DOPEG; in sharp contrast, the overflow of tritium evoked
by 10^{-3}M nicotine consists almost entirely of [^{3}H]DOPEG (Taube
et al., 1977). In conclusion, it seems very likely that in brain
slices nicotine, rather than activating nicotine receptors and
eliciting depolarization and calcium-dependent release, penetrates
into the nerve endings and displaces noradrenaline from storage
sites into the cytoplasm, where it is degraded by monoamine oxidase (Goodman, 1974; Gulati & Shah, 1977; Taube et al., 1977).

It has been stated briefly that acetylcholine excites cells in
the locus coeruleus (Bird & Kuhar, 1977), perhaps by activating
soma-dendritic nicotine receptors analogous to those of autonomic
ganglion cells. This makes the largely negative outcome of the
search for presynaptic nicotine receptors all the more surprising.
In the studies summarized above, the transmitter stores were
labelled by uptake of radioactive noradrenaline or metaraminol.
Could the negative results be due to the presence of the labelled
compound in the "reserve" rather than the "functional" pool (see
p.145)? A re-investigation with determination of endogenous or
newly synthesized noradrenaline might be fruitful.

According to Westfall (1974b), the potassium-evoked release of
noradrenaline in slices of rat cerebellum is reduced by 10^{-6} -
10^{-5}M acetylcholine. On the other hand, neither acetylcholine
nor the specific muscarinic agonist oxotremorine nor atropine had
any effect on the electrically or potassium-evoked release in
slices of occipital cortex or hypothalamus (Table 1). Thus, a
presynaptic muscarinic inhibitory mechanism equivalent to that in
the periphery remains equally doubtful.

GABA Receptors
GABA (10^{-4} - 3 x 10^{-3}M) accelerates the spontaneous loss of endogenous noradrenaline from incubated rat brain slices; the effect
is blocked by bicuculline, but not by picrotoxin (Yessaian,

Armenian & Buniatian, 1969; Yessaian, Demirjian & Tozalakian,
1977). The same concentrations of GABA increase the basal as well
as the electrically evoked overflow of tritium from superfused
brain slices preincubated with [^{3}H]noradrenaline (Taube *et al.*,
1977). No change of the potassium-evoked overflow was obtained
with the GABA transaminase inhibitor aminooxyacetic acid (Stoof &
Mulder, in press). More work is needed in order to establish whether GABA in fact, by interaction with specific presynaptic receptors, can release noradrenaline or facilitate its release by nerve
impulses. There are complementary *in vivo* observations. Philippu
et al. (1973a) demonstrated that local application of GABA augments
the outflow of previously stored [^{3}H]noradrenaline into push-pull
cannula superfusates of posterior hypothalamus of the cat. Moreover, aminooxyacetic acid and high doses of GABA increase the turnover of noradrenaline in several brain regions (Andén, 1974; Biswas
& Carlsson, 1977). The sites of action in these *in vivo* experiments are not known. The excitatory effects are unexpected since
GABA generally is an inhibitory neurotransmitter and in fact upon
iontophoretic application decreases the firing rate of locus
coeruleus cells (Cedarbaum & Aghajanian, 1977).

IV   REGULATION OF DOPAMINE RELEASE

Dopamine Receptors
In 1971, Farnebo and Hamberger reported that the dopaminergic
agonist apomorphine reduced, whereas the antagonists chlorpromazine and pimozide increased, the electrically evoked overflow of
tritium from rat striatal slices preincubated with [^{3}H]dopamine.
The results indicated that a presynaptic dopaminergic feedback
inhibition may control the release of dopamine, just as the
α-adrenergic loop controls the release of noradrenaline.

In contrast to the latter, however, the dopaminergic mechanism is
controversial: (1) Baldessarini (1975, p. 106; no details) and
Dismukes and Mulder (1977) did not observe any effect of apomorphine on the evoked overflow of tritium. (2) Three groups of
investigators found that several neuroleptic drugs produced a decrease rather than an increase (striatal slices and electrical
stimulation: Seeman & Lee, 1975; Dismukes & Mulder, 1977; striatal synaptosomes stimulated by protoveratrine: Iversen, Rogawski
& Miller, 1976), although Seeman and Lee (1975) and Dismukes and
Mulder (1977) replicated the method of Farnebo and Hamberger
(1971) as closely as feasible. (3) Even within these three
groups, however, results are not consistent. Seeman and Lee
(1975) calculated IC$_{50}$ values (concentrations that inhibited the
evoked overflow by 50%) for spiroperidol, haloperidol and chlorpromazine of about 10^{-8}, 10^{-7} and 7 x 10^{-7}M. On the other hand,
in the similar experiments of Dismukes and Mulder (1977) the
IC$_{50}$ of spiroperidol was about 10^{-6}M and that of haloperidol
2 x 10^{-6}M, while chlorpromazine at up to 10^{-5}M had no effect at
all. In the synaptosome preparation the IC$_{50}$ values were
2 x 10^{-6}, 2 x 10^{-6} and 10^{-6}M, respectively (Iversen *et al.*, 1976).
Fluphenazine behaved as a more potent inhibitor than haloperidol
in one laboratory (Seeman & Lee, 1975), but was inactive in
another (Dismukes & Mulder, 1977). Dismukes and Mulder (1977)
observed that a low concentration of haloperidol (2 x 10^{-7}M),

applied in the presence of cocaine, in fact caused a small and
marginally significant increase of the evoked overflow of tritium.
(4) Finally, Westfall, Besson, Giorguieff and Glowinski (1976a)
have been able to confirm the findings of Farnebo and Hamberger
(1971, 1973), using the technique of continuous superfusion of
striatal slices with [^{3}H]tyrosine. The potassium-evoked overflow
of [^{3}H]dopamine was augmented by 10^{-6}M fluphenazine as well as by
10^{-6}M benztropine. When both drugs were administered together,
their effects were additive, indicating different mechanisms of
action. Benztropine is thought to inhibit the re-uptake of dopamine, whereas fluphenazine, which is a weak uptake inhibitor
(Iversen *et al.*, 1976; Westfall *et al.*, 1976a) probably facilitates release. A confirmation of the facilitatory effect of
chlorpromazine is mentioned by Baldessarini in his review (1975,
p. 107; no details).

There is as yet no satisfactory explanation for these discrepancies, but the following points may be worth considering. (1) Generally speaking, some peculiarities were encountered even when
the fundamental properties of dopamine outflow from striatal
slices were studied (p.146). The inconsistencies in the effects
of dopaminergic drugs somehow may be related to these peculiarities. (2) More specifically, many neuroleptic drugs accelerate
the basal outflow of tritium from synaptosomes or slices preincubated with [^{3}H]dopamine (Seeman & Lee, 1974; Iversen *et al.*,
1976; Dismukes & Mulder, 1976). The threshold concentrations are
low in some cases, e.g., 10^{-7}M for haloperidol and pimozide. When
such concentrations are used in stimulation experiments, the
evoked overflow is superimposed on an elevated basal outflow, and
this may lead to false interpretation. The effect on basal outflow has another interesting aspect. As mentioned above (p.152),
a substantial part of the basal outflow of dopamine from striatal
slices appears to be due to impulse-evoked release. Could the
increase caused by neuroleptic drugs, at least at low concentrations, reflect interruption of dopaminergic feedback inhibition
on this ongoing active release? Admittedly, some points argue
against this view. For instance, low concentrations of haloperidol and pimozide also enhance the basal loss of dopamine from
striatal synaptosomes (Seeman & Lee, 1974) where a calcium-dependent release in the absence of external stimulation seems unlikely.
(3) Another potential reason for contradictory results was pointed
out by Dismukes and Mulder (1977). The release-modulating receptors might be located outside the dopaminergic nerve endings, influencing them through a chain of neurons. If so, the demonstration of dopaminergic modulation would be very dependent on the
integrity of these interneurons. Subtle differences in preparation, e.g., in the plane of cutting, might yield slices with
greatly differing properties.

Presynaptic dopamine receptors have been implicated not only in
the regulation of the release, but also in the regulation of the
biosynthesis of dopamine. A detailed discussion is beyond the
scope of this review (see Kehr, Carlsson, Lindqvist, Magnusson &
Atack, 1972; Iversen *et al.*, 1976; Walters & Roth, 1976; Westfall
et al., 1976a). In summary, dopaminergic agonists reduce the
rate of tyrosine hydroxylation in the corpus striatum. They do

so even after impulse flow in the nigro-striatal neurons has been
abolished. In agreement with a presynaptic, receptor-mediated
effect, the inhibition is also obtained in striatal synaptosomes
and slices, and is competitively antagonized by neuroleptic drugs.
The receptors may physiologically mediate a local negative feedback by which released dopamine inhibits further dopamine synthesis. The exact mechanism is not known, but it seems likely
that receptor activation leads to an increase in the sensitivity
of tyrosine hydroxylase to end-product inhibition by intraneuronal dopamine.

The unanimous acceptance of a presynaptic, receptor-mediated control of dopamine synthesis makes the case for the presynaptic
control of release less desperate. It is important to realize
that any dopaminergic modulation of release is not secondary to
changes in synthesis, since the secretion of exogenous dopamine
is also modified (Farnebo & Hamberger, 1971), and since the increases in synthesis and release produced by fluphenazine follow
different time courses (Westfall *et al.*, 1976a). The release-
modulating sites are distinct from α-adrenoceptors, because
neither phentolamine (Farnebo & Hamerger, 1971, 1973) nor clonidine (Baumann, personal communication) exerts any effect.

Systemic as well as iontophoretic application of dopaminergic
agonists decreases the electrical activity of units, presumably
the dopaminergic cells, in the zona compacta of the substantia
nigra. The depression is blocked by local injection of neuroleptic drugs (Aghajanian & Bunney, 1973, 1977; Dray & Straughan,
1976). The results indicate that dopamine receptors occur not
only near the terminals, but also in the soma-dendritic region of
dopaminergic neurons. No evidence for soma-dendritic α- or β-adrenoceptors was obtained (Aghajanian & Bunney, 1977).

Are the presynaptic and soma-dendritic receptors located on the
dopaminergic neurons themselves? Dopamine releases GABA from
slices of the substantia nigra of the rat; the effect is antagonized by neuroleptic drugs. Since GABA slows substantia nigra
cells, it seems possible that the dopaminergic inhibition of
these cells is mediated by GABA, and that the nigral "soma-dendritic" dopamine receptors are, at least in part, located on
GABAergic perikarya or terminals (Reubi, Iversen & Jessell, 1977).
An attempt to localize the presynaptic receptors has been made in
binding studies with membranes of the rat corpus striatum. The
specific binding of [^{3}H]dopamine was not changed after a lesion
by 6-hydroxydopamine that destroyed 90% of the dopaminergic nerve
terminals (Burt, Enna, Creese & Snyder, 1975). This experiment
failed to reveal binding to receptors on the dopaminergic nerve
endings. However, as discussed previously (p.146 and 151), it
does not rule out such receptors. Presynaptic, synthesis-inhibit-
ing, and soma-dendritic dopamine receptors may share a common
spectrum of drug sensitivities, and this spectrum may distinguish
them from postsynaptic dopamine receptors (Iversen *et al.*, 1976;
Walters & Roth, 1976; Aghajanian & Bunney, 1977). Such pharmalo-
gical similarity favours, but of course is not sound evidence for,
a common location on the dopaminergic cells.

Do presynaptic and soma-dendritic dopamine receptors play a
physiological role? There is little doubt that cerebral dopamine
receptors participate in the physiological control of dopaminergic
neurons. In agreement with this view, neuroleptic drugs increase
the synthesis, utilization (e.g., Carlsson & Lindqvist, 1963;
O'Keeffe, Sharman & Vogt, 1970; Kuschinsky & Hornykiewicz, 1974)
and probably release (Lloyd & Bartholini, 1975; Bartholini et al.,
1976) of dopamine in vivo, presumably because they remove a normal
dopaminergic inhibition. Moreover, systemically administered
neuroleptic agents increase the firing rate of substantia nigra
units (Aghajanian & Bunney, 1973). Apomorphine exerts the opposite biochemical and electrophysiological effects (e.g., Andén,
Rubenson, Fuxe & Hökfelt, 1967b; Aghajanian & Bunney, 1973).
Evidently, all these data match those of the α-adrenergic control
of noradrenaline neurons. The same holds good for the models
developed for interpretation (cf. Fig. 2). The classical hypothesis is that activation of postsynaptic dopamine receptors,
e.g., in the caudate nucleus, elicits a compensatory decrease of
the firing rate of the dopaminergic cells (cf. Fig. 2a); a likely
substrate for this feedback loop would be the striato-nigral
GABA pathway. However, dopamine may inhibit its own release
(cf. Fig. 2b) and synthesis (see above) also by a presynaptic
mechanism via receptors on the nerve endings. Or a physiological
inhibition may be mediated by axon collaterals and soma-dendritic
receptors as in Fig. 2c; these receptors may even be the target
of dopamine released from dendrites (Groves et al., 1975; Geffen,
Jessel, Cuello & Iversen, 1976). And there are further less obvious possibilities (cf. Fig. 2d).

At present it is difficult to weigh up these alternatives. Iontophoretic application of fluphenazine and chlorpromazine to substantia nigra cells, in contrast to systemic application, does
not accelerate their firing (Aghajanian & Bunney, 1973, 1977);
this is contrary to what one might expect if the antagonists
nullify a tonic soma-dendritic self-inhibition (cf. Fig. 2c). On
the other hand, evidence against a major role of postsynaptic
receptors comes from experiments by Chiara, Porceddu, Fratta and
Gessa (1977). Kainic acid, which after local application destroys
neuronal cell bodies but spares axons terminating in or passing
through the area, was injected unilaterally into the caudate nucleus of rats. The treatment led to a marked loss of neuronal perikarya; striatal dopamine-sensitive adenylate cyclase, which is
thought to be an essential part of the postsynaptic dopamine receptor, disappeared completely; dopamine levels were unchanged.
When haloperidol or fluphenazine were now administered systemically, they increased the rate of striatal dopamine metabolism at
least as much on the lesioned as on the control side. Similarly,
the inhibitory effect of apomorphine was augmented rather than
attenuated. If one accepts that the lesion had destroyed the
postsynaptic dopamine receptors, the drug effects must have been
mediated by other, most probably soma-dendritic or presynaptic,
sites. What is more important, these must be the crucial sites
for physiological dopaminergic control (cf. Fig. 2b and c).

Prostaglandin Receptors
Prostaglandins E_1 and E_2 slightly reduce the electrically evoked

release of dopamine in rat striatal slices, whereas prostaglandin
$F_{2\alpha}$ is inactive (Bergström, Farnebo & Fuxe, 1973; Farnebo &
Hamberger, 1973; Baldessarini, 1975, p. 107, without details).
An analogous presynaptic inhibition can be demonstrated *in vivo*:
infusion of prostaglandin E_2 into the corpus striatum retards the
dopamine depletion produced by blockade of tyrosine hydroxylase
(Bergström *et al.*, 1973).

Morphine Receptors

Simultaneously with the opiate-induced inhibition of cerebral
noradrenaline release, a similar modulation of the release of
dopamine was detected. Celsen and Kuschinsky (1974) preincubated
slices of the rat striatum with [^{14}C]dopamine and immediately
afterwards incubated them further in a tracer-free high-potassium
medium. Morphine (10^{-5} - 3×10^{-5}M) slightly but significantly
diminished the potassium-evoked loss of radioactivity from the
slices. The effect was blocked by naloxone. The observations
were confirmed by Loh, Brase, Sampath-Khanna, Mar and Way (1976)
who superfused slices preincubated with [^{3}H]dopamine and measured
the outflow of tritium into the superfusion fluid. Under these
conditions, the effect of morphine was more marked. In the presence of 10^{-5}M morphine, the potassium-evoked overflow was virtually abolished, and the IC_{50} was 2×10^{-6}M. Moreover, the endogenous ligand β-endorphin equally diminished the evoked overflow.
Methionine-enkephalin had no effect (Loh *et al.*, 1976), perhaps
because it was rapidly broken down. Morphine also reduces the
potassium-evoked release of dopamine from striatal synaptosomes
(Bosse, 1977) and in superfused striata of some strains of mice
(Sampath-Khanna, Brase, Loh & Way, 1976). The basal, non-stimu-
lated loss of dopamine from striatal synaptosomes is not changed
(Clouet & Williams, 1974).

Dopaminergic nerve endings appear to behave like noradrenergic
ones not only during acute, but also during chronic opiate treatment. When slices were prepared from the striata of morphine-
dependent rats either 42 hr after withdrawal, or 10 min after an
injection of naloxone, or when naloxone was added to such slices
in vitro, the potassium-evoked release of dopamine was enhanced
(Bosse & Kuschinsky, 1976). As discussed above for noradrenaline
and illustrated in Fig. 3, the dopamine-containing neurons ap-
apparently try to make up for the acute effect of morphine, i.e.,
depression of neurotransmission, by a compensatory facilitation
of the release process (cf. Kuschinsky, 1977).

In contrast to the locus coeruleus cells, most substantia nigra
units of the rat are accelerated by systemically injected morphine (Bunney, quoted by Lal, 1975; Chan, Lee & Wong, 1976;
Zieglgänsberger, personal communication). The effect is species-
dependent, since nigral neurons of mice uniformly respond with
depression (Bigler & Eidelberg, 1976). Unfortunately, microiontophoretic studies are lacking. It cannot be excluded that, like
the locus coeruleus cells, dopaminergic neurons also possess inhibitory soma-dendritic opiate receptors, but that in the rat the
inhibition is overcome by an excitation produced through receptors
outside the substantia nigra.

Where are the presynaptic opiate receptors. located? Pollard,
Llorens-Cortes and Schwartz (1977) recently studied the influence
of lesions of the nigro-striatal pathway on the specific binding
of [^{3}H]leucine-enkephalin and [^{3}H]naloxone to particles of rat
striatum. Three different types of lesions - electrolytic,
mechanical and chemical - all reduced the number of binding sites
by about 30%. This appears to be the first time that destruction
of central catecholamine neurons has been shown to result in a
loss of receptors. The data suggest at least that some, though
not all, striatal morphine receptors are located directly on the
dopaminergic nerve endings. On the other hand, the evidence is
not conclusive. As discussed by Pollard *et al.* (1977), the lesion
may have led to transsynaptic degeneration of neurons receiving a
dopaminergic input, and the lost fraction of receptors may have
been there. Nevertheless, the experiment doubtlessly gives
further support to the view that the term "presynaptic" is correct
also in a topographical sense.

There is no evidence for a physiological regulation of dopaminergic neurons by endorphins and opiate receptors. Opiate antagonists alone do not affect the turnover of dopamine (Gunne *et al.*,
1969; Smith *et al.*, 1972; Sugrue, 1974; Paalzow & Paalzow, 1975),
nor has an effect on the electrical activity of nigral cells or
the *in vitro* release of dopamine been reported.

Although exogenous opiate agonists do influence dopamine neurons
in vivo, they mainly act via other than presynaptic receptors.
These receptors are inhibitory. Narcotic analgesics, however,
consistently increase the turnover of dopamine in rats (Gunne
et al., 1969; Kuschinsky & Hornykiewicz, 1974; Sugrue, 1974;
Paalzow & Paalzow, 1975; Papeschi *et al.*, 1975; Gomes *et al.*,
1976) and mice (Smith *et al.*, 1972; Kuschinsky & Hornykiewicz,
1974). Furthermore, from the enhanced *in vitro* release during
withdrawal one might expect an increased turnover *in vivo*; again
the opposite was found (Gunne *et al.*, 1969; Gramsch, Bläsig &
Herz, 1977). *In vivo* indirect excitatory (acute administration)
or inhibitory (withdrawal) mechanisms apparently prevail. On the
other hand, some behavioural changes after acute injection of
opiates are difficult to reconcile with an overall activation of
dopamine neurons. Above all, rats become cataleptic, indicating
decreased rather than increased dopaminergic transmission. The
relation to the biochemical and electrophysiological findings is
still obscure (see Kuschinsky & Hornykiewicz, 1974; Lal, 1975;
Kuschinsky, 1977).

Cholinoceptors
Studies on the influence of cholinergic drugs on dopamine economics have yielded a complex picture. Nicotine (5 x 10^{-3}M) accelerates the outflow of [^{3}H]dopamine previously taken up by rat
striatal slices. The acceleration can be completely blocked by
hexamethonium (Westfall, 1974a). Similarly, acetylcholine (10^{-6}
- 10^{-5}M) increases the outflow of newly synthesized [^{3}H]dopamine.
However, its effect is only partly blocked by mecamylamine or
pempidine, thus indicating a non-nicotinic component (Besson *et
al.*, 1969; Giorguieff *et al.*, 1976, 1977). Indeed, not only nicotinic antagonists, but also atropine and scopolamine reduce the

effect of acetylcholine. The outflow of [3H]dopamine is also enhanced by oxotremorine, and this increase is entirely abolished
by atropine (Giorguieff *et al.*, 1977). Thus, there is a dual releasing mechanism, one mediated by nicotine receptors, the other
by muscarine receptors.

About 50% of the basal outflow of newly formed [3H]dopamine from
striatal slices seems to be due to action potential-evoked release (see p.143; Giorguieff *et al.*, 1977). Therefore, the
effects of acetylcholine and oxotremorine might reflect an increase in the amount of [3H]dopamine released per impulse, similar
to the angiotensin- or phentolamine-induced facilitation of noradrenaline release in the periphery. However, both the nicotinic
and the muscarinic components persist in the presence of tetrodotoxin which prevents action potentials (Giorguieff *et al.*, 1977).
Thus both release processes apparently are elicited *de novo* in
previously quiescent nerve endings. Moreover, both are calcium-
dependent (Giorguieff *et al.*, 1977).

Other presynaptic cholinergic effects have also been reported.
In his experiments with [3H]dopamine previously taken up, Westfall
(1974a, b) found that acetylcholine ($10^{-6} - 10^{-4}$M, but not 10^{-7}M)
reduced the overflow of transmitter evoked by nicotine (5×10^{-3}M)
as well as that evoked by electrical stimulation and high potassium. Inhibition was also obtained with methacholine which has
less nicotinic activity than acetylcholine. Although experiments
with anticholinergic drugs were not reported, the data suggest
that a muscarinic mechanism similar to that in the periphery can
inhibit calcium-dependent dopamine release in the striatum
(Westfall, 1974a, b; the author does not mention the influence of
acetylcholine on the basal outflow of [3H]dopamine. Possibly
there was no effect, because release originated from the "reserve"
pool. If so, it is not clear why under the same conditions nicotine did evoke release).

Taken together, these results suggest a threefold cholinergic action on dopaminergic nerve endings. The nicotinic releasing
effect and the muscarinic inhibition mirror analogous mechanisms
of postganglionic sympathetic fibres. On the other hand, the
muscarinic releasing effect has no peripheral parallel. In the
periphery, muscarinic inhibition requires markedly lower concentrations of acetylcholine than nicotinic excitation (Lindmar
et al., 1968). No such dissociation has been found in the corpus
striatum since muscarinic inhibition as well as dopamine release
were obtained with 10^{-6}M acetylcholine (see above).

The question of whether cholinoceptors exist in the soma-dendritic
region of nigral dopaminergic neurons is controversial. Aghajanian
and Bunney (1973) observed no effect of iontophoretically applied
acetylcholine on zona compacta units, whereas Dray and Straughan
(1976) found an excitation.

In autoradiographic binding studies the corpus striatum of the
rat was devoid of nicotine receptor sites, although muscarine
receptors are present in high density (Polz-Tejera, Schmidt &
Karten, 1975; see, however, Speth, Chen, Lindstrom, Kobayashi &

Yamamura, 1977). This is another example of functionally trace-
able presynaptic receptors in an area where binding assays could
not regularly detect receptors. The exact location of striatal
presynaptic cholinoceptors remains unknown.

Do the presynaptic cholinoceptors play a physiological role?
Systemic injection of oxotremorine or physostigmine increases the
rate of turnover of dopamine in the corpus striatum (Laverty &
Sharman, 1965; Andén & Wachtel, 1977). The increase is abolished
only by those antimuscarinic drugs that are able to cross the
blood-brain barrier (see Andén & Wachtel, 1977). Given alone,
antimuscarinic agents decrease dopamine turnover (O'Keeffe *et al.*,
1970; Bartholini & Pletscher, 1971). Moreover, intravenous oxotremorine enhances the outflow of dopamine into push-pull cannula
superfusates of the cat caudate nucleus (Bartholini & Stadler,
1975; Lloyd & Bartholini, 1975). These findings indicate that
central cholinoceptors help to regulate dopamine neurons *in vivo*,
their main influence being excitatory. On the other hand, experiments with local application of physostigmine and anticholinergic
drugs argue against a major role of presynaptic sites in this
physiological cholinergic control. Neither antimuscarinic nor
antinicotinic agents change the basal outflow of newly synthesized [^{3}H]dopamine from striatal slices. Moreover, locally administered physostigmine alone has no effect on the outflow of
[^{3}H]dopamine from the caudate nucleus *in vivo*. Antinicotinic
compounds tend to cause an increase, but this is probably unrelated to nicotine receptors (Giorguieff *et al.*, 1976, 1977).
Finally, intrastriatal injection of atropine does not change the
turnover of dopamine (Bartholini & Pletscher, 1971). The physiological regulation apparently operates via sites outside the
corpus striatum.

The possibility still remains that exogenous cholinergic agonists
enhance the turnover and release of dopamine through a presynaptic
mechanism. Indeed, exogenous acetylcholine and carbachol release
dopamine when they are directly applied to the caudate nucleus
in vivo. The effect is antagonized by antimuscarinic as well as
antinicotinic drugs (Bartholini & Stadler, 1975; Bartholini *et al.*,
1976; Giorguieff *et al.*, 1976). The observations can be explained
by the presynaptic nicotinic and muscarinic releasing effect. Yet,
after systemic administration other mechanisms possibly prevail.
Andén and Wachter (1977) recently showed that intraperitoneally
injected oxotremorine and physostigmine fail to accelerate the
turnover of dopamine when impulse traffic in the nigro-striatal
pathway is abolished. This is in contrast to the presynaptic
releasing effect, which persists in the absence of impulse flow
(see above; Giorguieff *et al.*, 1977). Apparently, the activation
of dopaminergic neurons after systemic injection *in vivo* and the
presynaptic effect are largely unrelated phenomena.

GABA Receptors
The *in vitro* presynaptic effects of GABA on dopaminergic neurons
are just beginning to be examined. Stoof and Mulder (in press)
investigated the influence of GABA and GABA transaminase inhibitors, including aminooxyacetic acid, on rat striatal slices preincubated with [^{3}H]dopamine or [^{14}C]tyrosine. GABA, at concen-

trations of up to 10^{-3}M, did not change the potassium-evoked overflow of labelled dopamine, but the transaminase inhibitors caused
an increase. The results are compatible with the view that endogenous GABA facilitates the depolarization-evoked release of dopamine,
and that this facilitation is enhanced when the enzymatic degradation of the amino acid is blocked. If so, however, the lack of effect of exogenous GABA is difficult to explain. The influence of
antagonists has not yet been reported. Whereas, according to an
earlier paper (Yessaian et al., 1969), GABA does not change the basal loss of endogenous dopamine from striatal slices, the basal outflow of newly synthesized [^{3}H]dopamine is accelerated (Giorguieff,
Kemel, Glowinski & Besson, quoted by Stoof & Mulder, in press).

These preliminary indications of a presynaptic facilitatory effect are surprising since previous in vivo experiments pointed
in the opposite direction. Some of these studies were discussed
above in order to illustrate the multiplicity of potential modes
of drug action in vivo (p.147). To repeat briefly, two sites of
GABAergic inhibition were found, namely the substantia nigra and
the corpus striatum. In the substantia nigra, GABA slows the
firing of the dopaminergic cells. The mechanism of the intrastriatal inhibition is less clear. One alternative is that GABA
acts on the dopaminergic nerve endings or on neighbouring structures which then inhibit the dopaminergic terminals. However,
this presynaptic mode of action is by no means certain. The .
facilitatory in vitro effect favours the view that the reduction
of dopamine release produced by intrastriatally applied GABA
in vivo is mediated by a neuronal loop projecting to the dopaminergic cell bodies. One substrate of this loop might be the
striato-nigral substance P pathway (Fig. 1).

Other biochemical studies support a GABAergic inhibition of dopamine neurons in vivo. After intracerebroventricular or systemic
administration of aminooxyacetic acid or high doses of GABA, the
brain content of dopamine increases, while its utilization declines (Andén, 1974; Biswas & Carlsson, 1977). The effect of
GABA is antagonized by picrotoxin (Biswas & Carlsson, 1977). The
main mechanism is probably a reduction of impulse flow, mediated
by soma-dendritic receptors in the substantia nigra. Interestingly, the biosynthesis of dopamine is simultaneously increased, presumably because with decreasing release and decreasing extracellular concentration of dopamine the receptor-mediated feedback inhibition of tyrosine hydroxylase ceases (p.164).

V   CONCLUDING REMARKS

The presently discussed presynaptic receptors of central catecholamine neurons are summarized in Table 2. Soma-dendritic receptors
are also included in order to give a coherent picture of potential
regulatory mechanisms. It must be emphasised again that the definition of "presynaptic" used here is functional rather than
topographical, and it should be noted that the exact location of
soma-dendritic receptors - directly on versus outside the respective cells, e.g., on adjoining dendrites of other neurons - is
also rarely, if ever, firmly established.

Table 2

SOMA-DENDRITIC AND PRESYNAPTIC RECEPTORS OF CENTRAL NORADRENERGIC AND DOPAMINERGIC NEURONS

Receptor	Noradrenergic Neurons		Dopaminergic Neurons	
	Soma-dendritic	Presynaptic	Soma-dendritic	Presynaptic
α-Adrenoceptor	-	-	0	0
β-Adrenoceptor	0	0	0	0
Dopamine receptor	0	0	-	-
Prostaglandin receptor	-	-	-	-
Morphine receptor	-	-	-	-
Cholinoceptors	(+)	(+ or -)	(+)	+ or -
GABA receptor	-	(+)	-	(+ or -)
Histamine receptor		(-)		
Serotonin receptor		0		
Angiotensin receptor		0		
Substance P receptor	+	0	+	

+, Excitatory receptor (mediating increase of electrical or secretory activity).
-, Inhibitory receptor (mediating decrease of electrical or secretory activity).
0 Indicates that attempts to detect the receptor failed.
Brackets indicate that the evidence is contradictory or very preliminary.
For presynaptic effects of histamine, serotonin, angiotensin and substance P - see Table 1; for histamine see also Subramanian and Mulder (1977).
Presynaptic effects of cyclic nucleotides are not included (see Dismukes & Mulder, 1976; Patrick & Barchas, 1976; Westfall, Kitay & Wahl, 1976b).
Substance P receptors in the locus coeruleus according to Aghajanian (personal communication)

Presynaptic regulation

Three potential physiological functions of presynaptic receptors
have been distinguished (Starke, 1977). They may be sites of
action of blood-borne agents, of substances derived from adjacent
cells, and of the neuron's own transmitter. For central presynaptic receptors, the first function seems unlikely, both because
the blood rarely contains appreciable levels of the endogenous
agonists and because the blood-brain barrier would impede their
access. The second function, on the other hand, seems possible.
For instance, presynaptic receptors near noradrenergic nerve
endings may mediate inhibition by prostaglandins, endorphins and
histamine and facilitation by GABA. Presynaptic receptors near
dopaminergic nerve endings may mediate inhibition by prostaglandins and endorphins and facilitation (or perhaps inhibition)
by acetylcholine and GABA. Admittedly, experimental support for
a physiological operation of any of these mechanisms is either
lacking or incomplete. However, the research in this field is
recent and future studies using individual catecholaminergic pathways, species other than the extensively used rat, and diverse
experimental conditions, may well reveal a physiological role.

The inhibition of catecholamine release by neighbouring neurotransmitters may be a biochemical phenomenon parallel to the
electrophysiological phenomenon called "presynaptic" or "remote"
inhibition. Mostly from studies in the spinal cord it has been
concluded that in some cases of inhibition of synaptic transmission the inhibitory compound acts not on the postsynaptic cell
to make it less excitable but rather on the presynaptic excitatory nerve terminals to reduce the release of transmitter. For
instance, afferent fibres from primary muscle spindle endings release an unknown excitatory transmitter onto the homonymous moto-
neurons. The release appears to be inhibited by certain other
afferent fibres, presumably via axo-axonic synapses (see Schmidt,
1971). This interpretation of the electrophysiological "presynaptic inhibition" is controversial (see Ryall, 1975). However, it
cannot be excluded that the biochemical and electrophysiological
studies, performed on different neuron systems, in fact basically
deal with the same phenomenon.

The most extensive evidence has been gathered for the third function, namely for presynaptic receptors being targets of the transmitter itself. Following the description of α-adrenoceptors near
noradrenergic nerve endings, and of dopamine receptors near dopaminergic nerve endings, these receptors were also found in the
soma-dendritic region. Carlsson (1975) proposed that all receptors of a neuron for its own transmitter should be called "autoreceptors". The term must be used with the reservation that a
neuron may possess more than one type of autoreceptor. For instance, some peripheral noradrenergic nerve endings are endowed
not only with α-, but also with β- and dopamine receptors. For
those central neurons that have been studied, the situation seems
simpler, since only α-adrenoceptors have been found near noradrenergic, and only dopamine receptors near dopaminergic neurons. If
we assume that these in fact are the only or at least prevailing
autoreceptors, the unifying concept emerges that central catecholamine neurons are surrounded all over by receptor mechanisms which
dampen their function and perhaps protect them against excessive

electrical and secretory activity.

VI REFERENCES

Aghajanian, G.K. & Bunney, B.S. (1973). Central dopaminergic neurons: Neurophysiological identification and responses to drugs. In: *Frontiers in Catecholamine Research* (eds.) E. Usdin & S.H. Snyder, Pergamon Press, New York, pp. 643-648.

Aghajanian, G.K. & Bunney, B.S. (1977). Dopamine "autoreceptors": Pharmacological characterization by microiontophoretic single cell recording studies. *Naunyn-Schmiedeberg's Arch. Pharmacol.* 297, 1-7.

Aghajanian, G.K., Cedarbaum, J.M. & Wang, R.Y. Evidence for norepinephrine-mediated collateral inhibition of locus coeruleus neurons. *Brain Res.*, in press.

Andén, N.E. (1974). Inhibition of the turnover of the brain dopamine after treatment with the gammaaminobutyrate: 2-oxyglutarate transaminase inhibitor aminooxyacetic acid. *Naunyn-Schmiedeberg's Arch. Pharmacol.* 283, 419-424.

Andén, N.E., Corrodi, H., Fuxe, K. & Hökfelt, T. (1967a). Increased impulse flow in bulbospinal noradrenaline neurons produced by catecholamine receptor blocking agents. *Eur. J. Pharmacol.* 2, 59-64.

Andén, N.E., Grabowska, M. & Strömbom, U. (1976). Different alpha-adrenoceptors in the central nervous system mediating biochemical and functional effects of clonidine and receptor blocking agents. *Naunyn-Schmiedeberg's Arch. Pharmacol.* 292, 43-52.

Andén, N.E., Rubenson, A., Fuxe, K. & Hökfelt, T. (1967b). Evidence for dopamine receptor stimulation by apomorphine. *J. Pharm. Pharmacol.* 19, 627-629.

Andén, N.E. & Wachtel, H. (1977). Increase in the turnover of brain dopamine by stimulation of muscarinic receptors outside the dopamine nerve terminals. *J. Pharm. Pharmacol.* 29, 435-437.

Bacq, Z.M. (1976). Les contrôles de la libération des médiateurs aux terminaisons des nerf adrénergiques. *J. Physiol.* [*Paris*], 72, 371-542.

Baldessarini, R.J. (1975). Release of catecholamines. In: *Handbook of Psychopharmacology* Vol. 3 (eds.) L.L. Iversen, S.D. Iversen & S.H. Snyder, Plenum Press, New York - London, pp. 37-137.

Balfour, D.J.K. (1973). Effects of nicotine on the uptake and retention of ^{14}C-noradrenaline and ^{14}C-5-hydroxytryptamine by rat brain homogenates. *Eur. J. Pharmacol.* 23, 19-26.

Barker, K.A., Harper, B. & Hughes, I.E. (1977). Possible sub-
divisions among α-adrenoceptors in various isolated tissues.
J. Pharm. Pharmacol. 29, 129-134.

Bartholini, G. & Pletscher, A. (1971). Atropine-induced changes
of cerebral dopamine turnover. *Experientia* 27, 1302-1303.

Bartholini, G. & Stadler, H. (1975). Cholinergic and GABAergic
influence on the dopamine release in extrapyramidal centers.
In: *Chemical Tools in Catecholamine Research* Vol. 2 (eds.)
O. Almgren, A. Carlsson & J. Engel, North-Holland, Amsterdam-
Oxford, pp. 235-241.

Bartholini, G., Stadler, H., Gadea Ciria, M. & Lloyd, K.G. (1976).
The use of the push-pull cannula to estimate the dynamics of
acetylcholine and catecholamines within various brain areas.
Neuropharmacology 15, 515-519.

Baumann, P.A. & Maître, L. (1978). Blockade of presynaptic α-
receptors and of amine uptake in the rat brain by the antidepressant mianserine. *Naunyn-Schmiedeberg's Arch. Pharmacol.*,
in press.

Beaudet, A. & Descarries, L. (1976). Quantitative data on serotonin nerve terminals in adult rat neocortex. *Brain Res.* 111,
301-309.

Bennett, M.R. & Florin, T. (1975). An electrophysiological
analysis of the effect of Ca ions on neuromuscular transmission in the mouse vas deferens. *Br. J. Pharmacol.* 55,
97-104.

Bergström, S., Farnebo, L.O. & Fuxe, K. (1973). Effect of
prostaglandin E_2 on central and peripheral catecholamine
neurons. *Eur. J. Pharmacol.* 21, 362-368.

Besson, M.J., Cheramy, A., Feltz, P. & Glowinski, J. (1969).
Release of newly synthesized dopamine from dopamine-containing
terminals in the striatum of the rat. *Proc. Nat. Acad. Sci.*
[*U.S.A.*] 62, 741-748.

Bigler, E.D. & Eidelberg, E. (1976). Nigrostriatal effects of
morphine in two mouse strains. *Life Sci.* 19, 1399-1406.

Bird, S.J. & Kuhar, M.J. (1977). Iontophoretic application of
opiates to the locus coeruleus. *Brain Res.* 122, 523-533.

Biswas, B. & Carlsson, A. (1977). The effect of intracerebro-
ventricularly administered GABA on brain monoamine metabolism.
Naunyn Schmiedeberg's Arch. Pharmacol. 299, 41-46.

Borowski, E., Starke, K., Ehrl, H. & Endo, T. (1977). A comparison of pre- and postsynaptic effects of α-adrenolytic drugs
in the pulmonary artery of the rabbit. *Neuroscience* 2, 285-
296.

Bosse, A. (1977). *In vitro* studies in synaptosomes of rat stria-
tum about the effects of morphine on uptake and release of
C-14-dopamine. *Naunyn-Schmiedeberg's Arch. Pharmacol.* 297,
R52.

Bosse, A. & Kuschinsky, K. (1976). Alterations of dopaminergic
neurotransmission after chronic morphine treatment: Pre- and
postjunctional studies in striatal tissue. *Naunyn-Schmiedeberg's Arch. Pharmacol.* 294, 17-22.

Bradford, H.F. (1975). Isolated nerve terminals as an *in vitro*
preparation for the study of dynamic aspects of transmitter
metabolism and release. In: *Handbook of Psychopharmacology*
Vol. 1 (eds.) L.L. Iversen, S.D. Iversen & S.H. Snyder,
Plenum Press, New York - London, pp. 191-252.

Bryant, B.J., McCulloch, M.W., Rand, M.J. & Story, D.F. (1975).
Release of ^{3}H-(-)-noradrenaline from guinea-pig hypothalamic
slices: effects of adrenoceptor agonists and antagonists.
Br. J. Pharmacol. 53, 454P.

Burt, D.R., Enna, S.J., Creese, I. & Snyder, S.H. (1975).
Dopamine receptor binding in the corpus striatum of mammalian
brain. *Proc. Nat. Acad. Sci.* [*U.S.A.*] 72, 4655-4659.

Cardenas, H.L. & Ross, D.H. (1976). Calcium depletion of synaptosomes after morphine treatment. *Br. J. Pharmacol.* 57, 521-
526.

Carlsson, A. (1975). Dopaminergic autoreceptors. In: *Chemical
Tools in Catecholamine Research* Vol. 2 (eds.) O. Almgren,
A. Carlsson & J. Engel, North-Holland, Amsterdam - Oxford,
pp. 219-225.

Carlsson, A. & Lindqvist, M. (1963). Effect of chlorpromazine or
haloperidol on formation of 3-methoxytyramine and normetanephrine in mouse brain. *Acta Pharmacol. Toxicol.* 20, 140-144.

Cedarbaum, J.M. & Aghajanian, G.K. (1977). Catecholamine receptors on lôcus coeruleus neurons: Pharmacological characterization. *Eur. J. Pharmacol.* 44, 375-385.

Celsen, B. & Kuschinsky, K. (1974). Effects of morphine on
kinetics of ^{14}C-dopamine in rat striatal slices. *Naunyn-
Schmiedeberg's Arch. Pharmacol.* 284, 159-165.

Chan, S.H.H., Lee, C.M. & Wong, P.C.L. (1977). Suppression of
caudate neuron activities by morphine and the involvement of
dopaminergic neurotransmission. *Fed. Proc.* 36, 395.

Cheramy, A., Nieoullon, A. & Glowinski, J. (1977). Effects of
peripheral and local administration of picrotoxin on the release of newly synthesized ^{3}H-dopamine in the caudate nucleus
of the cat. *Naunyn-Schmiedeberg's Arch. Pharmacol.* 297, 31-37.

Chiara, G. di, Porceddu, M.L., Fratta, W. & Gessa, G.L. (1977).
Postsynaptic receptors are not essential for dopaminergic
feedback regulation. *Nature* [*Lond.*] 267, 270-272.

Clarenbach, P., Raffel, G., Meyer, D.K. & Hertting, G. (1976).
Inhibition by indomethacin and niflumic acid of catecholamine-
uptake into rat hypothalamic and striatal synaptosomes. *Arch.
Int. Pharmacodyn. Ther.* 219, 79-86.

Clouet, D.H. & Williams, N. (1974). The effect of narcotic analgesic drugs on the uptake and release of neurotransmitters in
isolated synaptosomes. *J. Pharmacol. Exp. Ther.* 188, 419-428.

Collier, H.O.J., McDonald-Gibson, W.J. & Saeed, S.A. (1974).
Morphine and apomorphine stimulate prostaglandin production
by rabbit brain homogenate. *Br. J. Pharmacol.* 52, 116P.

Crossman, A.R., Walker, R.J. & Woodruff, G.N. (1973). Picrotoxin
antagonism of γ aminobutyric acid inhibitory responses and
synaptic inhibition in the rat substantia nigra. *Br. J.
Pharmacol.* 49, 696-698.

Dismukes, K., de Boer, A.A. & Mulder, A.H. (1977). On the
mechanism of alpha-receptor mediated modulation of ^{3}H-nor-
adrenaline release from slices of rat brain neocortex.
Naunyn-Schmiedeberg's Arch. Pharmacol. 299, 115-122.

Dismukes, R.K. & Mulder, A.H. (1976). Cyclic AMP and α-receptor-
mediated modulation of noradrenaline release from rat brain
slices. *Eur. J. Pharmacol.* 39, 383-388.

Dismukes, K. & Mulder, A.H. (1977). Effects of neuroleptics on
release of ^{3}H-dopamine from slices of rat corpus striatum.
Naunyn-Schmiedeberg's Arch. Pharmacol. 297, 23-29.

Dray, A. & Straughan, D.W. (1976). Synaptic mechanisms in the
substantia nigra. *J. Pharm. Pharmacol.* 28, 400-405.

Endo, T., Starke, K., Bangerter, A. & Taube, H.D. (1977). Presynaptic receptor systems on the noradrenergic neurones of the
rabbit pulmonary artery. *Naunyn-Schmiedeberg's Arch. Pharmacol.* 296, 229-247.

Farah, M.B., Adler-Graschinsky, E. & Langer, S.Z. (1977).
Possible physiological significance of the initial step in
the catabolism of noradrenaline in the central nervous system
of the rat. *Naunyn-Schmiedeberg's Arch. Pharmacol.* 297,
119-131.

Farnebo, L.O. (1971). Histochemical demonstration of transmitter
release from noradrenaline, dopamine and 5-hydroxytryptamine
nerve terminals in field stimulated rat brain slices. *Z. Zellforsch.* 122, 503-519.

Farnebo, L.O. & Hamberger, B. (1970). Effects of desipramine, phentolamine and phenoxybenzamine on the release of noradrenaline from isolated tissues. *J. Pharm. Pharmacol.* 22, 855-857.

Farnebo, L.O. & Hamberger, B. (1971). Drug-induced changes in the release of 3H-monoamines from field stimulated rat brain slices. *Acta Physiol. Scand.*, Suppl. 371, 35-44.

Farnebo, L.O. & Hamberger, B. (1973). Catecholamine release and receptors in brain slices. In: *Frontiers in Catecholamine Research* (eds.) E. Usdin & S.H. Snyder, Pergamon Press, New York, pp. 589-593.

Geffen, L.B., Jessell, T.M., Cuello, A.C. & Iversen, L.L. (1976). Release of dopamine from dendrites in rat substantia nigra. *Nature [Lond.]* 260, 258-260.

Giorguieff, M.F., Le Floc'h, M.L., Glowinski, J. & Besson, M.J. (1977). Involvement of cholinergic presynaptic receptors of nicotinic and muscarinic types in the control of the spontaneous release of dopamine from striatal dopaminergic terminals in the rat. *J. Pharmacol. Exp. Ther.* 200, 535-544.

Giorguieff, M.F., Le Floc'h, M.L., Westfall, T.C., Glowinski, J. & Besson, M.J. (1976). Nicotinic effect of acetylcholine on the release of newly synthesized [3H]dopamine in rat striatal slices and cat caudate nucleus. *Brain Res.* 106, 117-131.

Glowinski, J. (1975). Properties and functions of intraneuronal monoamine compartments in central aminergic neurons. In: *Handbook of Psychopharmacology* Vol. 3 (eds.) L.L. Iversen, S.D. Iversen & S.H. Snyder, Plenum Press, New York - London, pp. 139-167.

Gomes, C., Svensson, T.H. & Trolin, G. (1976). Effects of morphine on central catecholamine turnover, blood pressure and heart rate in the rat. *Naunyn-Schmiedeberg's Arch. Pharmacol.* 294, 141-147.

Goodman, F.R. (1974). Effects of nicotine on distribution and release of 14C-norepinephrine and 14C-dopamine in rat brain striatum and hypothalamus slices. *Neuropharmacology* 13, 1025-1032.

Gramsch, C. & Bläsig, J. (1976). Changes in brain catecholamine turnover during precipitated morphine withdrawal in the rat. *Naunyn-Schmiedeberg's Arch. Pharmacol.* 293, R9.

Gramsch, C., Bläsig, J. & Herz, A. (1977). Changes in striatal dopamine metabolism during precipitated morphine withdrawal. *Eur. J. Pharmacol.* 44, 231-240.

Groves, P.M., Wilson, C.J., Young, S.J. & Rebec, G.V. (1975). Self-inhibition by dopaminergic neurons. *Science* 190, 522-529.

Gulati, O.D. & Shah, N.S. (1977). Amine releasing action of nicotine from rat hypothalamus *in vitro*. *Res. Commun. Chem. Pathol. Pharmacol.* 16, 565-568.

Gunne, L.M., Jonsson, J. & Fuxe, K. (1969). Effects of morphine intoxication on brain catecholamine neurons. *Eur. J. Pharmacol.* 5, 338-342.

Hall, G.H. & Turner, D.M. (1972). Effects of nicotine on the release of ^{3}H-noradrenaline from the hypothalamus. *Biochem. Pharmacol.* 21, 1829-1838.

Harris, R.A., Yamamoto, H., Loh, H.H. & Way, E.L. (1977). Discrete changes in brain calcium with morphine analgesia, tolerance-dependence, and abstinence. *Life Sci.* 20, 501-506.

Hedqvist, P. (1977). Basic mechanisms of prostaglandin action on autonomic neurotransmission. *Ann. Rev. Pharmacol. Toxicol.* 17, 259-279.

Hökfelt, T., Fuxe, K., Goldstein, M. & Johansson, O. (1974). Immunohistochemical evidence for the existence of adrenaline neurons in the rat brain. *Brain Res.* 66, 235-251.

Höllt, V., Haarmann, I. & Herz, A. (1976). Identification of opiate/receptor binding *in vivo*. *Arzneim.-Forsch.* 26, 1102-1104.

Iversen, L.L., Rogawski, M.A. & Miller, R.J. (1976). Comparison of the effects of neuroleptic drugs on pre- and postsynaptic dopaminergic mechanisms in the rat striatum. *Mol. Pharmacol.* 12, 251-262.

Jones, D.G. (1975). *Synapses and Synaptosomes - Morphological Aspects*, Chapman & Hall, London.

Kanazawa, I., Emson, P.C. & Cuello, A.C. (1977). Evidence for the existence of substance P-containing fibres in striato-nigral and pallido-nigral pathways in rat brain. *Brain Res.* 119, 447-453.

Katz, R.I. & Chase, T.N. (1970). Neurohumoral mechanisms in the brain slice. *Adv. Pharmacol. Chemother.* 8, 1-30.

Kehr, W., Carlsson, A., Lindqvist, M., Magnusson, T. & Atack, C. (1972). Evidence for a receptor-mediated feedback control of striatal tyrosine hydroxylase activity. *J. Pharm. Pharmacol.* 24, 744-747.

Korf, J., Bunney, B.S. & Aghajanian, G.K. (1974). Noradrenergic neurons: Morphine inhibition of spontaneous activity. *Eur. J. Pharmacol.* 25, 165-169.

Kuhar, M.J., Pert, C.B. & Snyder, S.H. (1973). Regional distribution of opiate receptor binding in monkey and human brain. *Nature [Lond.]* 245, 447-450.

Kuschinsky, K. (1977). Opiate dependence. *Progress Pharmacol.*
1 (2).

Kuschinsky, K. & Hornykiewicz, O. (1974). Effects of morphine on
striatal dopamine metabolism: Possible mechanism of its opposite effect on locomotor activity in rats and mice. *Eur. J.
Pharmacol.* 26, 41-50.

Lal, H. (1975). Narcotic dependence, narcotic action and dopamine receptors. *Life Sci.* 7, 483-496.

Langer, S.Z. (1974). Presynaptic regulation of catecholamine
release. *Biochem. Pharmacol.* 23, 1793-1800.

Lapierre, Y., Beaudet, A., Demianczuk, N. & Descarries, L.
(1973). Noradrenergic axon terminals in the cerebral cortex
of rat. II. Quantitative data revealed by light and electron
microscope radioautography of the frontal cortex. *Brain Res.*
63, 175-182.

Laverty, R. & Sharman, D.F. (1965). Modification by drugs of the
metabolism of 3,4-dihydroxyphenylethylamine, noradrenaline and
5-hydroxytryptamine in the brain. *Br. J. Pharmacol.* 24, 759-
772.

Lindmar, R., Löffelholz, K. & Muscholl, E. (1968). A muscarinic
mechanism inhibiting the release of noradrenaline from peripheral adrenergic nerve fibres by nicotinic agents. *Br. J.
Pharmacol.* 32, 280-294.

Lloyd, K.G. & Bartholini, G. (1975). The effect of drugs on the
release of endogenous catecholamines into the perfusate of
discrete brain areas of the cat *in vivo*. *Experientia* 31, 560-
561.

Löffelholz, K. (1970). Autoinhibition of nicotinic release of
noradrenaline from postganglionic sympathetic nerves. *Naunyn-
Schmiedeberg's Arch. Pharmacol.* 267, 49-63.

Loh, H.H., Brase, D.A., Sampath-Khanna, S., Mar, J.B. & Way, E.L.
(1976). β-Endorphin *in vitro* inhibition of striatal dopamine
release. *Nature [Lond.]* 264, 567-568.

Montel, H., Starke, K. & Taube, H.D. (1975a). Morphine tolerance
and dependence in noradrenaline neurones of the rat cerebral
cortex. *Naunyn-Schmiedeberg's Arch. Pharmacol.* 288, 415-426.

Montel, H., Starke, K. & Taube, H.D. (1975b). Influence of morphine and naloxone on the release of noradrenaline from rat
cerebellar cortex slices. *Naunyn-Schmiedeberg's Arch. Pharmacol.* 288, 427-433.

Montel, H., Starke, K. & Weber, F. (1974a). Influence of morphine and naloxone on the release of noradrenaline from rat
brain cortex slices. *Naunyn-Schmiedeberg's Arch. Pharmacol.*
283, 357-369.

Montel, H., Starke, K. & Weber, F. (1974b). Influence of fentanyl, levorphanol and pethidine on the release of noradrenaline from rat brain cortex slices. *Naunyn-Schmiedeberg's Arch. Pharmacol.* 283, 371-377.

Nieoullon, A., Cheramy, A. & Glowinski, J. (1977). An adaptation of the push-pull cannula method to study the *in vivo* release of [^{3}H]dopamine synthesized from [^{3}H]tyrosine in the cat caudate nucleus: Effects of various physical and pharmacological treatments. *J. Neurochem.* 28, 819-828.

O'Keeffe, R., Sharman, D.F. & Vogt, M. (1970). Effect of drugs used in psychoses on cerebral dopamine metabolism. *Br. J. Pharmacol.* 38, 287-304.

Orrego, F. & Miranda, R. (1977). Effects of tetrodotoxin, elevated calcium and calcium antagonists on electrically induced ^{3}H-noradrenaline release from brain slices. *Eur. J. Pharmacol.* 44, 275-278.

Paalzow, G. & Paalzow, L. (1975). Morphine-induced inhibition of different pain responses in relation to the regional turnover of rat brain noradrenaline and dopamine. *Psychopharmacologia* [*Berl.*] 45, 9-20.

Papeschi, R., Theiss, P. & Herz, A. (1975). Effects of morphine on the turnover of brain catecholamines and serotonin in rats - acute morphine administration. *Eur. J. Pharmacol.* 34, 253-261.

Patrick, R.L. & Barchas, J.D. (1976). Dopamine synthesis in rat brain striatal synaptosomes. II. Dibutyryl cyclic adenosine 3':5'-monophosphoric acid and 6-methyltetrahydropterine-induced synthesis increases without an increase in endogenous dopamine release. *J. Pharmacol. Exp. Ther.* 197, 97-104.

Philippu, A., Przuntek, H. & Roensberg, W. (1973a). Superfusion of the hypothalamus with gamma-aminobutyric acid. Effect on release of noradrenaline and blood pressure. *Naunyn-Schmiedeberg's Arch. Pharmacol.* 276, 103-118.

Philippu, A., Roensberg, W. & Przuntek, H. (1973b). Effects of adrenergic drugs on pressor responses to hypothalamic stimulation. *Naunyn-Schmiedeberg's Arch. Pharmacol.* 278, 373-386.

Pollard, H., Llorens-Cortes, C. & Schwartz, J.C. (1977). Enkephalin receptors on dopaminergic neurones in rat striatum. *Nature* [*Lond.*] 268, 745-747.

Polz-Tejera, G., Schmidt, J. & Karten, H.J. (1975). Autoradiographic localisation of α-bungarotoxin-binding sites in the central nervous system. *Nature* [*Lond.*] 258, 349-351.

Rand, M.J., McCulloch, M.W. & Story, D.F. (1975). Pre-junctional modulation of noradrenergic transmission by noradrenaline, dopamine and acetylcholine. In: *Central Action of Drugs in Blood Pressure Regulation* (eds.) D.S. Davies & J.L. Reid, Pitman Medical Publishing, Tunbridge Wells, pp. 94-132.

Reubi, J.C., Iversen, L.L. & Jessell, T.M. (1977). Dopamine selectively increases ^{3}H-GABA release from slices of rat substantia nigra *in vitro*. *Nature [Lond.]* 268, 652-654.

Ryall, R.W. (1975). Amino acid receptors in CNS. I. GABA and glycine in spinal cord. In: *Handbook of Psychopharmacology*, Vol. 4 (eds.) L.L. Iversen, S.D. Iversen & S.H. Snyder, Plenum Press, New York - London, pp. 83-128.

Sampath-Khanna, S., Brase, D.A., Loh, H.H. & Way, E.L. (1976). Opiate inhibition of ^{3}H-dopamine release from striatal tissue. *Pharmacologist* 18, 213.

Schmidt, R.F. (1971). Presynaptic inhibition in the vertebrate central nervous system. *Rev. Physiol. Biochem. Pharmacol.* 63, 20-101.

Seeman, P. & Lee, T. (1974). The dopamine-releasing actions of neuroleptics and ethanol. *J. Pharmacol. Exp. Ther.* 190, 131-140.

Seeman, P. & Lee, T. (1975). Antipsychotic drugs: Direct correlation between clinical potency and presynaptic action on dopamine neurons. *Science* 188, 1217-1219.

Smith, C.B., Sheldon, M.I., Bednarczyk, J.H. & Villarreal, J.E. (1972). Morphine-induced increases in the incorporation of ^{14}C-tyrosine into ^{14}C-dopamine and ^{14}C-norepinephrine in the mouse brain: Antagonism by naloxone and tolerance. *J. Pharmacol. Exp. Ther.* 180, 547-557.

Snyder, S.H. & Simantov, R. (1977). The opiate receptor and opioid peptides. *J. Neurochem.* 28, 13-20.

Speth, R.C., Chen, F.M., Lindstrom, J.M., Kobayashi, R.M. & Yamamura, H.I. (1977). Nicotinic cholinergic receptors in rat brain identified by [^{125}I] Naja naja siamensis α-toxin binding. *Brain Res.* 131, 350-355.

Starke, K. (1972). Alpha sympathomimetic inhibition of adrenergic and cholinergic transmission in the rabbit heart. *Naunyn-Schmiedeberg's Arch. Pharmacol.* 274, 18-45.

Starke, K. (1977). Regulation of noradrenaline release by presynaptic receptor systems. *Rev. Physiol. Biochem. Pharmacol.* 77, 1-124.

182   K. Starke

Starke, K., Endo, T. & Taube, H.D. (1975a). Relative pre- and
    postsynaptic potencies of α-adrenoceptor agonists in the
    rabbit pulmonary artery. *Naunyn-Schmiedeberg's Arch. Pharma-
    col.* 291, 55-78.

Starke, K., Endo, T., Taube, H.D. & Borowski, E. (1975b). Pre-
    synaptic receptor systems on noradrenergic nerves. In:
    Chemical Tools in Catecholamine Research, Vol. 2 (eds.)
    O. Almgren, A. Carlsson & J. Engel, North-Holland, Amsterdam-
    Oxford, pp. 193-200.

Starke, K. & Montel, H. (1973a). Involvement of α-receptors in
    clonidine-induced inhibition of transmitter release from
    central monoamine neurónes. *Neuropharmacology* 12, 1073-1080.

Starke, K. & Montel, H. (1973b). Alpha-receptor-mediated modu-
    lation of transmitter release from central noradrenergic
    neurones. *Naunyn-Schmiedeberg's Arch. Pharmacol.* 279, 53-60.

Starke, K. & Montel, H. (1973c). Interaction between indometha-
    cin, oxymetazoline and phentolamine on the release of [^{3}H]nor-
    adrenaline from brain slices. *J. Pharm. Pharmacol.* 25, 758-
    759.

Stjärne, L. (1975). Basic mechanisms and local feedback control
    of secretion of adrenergic and cholinergic neurotransmitters.
    In: *Handbook of Psychopharmacology*, Vol. 6 (eds.)
    L.L. Iversen, S.D. Iversen & S.H. Snyder, Plenum Press, New
    York - London, pp. 179-233.

Stoof, J.C. & Mulder, A.H. (1978). Increased dopamine release
    from rat striatal slices by inhibitors of GABA-aminotrans-
    ferase. *Eur. J. Pharmacol.*, in press.

Subramanian, N. & Mulder, A.H. (1977). Modulation by histamine
    of the efflux of radiolabeled catecholamines from rat brain
    slices. *Eur. J. Pharmacol.* 43, 143-152.

Sugrue, M.F. (1974). The effects of acutely administered anal-
    gesics on the turnover of noradrenaline and dopamine in
    various regions of the rat brain. *Br. J. Pharmacol.* 52,
    159-165.

Svensson, T.H., Bunney, B.S. & Aghajanian, G.K. (1975). Inhibi-
    tion of both noradrenergic and serotonergic neurons in brain
    by the α-adrenergic agonist clonidine. *Brain Res.* 92, 291-306.

Taube, H.D., Borowski, E., Endo, T. & Starke, K. (1976). Enkepha-
    lin: A potential modulator of noradrenaline release in rat
    brain. *Eur. J. Pharmacol.* 38, 377-380.

Taube, H.D., Starke, K. & Borowski, E. (1977). Presynaptic re-
    ceptor systems on the noradrenergic neurones of rat brain.
    Naunyn-Schmiedeberg's Arch. Pharmacol. 299, 123-141.

U'Prichard, D.C., Greenberg, D.A. & Snyder, S.H. (1977). Binding characteristics of a radiolabeled agonist and antagonist at central nervous system alpha noradrenergic receptors. *Mol. Pharmacol.* 13, 454-473.

Walker, R.J., Kemp, J.A., Yajima, H., Kitagawa, K. & Woodruff, G.N. (1976). The action of substance P on mesencephalic reticular and substantia nigral neurones of the rat. *Experientia* 32, 214-215.

Walters, J.R. & Roth, R.H. (1976). Dopaminergic neurons: An *in vivo* system for measuring drug interactions with presynaptic receptors. *Naunyn-Schmiedeberg's Arch. Pharmacol.* 296, 5-14.

Westfall, T.C. (1974a). Effect of nicotine and other drugs on the release of ^{3}H-norepinephrine and ^{3}H-dopamine from rat brain slices. *Neuropharmacology* 13, 693-700.

Westfall, T.C. (1974b). Effect of muscarinic agonists on the release of ^{3}H-norepinephrine and ^{3}H-dopamine by potassium and electrical stimulation from rat brain slices. *Life Sci.* 14, 1641-1652.

Westfall, T.C., Besson, M.J., Giorguieff, M.F. & Glowinski, J. (1976a). The role of presynaptic receptors in the release and synthesis of ^{3}H-dopamine by slices of rat striatum. *Naunyn-Schmiedeberg's Arch. Pharmacol.* 292, 279-287.

Westfall, T.C., Kitay, D. & Wahl, G. (1976b). The effect of cyclic nucleotides on the release of ^{3}H-dopamine from rat striatal slices. *J. Pharmacol. Exp. Ther.* 199, 149-157.

Yessaian, N.H., Armenian, A.R. & Buniatian, H.C. (1969). Effect of γ-aminobutyric acid on brain serotonin and catecholamines. *J. Neurochem.* 16, 1425-1433.

Yessaian, N.H., Demirjian, A.H. & Tozalakian, B.V. (1977). Effect of GABA, picrotoxin and bicuculline on loss of noradrenaline and serotonin from rat brain mesodiencephalic region *in vitro*. *J. Neurochem.* 28, 1151-1153.

Young, W.S., Bird, S.J. & Kuhar, M.J. (1977). Iontophoresis of methionine-enkephalin in the locus coeruleus area. *Brain Res.* 129, 366-370.

MODIFICATION OF RELEASE BY ADRENERGIC NEURON BLOCKING AGENTS AND AGENTS THAT ALTER THE ACTION POTENTIAL

G. Häusler and W. Haefely

I   INTRODUCTION

This chapter describes the modification by various groups of agents of the evoked release of noradrenaline from noradrenergic nerve terminals. Adrenergic neuron blockers are drugs whose main pharmacological property is to inhibit the release of noradrenaline. In view of the vast literature on this subject, it was impossible to quote all the papers that deal in a descriptive manner with adrenergic neuron blocking agents. We have, therefore, selected those papers which we considered to be relevant mainly for an understanding of their mode of action. A few examples of drugs are also given which possess adrenergic neuron blocking properties, but which are not used for this purpose. Another section of this chapter deals with agents and ions which are known to modify the action potential of various neurons and whose action on the evoked release of noradrenaline is of purely basic interest. These agents include the local anesthetics; their depressant effect on adrenergic nerve terminals is of special interest when compared to that of adrenergic neuron blocking agents. Tetraethylammonium and several cations facilitate the evoked release of noradrenaline by affecting the first step in the excitation secretion coupling. An opposite effect in this step is thought to underly the inhibitory effect of veratrum alkaloids as well as of nickel and potassium ions.

II   CLASSICAL ADRENERGIC NEURON BLOCKING AGENTS

The term adrenergic neuron blocking drugs defines a group of agents which have in common the property of inhibiting the evoked release of the transmitter noradrenaline from adrenergic nerve endings in concentrations that do not affect the release of other neurotransmitters. Although a systematic comparison has not been made, it appears that the adrenergic nerves of all peripheral organs are equally sensitive to the action of adrenergic neuron blocking drugs and it does not matter whether the innervation is through long or short adrenergic neurons. The release of noradrenaline or adrenaline from chromaffin cells of the adrenal medulla is, however, barely influenced by adrenergic neuron blocking agents (Cass & Spriggs, 1961; Athos, McHugh, Fineberg & Hilton, 1962; Abercrombie & Davies, 1963).

Since all adrenergic neuron blocking agents are highly polar molecules which do not readily penetrate the blood-brain barrier,

their effects on central adrenergic neurons cannot be assessed
when peripheral routes of drug administration are used. Direct
exposure of central adrenergic neurons to these blocking agents,
for example during push-pull perfusion of the hypothalamus with
bretylium (Przuntek, Guimarães & Philippu, 1971), indicates that
central adrenergic neurons may also be susceptible to the action
of adrenergic neuron blocking drugs.

Adrenergic neuron blocking agents show marked similarities in
chemical structure by possessing either a quaternary nitrogen
(e.g. xylocholine and bretylium) or a guanidine group (e.g.
guanethidine, bethanidine and guanoxan) (Fig. 1). In debrisoquine, the guanidine group is part of the isoquinoline ring
system (Fig. 1). Due to the guanidine moiety or the quaternary
nitrogen, the adrenergic neuron blocking agents are strongly
basic molecules and thus readily form highly water soluble salts.

A   Pharmacological Properties

The synthesis of choline 2,6-xylyl ether bromide (TM 10, xylocholine) (Fig. 1) and the description of its pharmacological
properties (Hey & Willey, 1954; Exley, 1957; Willey, 1957) initiated the development of adrenergic neuron blocking agents. The
properties of xylocholine gave rise to the belief that compounds
could be found that selectively impair the function of adrenergic
nerves without antagonizing the actions of noradrenaline and
adrenaline. This expectation was fulfilled when, among a number
of quaternary benzylammonium salts, bretylium proved to specifically block the effects of adrenergic nerve stimulation without
producing the parasympathomimetic effects of xylocholine (Boura,
Copp & Green, 1959; Boura & Green, 1959).

Bretylium, guanethidine, debrisoquine and bethanidine are those
adrenergic neuron blocking agents that have been investigated
most extensively and, in the present article, reference will be
made in general to these agents. Of these four compounds, only
the latter three are still in therapeutic use. Bretylium was
the first clinically employed representative of the group of
adrenergic neuron blocking agents; it was soon followed by guanethidine (Maxwell, Plummer, Schneider, Povalski & Daniel, 1960;
Page & Dustan, 1959; Freis, 1965). The prevailing therapeutic
use of these drugs is in moderate to severe arterial hypertension.

The main pharmacologic property of adrenergic neuron blocking
drugs is the <u>inhibition of the noradrenaline release from adrenergic nerves</u> (Boura & Green, 1959; Maxwell *et al.*, 1960; Cass &
Spriggs, 1961; Hertting, Axelrod & Patrick, 1962; Abercrombie &
Davies, 1963). They not only depress the release of noradrenaline in response to spontaneous or evoked action potentials invading the terminal part of adrenergic neurons but also the
release in response to various chemical stimuli. There can be
little doubt that impairment of adrenergic nerve function by
adrenergic neuron blocking drugs is intimately related to the
high affinity of these agents for adrenergic nerves which is
clearly indicated by their accumulation in these structures

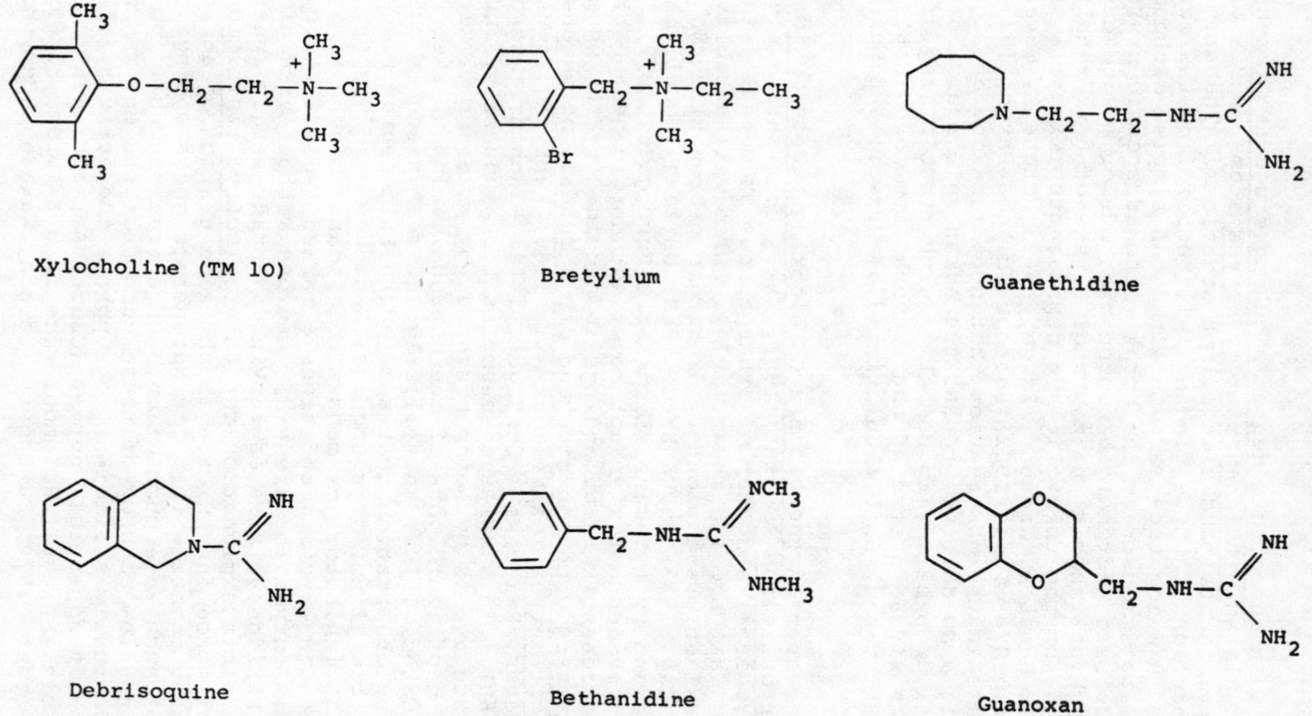

Fig. 1. Structural formulae of several adrenergic neuron blocking drugs.

(Boura, Copp, Duncombe, Green & McCoubrey, 1960; Boura, Duncombe
& McCoubrey, 1961; Mitchell & Oates, 1970; Shah, Premanand,
Jariwala & Gulati, 1974).

The evidence that adrenergic neuron blocking drugs are taken up
into and accumulated within adrenergic nerves stems from a wide
variety of experimental and clinical observations. The enumera-
tion and discussion of these findings will not follow the chrono-
logical order in which they were obtained. A simple, although
indirect, way to demonstrate the uptake into adrenergic neurons
is the prevention of adrenergic neuron blockade or its reversal
by compounds which inhibit the neuronal uptake of noradrenaline,
e.g. by cocaine or the tricyclic antidepressants (Mitchell, Arias
& Oates, 1967; Hanahoe, Ireson & Large, 1969; Mitchell, Cavanaugh,
Arias & Oates, 1970; Toda, 1972; Huston, Golko & Paton, 1977).
Related to this is the observation that noradrenaline at high concentrations is also able to prevent the adrenergic neuron blocking
action, in all probability by competing with the blocking drugs
for the uptake sites located at the neuronal membrane (Mitchell
& Oates, 1970; Prasad, Shah & Gulati, 1973; Maxwell & Eckhardt,
1975).

For the same reason adrenergic neuron blocking agents inhibit the
uptake of noradrenaline (Foster, 1967; Koe & Constantine, 1972;
Huston *et al.*, 1977) and that of other amines or mutually inhibit
their uptake (Gaitondé & Nimbkar, 1973). Also well established
is the reversal or prevention of adrenergic neuron blockade by
amphetamine (Day, 1962; Day & Rand, 1963; Gerkens, McCulloch &
Wilson, 1969) and by tyramine (Kirpekar & Furchgott, 1972). Further indirect evidence for an uptake of adrenergic neuron blocking
agents into adrenergic nerve endings is provided by the observation that adrenergic neuron blocking drugs release noradrenaline
from adrenergic nerves (Maxwell *et al.*, 1960; Hertting *et al.*,
1962; Moe, Bates, Palkoski & Banziger, 1964; Pluchino, Muskus &
Pluchino, 1969). This release resembles that induced by indirect
sympathomimetic agents by being prevented by prior or simultaneous
administration of inhibitors of the neuronal amine uptake
(Mitchell & Oates, 1970). A similarly indirect piece of evidence
stems from the observation that some adrenergic neuron blocking
agents (e.g. bretylium, debrisoquine), which under *in vitro* conditions are weak inhibitors of monoamine oxidase (Giachetti & Shore,
1967), show under *in vivo* conditions a marked and selective inhibition of this enzyme in adrenergic neurons without affecting its
activity in peripheral tissues lacking a noradrenergic innervation.
The most plausible explanation for this selective inhibition of
intraneuronal monoamine oxidase is the accumulation of adrenergic
neuron blocking agents within the adrenergic nerve endings. In
the course of such an accumulation, concentrations build up which,
in spite of the low potency of these compounds for enzyme inhibition, are eventually sufficient to suppress the activity of monoamine oxidase in adrenergic nerves (Clarke & Leach, 1968;
Pettinger, Korn, Spiegel, Solomon, Pocelinko & Abrams, 1969;
Malmfors & Abrams, 1970; Furchgott, Garcia, Wakade & Cervoni,
1971).

That adrenergic neuron blocking drugs are taken up into and probably stored within adrenergic nerve endings can also be inferred
from the observation that these agents are released by adrenergic
nerve stimulation. This has been reported for guanethidine by
Boullin, Costa and Brodie (1966) and for guanethidine and bethanidine by Shrand, Morgan and Oates (1973).

Human blood platelets, which in several respects can be considered
as a model of adrenergic nerve endings, also take up and accumulate adrenergic neuron blocking agents (Boullin & O'Brien, 1969;
Pocelinko & Solomon, 1970), probably through the uptake system
for 5-hydroxytryptamine (O'Brien & Boullin, 1972); moreover, the
uptake of biogenic amines into blood platelets is inhibited by
adrenergic neuron blocking agents (Solomon, Ashley, Spirt &
Abrams, 1969). Furthermore, adrenergic neuron blocking agents
inhibit the monoamine oxidase activity of blood platelets by a
similarly selective accumulation (Solomon *et al.*, 1969) as described above for adrenergic nerve endings.

If adrenergic neuron blocking agents share with noradrenaline the
uptake system at the neuronal membrane, one could expect that
measures which inactivate this uptake system, e.g. exposure of
tissues to low temperature, to sodium-free media or to ouabain,
would prevent the uptake of adrenergic neuron blocking agents into
adrenergic nerve endings and the development of blockade. The
results obtained so far are not uniform. An inhibition of uptake
of adrenergic neuron blocking agents by low temperature, sodium
deficiency or ouabain have been reported by Gulati and Jaykar
(1971); Gaitondé and Nimbkar (1973); Shah *et al.* (1974), Ross and
Kelder (1976); Hosotani and Misu (1977). Toda (1972) reported
that adrenergic neuron blockade produced by bretylium in rabbit
atria and aortae was not antagonized in solutions with reduced
sodium concentration (103 mM) or containing ouabain (2×10^{-7}M),
although cocaine and desipramine prevented or reversed the action
of bretylium. Prasad *et al.* (1973) found that low temperature
(0°C) prevented the neuron blocking action of xylocholine, bretylium, guanethidine and debrisoquine but was not able to reverse
the blockade induced by any of these blockers. Sodium deprivation partially prevented the effect of guanethidine but not that
of the other three blockers.

The most convincing piece of evidence for neuronal uptake is the
finding that adrenergic neuron blocking drugs (radioactively
labelled or unlabelled) are accumulated in sympathetic ganglia,
their postganglionic nerves and, in general, in organs with an
intact adrenergic innervation, but not after adrenergic denervation, and that this accumulation is prevented by uptake inhibition
(Boura *et al*, 1960; Boura *et al.*, 1961; Mitchell & Oates, 1970;
Giachetti & Hollenbeck, 1976; Almgren & Lundberg, 1976; Eckhardt,
Maxwell & Copp, 1977).

From the vast amount of experimental results presented in the
literature, it appears safe to conclude that uptake of adrenergic
neuron blocking agents into adrenergic nerve endings and accumulation within these structures is a well-established fact.

Another pharmacological property which appears to be common to
all adrenergic neuron blocking agents is the ability to produce
local anesthetic (membrane stabilizing) effects when used at high
concentrations. Although, at first glance, this property seems
to be of minor biological significance, it is essential for one
of the theories on the mechanism of action of adrenergic neuron
blocking drugs (see below). Xylocholine was reported early to
possess local anesthetic properties (Hey & Willey, 1954). Topi-
cal application of bretylium to adrenergic nerve trunks and other
types of nerves caused a conduction block; adrenergic nerves and
sensory nerves were more sensitive than heavily myelinated fibres
(Boura & Green, 1959; Boura et al., 1960). The experiments
allowed no clear-cut decision whether the nonuniform sensitivity
was due to penetration barriers for bretylium, related to the
different myelinisation of the nerves, or to the presence and absence, respectively, of an amine uptake system in the nerve
trunks. The findings of other authors have confirmed the local
anesthetic properties of xylocholine (Exley, 1957, 1960) and
bretylium (Exley, 1960; Boyd, Chang & Rand, 1961) and provided
evidence that the impairment of adrenergic nerve function by
those agents is not related to a conduction block in adrenergic
nerve trunks but rather to an action on the terminal part of the
adrenergic neuron (Exley, 1957; 1960; Boyd et al., 1961). There
are other reports on the local anesthetic effects of bretylium
(Haeusler, Haefely & Huerlimann, 1969a) and guanethidine (Rand &
Wilson, 1967). Guanethidine, debrisoquine and bretylium have a
similar local anesthetic potency (Haeusler, unpublished) when
studied on carotid baroreceptors with the same method as described
by Haeusler et al. (1969a).

    B   Mechanism of Action

The theories on the mechanism of action of adrenergic neuron
blocking agents may be divided into those (a) which relate the
neuronal blockade to depletion of noradrenaline or of a functionally important fraction of the noradrenaline stores in adrenergic nerve endings and (b,c) into those which ascribe the blockade to altered properties of the neuronal terminal membrane.
Among the authors who favour the latter view, some believe that
the inhibition of transmitter release results from (b) a depolarization of the membrane of the adrenergic nerve terminals, while
others claim that the blockade may be caused by (c) a stabilization
of the neuronal membrane due to the well-established local anesthetic properties of adrenergic neuron blocking drugs.

(a) Depletion of Noradrenaline
Adrenergic neuron blockade is in general preceded by a sympathomimetic effect due to the release of noradrenaline (Maxwell et al.,
1960; Moe et al., 1964; Abbs, 1966). This sympathomimetic effect
is more sustained after guanethidine and debrisoquine than after
bretylium. Guanethidine (Sheppard & Zimmermann, 1959; Cass,
Kuntzman & Brodie, 1960; Moe et al., 1964) and debrisoquine
(Haeusler, Lorez, Bartholini, Kettler & Tranzer, 1974) cause a
pronounced depletion of noradrenaline in adrenergically innervated
organs, and it was logical to consider the possibility that the
loss of adrenergic function after guanethidine is attributable to

the loss of the amine from the nerve endings (Cass *et al.*, 1960). However, this explanation is unsatisfactory because the noradrenaline content of tissues is little affected by guanethidine at the time when the adrenergic neuron blockade is already established (Cass & Spriggs, 1961; Gaffney, Chidsey & Braunwald, 1963; Spriggs, 1966).

Chang, Chang and Su (1967) confirmed the absence of any change of the total content of noradrenaline in the heart and vas deferens of rats 30 min after the administration of guanethidine but found a significant decrease in noradrenaline of the particulate fraction at this time. The noradrenaline content of the supernatant fraction was unaltered. The fractions were obtained by sucrose density gradient centrifugation of the tissue homogenates. Five hours after the administration of guanethidine, noradrenaline in the supernatant was also markedly reduced whereas the amine depletion in the particulate fraction was not much more marked than after 30 min. Amphetamine prevented the depletion of noradrenaline by guanethidine in both the particulate and the supernatant fraction. In contrast to guanethidine, bretylium did not cause any change in the pattern of the subcellular distribution of noradrenaline. Abbs and Robertson (1970) used a different method of subcellular fractionation of the cat spleen and found that 15 min after the administration of bretylium, i.e. at a time when adrenergic neuron blockade was evident, depletion of noradrenaline occurred only in the supernatant fraction of the homogenate. This depletion remained apparent up to 18 hours but disappeared 7 days after the administration of bretylium, when nerve function was also restored. (+)-Amphetamine prevented or reversed the effects of bretylium on both nerve function and noradrenaline content in the supernatant fraction. There was also a reduction of noradrenaline in other subcellular fractions - especially the high-speed particulate fraction - but the authors concluded that this was unassociated with adrenergic neuron blockade. The authors assumed that bretylium releases noradrenaline from a compartment which is essential for the proper functioning of adrenergic nerves and that refilling of this compartment is prevented by bretylium. In a later publication Abbs and Pycock (1973) reported similar findings with the rat heart; they observed a correlation in time between the bretylium-induced depletion of noradrenaline from the microsomal fraction and adrenergic neuron blockade. Using the cat spleen Abbs and Dodd (1974) found that low doses of (-)-N-(1-phenylethyl) guanidine and debrisoquine produced a decrease of similar magnitude in the noradrenaline content of the high-speed particulate and supernatant fractions; this decrease was temporally correlated with the adrenergic neuron blocking action of the compounds. Guanethidine, in contrast, caused a marked progressive loss of the transmitter from all subcellular fractions. When the doses of the adrenergic neuron blocking drugs were increased, the pattern of depletion from the subcellular fractions changed.

The above studies have doubtlessly revealed significant changes in the intraneuronal distribution of noradrenaline by adrenergic neuron blocking agents. However, the various adrenergic neuron blocking drugs seem to cause different patterns of noradrenaline depletion in the various subcellular fractions in spite of the final outcome which is neuron blockade. Furthermore, it is

difficult to assign a functional role to subcellular fractions
of tissue homogenates since they may not correspond to functional
compartments or sites existing in intact tissues.

(b) Depolarization of the Neuronal Terminal Membrane by Adrenergic Neuron Blocking Drugs

Chang, Costa and Brodie (1965) and Brodie, Chang and Costa (1965)
proposed that guanethidine elicits a persistent depolarization
of the membrane of adrenergic nerve terminals. According to this
view, drug-induced depolarization does not only render the nerve
endings unresponsive to nerve impulses but is also responsible
for the progressive loss of noradrenaline from the terminals.
Since bretylium does not deplete tissue noradrenaline, the authors
assumed that this adrenergic neuron blocking drug had a different
mode of action. The experimental evidence for this concept is
only indirect.

More recent findings by Kubo and Misu (1974) appear to be partially
related to the theory of a depolarisation of the neuronal terminal
membrane. These authors claim that guanethidine increases the
permeability of the membrane of the adrenergic nerve endings to
sodium and thereby produces adrenergic neuron blockade. The conclusion is based on the observation that an established adrenergic neuron blockade in isolated rabbit hearts is moderately
diminished after a change of the perfusion from a normal to a
low sodium (86 mM) solution, while perfusion with a high sodium
(286 mM) solution accentuates the blockade. A similar observation has been made by the same authors for bretylium (Misu &
Kubo, 1974). According to Kubo and Misu (1974) adrenergic neuron
blockade results from an increase in the sodium permeability of
the membrane of the adrenergic nerve terminals leading to a higher
intracellular sodium concentration and consequently to a competition between sodium and calcium at sites that are essential for
transmitter release. The results obtained by Kubo and Misu (1974)
and Misu and Kubo (1974) are open to interpretation in at least
two other ways. It seems to be well established that a sodium-
calcium exchange mechanism in the cell membrane (Baker, Blaustein,
Hodgkin & Steinhardt, 1969; Glitsch, Reuter & Scholz, 1970;
Brinley, Spangler & Mullins, 1975; Blaustein & Ector, 1976;
Blaustein, 1977) operating in various tissues, including nerves,
participates in the maintenance of a low intracellular calcium
concentration. According to this concept calcium is extruded
from the cell in exchange to sodium which enters the cell. The
driving force for the exchange mechanism is provided by the
sodium gradient across the cell membrane; the gradient is maintained by the activity of the membrane ATPase. The results of
Misu and Kubo (1974) can be perfectly explained on the grounds
of such a sodium-calcium exchange mechanism. A reduction of
external sodium decreases the driving force for the sodium-calcium
exchange, i.e. it diminishes calcium extrusion, and thereby
favours the net gain of intracellular calcium. In this condition
transmitter release would be improved. An alternative or an
additional explanation is provided by the well-known fact that
the uptake mechanism of adrenergic nerves for monoamines (and
adrenergic neuron blocking drugs) is impaired in low sodium solution. The loss of guanethidine (after it had accumulated during

perfusion with a normal physiological salt solution) from the
adrenergic nerve endings due to passive efflux of the drug would
then no longer be compensated by an efficient reuptake (see below
for detailed discussion).

(c) Stabilization of the Neuronal Terminal Membrane Resulting from Accumulation of Adrenergic Neuron Blocking Drugs Within Adrenergic Nerve Terminals

Starting from two well-established properties of adrenergic neuron
blocking drugs - their uptake and accumulation within adrenergic
nerve terminals and their moderate local anesthetic effects -
Haeusler *et al.* (1969a) have provided evidence for the following
concept of the mechanism of action. The adrenergic neuron
blocking drugs accumulate within adrenergic nerve terminals to
such a degree to reach concentrations that are sufficient to
produce stabilization of the membrane. Action potentials propagated in a normal way along the large nerve trunks of postganglionic sympathetic nerves would then be prevented from invading
the nerve terminals and from releasing transmitter. A prerequisite for testing this concept experimentally is the possibility
of obtaining information on the excitability of the membrane of
adrenergic nerve terminals. Haeusler *et al.* (1969a) took advantage of earlier observations (Ferry, 1963) that acetylcholine and
other agents elicit in the terminal parts of neurons action potentials which are conducted antidromically and, thus, can be
recorded from fine strands of nerves. Evidently, this process
is not restricted to adrenergic nerves and can be equally well
elicited in sensory fibres (Douglas & Gray, 1953; Douglas &
Ritchie, 1960). It was, however, found that the inferior cardiac
nerve of the·cat heart consists virtually exclusively of adrenergic fibres. For instance, after destruction of cardiac adrenergic nerve terminals with 6-hydroxydopamine in a large number
of cats it was never possible to record antidromic discharges from
the inferior cardiac nerve in response to acetylcholine injected
into the perfusion system of the isolated heart (Haeusler, Thoenen,
Haefely & Huerlimann, 1968a; Haeusler, 1971). These experiments
provided also evidence that the antidromically conducted discharges indeed originated in the terminal part of the adrenergic
neuron since electron microscopic studies had shown that only
this part of the adrenergic neuron is affected by 6-hydroxydopa-
mine (Thoenen & Tranzer, 1968). Besides the presence of a pure
adrenergic nerve, the isolated perfused cat heart offers the
possibility of measuring the effect of sympathetic nerve stimulation on cardiac rate and contractile force. It is, therefore, a
good model to study the relationship between the degree of adrenergic neuron blockade and changes in the excitability of the
terminal membrane of adrenergic nerves.

Using this model Haeusler *et al.* (1969a) found for bretylium a
direct correlation between the inhibition of the effects of sympathetic nerve stimulation on heart rate and the suppression of
acetylcholine- or KCl-induced antidromic discharges with regard
to both intensity and time course. The interval between the
onset of the perfusion with bretylium and the disappearance of
evoked antidromic discharges coupled with adrenergic neuron
blockade was inversely correlated with the concentration of

bretylium in the perfusion medium; in all probability, it reflects the time necessary for the build-up of a concentration of brety-lium producing membrane stabilization within the adrenergic nerve terminal. After the full establishment of the bretylium-induced neuron blockade the perfusion of the heart with drug-free solution for up to 3 hours did not lead to the reappearance of either evoked discharges or the effect of sympathetic nerve stimulation. Apparently, the uptake mechanism for amines maintained sufficient-ly high concentrations of bretylium within the adrenergic nerve endings by recapturing drug molecules which leaked out of the nerve endings.

If neuronal blockade is related to the local anesthetic property of adrenergic neuron blocking agents, one would expect that clas-sical local anesthetics would produce similar effects except that the onset and disappearance of their action would not be governed by the uptake mechanism for amines but rather by diffusion and penetration processes. This was in fact observed for the iso-lated cat heart (Haeusler et al., 1969a).

Perfusion of the heart with a medium containing tetracaine reduced within a few minutes the evoked discharges in the inferior cardiac nerve and the effect of sympathetic nerve stimulation in a con-centration-dependent manner. This inhibitory effect on both para-meters was fully reversible when the heart was perfused for 10-15 min with tetracaine-free solution.

Another possibility to validate the proposed mechanism of action is a comparison of the effects of adrenergic neuron blocking drugs and local anesthetics on sensory nerve endings which are devoid of an uptake mechanism for monoamines. Haeusler et al. (1969a) used the baroreceptors of the carotid sinus as an example of sensory nerve endings. Discharges from the baroreceptors were elicited by artificial, well-controlled pressure increases in the in situ perfused carotid sinus of the cat and were recorded from the carotid sinus nerve. While the concentration of tetracaine necessary to abolish pressure-induced discharges from the baro-receptors and KCl-elicited discharges from adrenergic nerve end-ings was identical, more than 1000 fold higher concentrations of bretylium were required for the inhibition of baroreceptor dis-charges than for the suppression of evoked discharges from adrenergic nerve endings. This huge difference in the effective concentrations of bretylium for the two types of nerve endings illustrates the important role of the uptake mechanism for the action of adrenergic neuron blocking drugs. In contrast to the adrenergic nerve endings the inhibitory effect of bretylium on the baroreceptors was at least partially reversible within short time and this illustrates the role of the uptake mechanism for the duration of action of adrenergic neuron blocking drugs.

Basically similar results as just described for bretylium have been obtained with guanethidine (Haeusler, Thoenen, Haefely & Huerlimann, 1968b; Haeusler, Haefely & Huerlimann, 1969b) and debrisoquine (Haeusler, unpublished results). After the adren-ergic nerve function had been impaired by bretylium, guanethidine or debrisoquine, exposure of the cat heart to amphetamine restored

not only the adrenergic nerve function but also the acetylcholine-
or KCl-evoked discharges recorded from the inferior cardiac nerve
(Haeusler, unpublished results). Apparently amphetamine displaced
the adrenergic neuron blocking agents from the adrenergic nerve
endings, the concentrations of these drugs fell below the level
necessary for local anesthesia and in this way the adrenergic
nerve endings regained their sensitivity to acetylcholine or KCl
(reappearance of evoked antidromic discharges) and were able to
respond to orthodromically conducted action potentials with transmitter release (reappearance of the effect of sympathetic nerve
stimulation).

Davey, Hayden and Scholfield (1968) found that at a time when
bretylium had blocked the acetylcholine-induced release of noradrenaline from the cat spleen, acetylcholine still induced antidromic firing in splenic C-fibres and they concluded that bretylium
impairs stimulus-transmitter release coupling. Similar observations were made by Haeusler *et al*. (1969a). These authors have,
however, provided evidence that besides adrenergic C-fibres the
spleen also contains non-adrenergic C-fibres - probably sensory
fibres - which are not affected by bretylium at concentrations
that block adrenergic neurons.

The proposed mechanism of action of adrenergic neuron blocking
drugs based on their local anesthetic activity is compatible with
the observation that local anesthetic agents act in their charged
form at the inside of the cell membrane as was convincingly demonstrated by the investigations of Narahashi, Frazier and Yamada
(1970); Frazier, Narahashi and Yamada (1970) and Narahashi and
Frazier (1975). After adrenergic neuron blocking drugs are taken
up into adrenergic nerve endings they have access to this postulated site of action.

Bretylium which apparently does not enter the amine storage vesicles of adrenergic nerve endings as well as guanethidine and
debrisoquine, which both are stored in these vesicles, produces a
similar inhibition of adrenergic nerve function and suppresses
the ability of adrenergic nerve endings to respond to acetylcholine
or KCl with asynchronous antidromically conducted discharges. It
seems that a fraction of adrenergic neuron blocking drug not bound
to intracellular storage organelles and freely diffusible in the
neuroplasm is responsible for the impairment of adrenergic function. This fraction tends to leave the adrenergic nerve ending
by diffusion along the concentration gradient which is established
by the amine pump. After leakage from the adrenergic nerve
endings the drug molecules are, however, taken up again by the
membrane. Due to this cycle rather high amounts of adrenergic
neuron blocking drugs may be permanently present within or in the
immediate vicinity of the membrane of the adrenergic nerve endings.
Maxwell and Eckhardt (1975); Eckhardt *et al*. (1977) and Huston
et al. (1977) have provided evidence for such a recycling.

In the light of the proposed hypothesis on the mode of action,
minor differences between the effects of various adrenergic neuron
blocking agents are conceivable. They could be related to differences in the local anesthetic potency, in the affinity to the

amine pump, in the equilibrium between free and bound drug within
the adrenergic nerve endings and in differences with regard to
blockade of intraneuronal monoamine oxidase.

(d) Concluding Remarks on Classical Adrenergic Neuron Blocking Drugs

From the data obtained so far, it seems safe to conclude that
adrenergic neuron blocking drugs are taken up into and accumulated within adrenergic nerve endings. As a result of this, the
membrane of the endings loses its ability both to become excited
by orthodromically conducted action potentials and to generate
antidromically conducted action potentials. The ionic permeability changes of the membrane which underly this inexcitability are
not yet elucidated. Some experimental findings (see section B(b))
have been explained by assuming that guanethidine increases the
sodium permeability of the neuronal terminal membrane and, thereby, produces depolarization. Haeusler and associates favoured
the interpretation of a membrane stabilizing action of adrenergic
neuron blocking agents (see preceding section) It has to be
considered that both stabilization and depolarization of the
neuronal terminal membrane finally lead to its inexcitability and
that some of the results described in the preceding section are
open to interpretation in both ways. However, neither bretylium
(Haeusler *et al.*, 1969a) nor guanethidine or debrisoquine
(Haeusler, unpublished results) evoked by themselves antidromically conducted discharges in adrenergic nerves as one would
expect if these agents caused depolarization of adrenergic nerve
terminals. Furthermore, these agents at no time after their
administration increased the amplitude of evoked antidromic discharges; a slight depolarization should increase the number of
terminals that are excited by a submaximal concentration of chemical stimulants and, hence, increase the amplitude of antidromic
mass action potentials in a sympathetic nerve. Finally, when
bretylium had blocked the antidromic firing induced by a low concentration of acetylcholine, this blockade was overcome by increasing the concentration of acetylcholine; such a finding is
compatible with a membrane stabilizing or hyperpolarizing action
of bretylium, but not with a depolarizing effect. In the absence
of bretylium such high concentrations of acetylcholine produce
only a transient firing followed by electrical silence. The
latter is at least initially due to a depolarization of the membrane of the adrenergic nerve endings (Haeusler *et al.*, 1968a).
Similar results have been obtained with guanethidine and debrisoquine. From an electrophysiological point of view these observations make it unlikely that adrenergic neuron blocking drugs
induce depolarization of the membrane of adrenergic nerve endings.
Furthermore, in cardiac muscle there is no indication for a depolarizing action of bretylium (Wit, Steiner & Damato, 1970;
Bigger & Jaffe, 1971) or guanethidine (Misu & Nishio, 1973).

It has been reported that elevation of the calcium concentration
to 11 mM or 50 mM reduces an established adrenergic neuron blockade produced by bretylium or guanethidine (Burn & Welsh, 1967;
Kirpekar *et al.*, 1969; Chang, Lai & Chiueh, 1971). Such a reversal of adrenergic neuron blockade is not incompatible with the
theory of a membrane stabilization of the adrenergic nerve

endings.   It is generally agreed that influx of calcium during the
action potential is essential for the release of noradrenaline in
response to nerve stimulation.   Under the influence of adrenergic
neuron blocking drugs and due to their membrane stabilizing effect
the adrenergic nerve terminals may be reached only by abortive
spikes or by electronic spread of excitation.   At a normal calcium
concentration these would not allow sufficient calcium to enter
for triggering the release of adrenaline but may do so when the
extracellular calcium concentration is increased.   This explanation fits in with the observation that after re-lowering of an
elevated calcium concentration the adrenergic neuron blockade
reappears (Burn & Welsh, 1967).   There seems to be no need to
claim a competition between calcium ions and guanethidine for a
particular site in the adrenergic nerve endings as proposed by
Kirpekar *et al.* (1969).

Thus, the concept that adrenergic neuron blocking drugs are accumulated in adrenergic nerve endings resulting in a stabilization
of the terminal membrane is compatible with virtually all experimental findings obtained so far and seems to explain best the
mode of action of this class of drugs.

III   MISCELLANEOUS AGENTS WITH ADRENERGIC NEURON BLOCKING
        PROPERTIES

Adrenergic neuron blockade has also been observed with various
agents that are not used for this purpose.   Their action on noradrenergic neurons is either their main pharmacological property
or represents a side effect.   A few examples of such agents are
given below.

    A   Coumaran Derivatives

Fielden *et al.* (1964) reported on a series of coumaran (2,3-di-
hydrobenzofuran) derivatives bearing some structural similarities
with xylocholine.   They rather selectively blocked the evoked
release of noradrenaline in different sympathetically innervated
organs; the depleting effect on cardiac noradrenaline stores and
the sympathomimetic activity of some of these compounds were considerably less marked than those of guanethidine.

    B   Emetine and Dehydroemetine

Because of the frequent occurrence of diarrhoea and arterial
hypotension in patients treated with emetine for amoebiasis, Ng
(1966) examined its effect and that of dehydroemetine (Ng & Ng,
1970) on adrenergic transmission.   In various sympathetically
innervated organs *in vitro*, the two compounds blocked the inhibitory or motor response to sympathetic nerve stimulation without
affecting the response to exogenous noradrenaline.   In the cat
nictitating membrane *in vivo*, emetine produced only a slight
adrenergic neuron blockade in a subtoxic dose (10 mg/kg i.v.).
At higher concentrations than required for adrenergic neuron
blockade, emetine blocked neuromuscular transmission in the isolated rat diaphragm.   The adrenergic neuron blockade produced by

emetine was not reversed by amphetamine. It appears questionable
whether emetine and dehydroemetine produce a relevant adrenergic
neuron block at doses that are tolerated by animals and man.

    C   Dehydrocorydaline

Dehydrocorydaline is one of the active principles of the *corydalis
bulbosa* and belongs to the class of protoberberine alkaloids. In
concentrations of 10 to 50 mM it inhibited the relaxation and the
concomitant release of noradrenaline in the guinea-pig taenia
caeci in response to electrical perivascular nerve stimulation,
as well as the contraction and noradrenaline release of the isolated rabbit pulmonary artery in response to sympathetic nerve
stimulation (Kurahashi & Fujiwara, 1976). Since the response to
exogenous noradrenaline remained unaffected at these concentrations, an adrenergic neuron blocking effect appears likely.

    IV   AGENTS AND IONS AFFECTING THE ACTION POTENTIAL

    A   Local Anesthetics

In the present context, local anesthetics may be defined as agents
that block the chemically and electrically controlled channels
for sodium and other cations in various excitable membranes to
roughly the same degree, provided that their access to the membranes is not blocked by special structures, and for which there
does not exist a specific transport mechanism resulting in the
accumulation of the agents in some cells but not in others. The
characteristic effects of local anesthetics on the evoked release
of noradrenaline as opposed to those of adrenergic neuron blocking
agents were considered in the preceding paragraph. A systematic
study of the effects of local anesthetics on the release of noradrenaline has not been carried out, but it appears from the few
available studies (e.g. Bentley, 1966) that their order of potency
in depressing the evoked release roughly parallels their local
anesthetic potency on somatic nerves. This statement does not
hold true for the effect of local anesthetics on responses of
target organs to sympathetic nerve stimulation, since some local
anesthetics, in addition to blocking the action potential, also
inhibit the neuronal uptake of noradrenaline. Local anesthetics
achieve a rapid concentration-dependent plateau of their effect
on noradrenergic endings, as opposed to the adrenergic blocking
agents (Haeusler *et al*., 1969a), and the inhibitory effect of
local anesthetics on the evoked release of noradrenaline is not
reversed by amphetamine (Bentley, 1966).

Since local anesthetics block sodium and calcium channels at
similar concentrations, they depress electrosecretory coupling in
noradrenergic nerve terminals in a twofold way, namely by abol-
ishing the sodium-mediated depolarization which normally triggers
the inflow of calcium as well as by closing the calcium channel
directly. In this respect they differ from agents affecting exclusively the sodium channel, e.g. tetrodotoxin.

B   Tetrodotoxin

Tetrodotoxin very potently and selectively blocks the sodium
channel regulated by the membrane potential, but not the chemically regulated sodium channel. It is safe to assume that tetrodotoxin affects noradrenergic nerve terminals in the same way as
their cell bodies; noradrenergic ganglion cells in the cat superior cervical ganglion no longer produce action potentials but are
still depolarized in response to dimethylphenylpiperazinium and
KCl in the presence of tetrodotoxin (Haefely, 1974).

In concentrations of 0.1 to 0.5 µg/ml, tetrodotoxin blocked the
relaxation of the isolated taenia coli muscle induced by electrical stimulation of periarterial nerves, the contraction of the
isolated vas deferens in response to transmural nerve stimulation,
and the constriction of the isolated rabbit ear artery by transmural stimulation of sympathetic nerves (Bell, 1968). In the
anesthetized cat, tetrodotoxin 10 µg i.v. abolished the pressor
response to electrical stimulation of the left thoracic sympathetic chain and of the postganglionic cardiac nerve (Feinstein &
Paimre, 1968). Tetrodotoxin perfused through the isolated perfused cat heart in a concentration of 10 nM abolished antidromic
asynchronous discharges in cardiac sympathetic nerve fibres
induced by acetylcholine, but had little effect on the acetylcholine-induced release of noradrenaline (Haeusler *et al.*, 1968a).

C   Veratrum Alkaloids

Veratrum alkaloids have prominent effects on the properties of
excitable membranes. Most important, they retard the inactivation
of the sodium-carrying system which is responsible for the ascending phase of the action potential spike, and they increase the
sodium and potassium permeability (Ulbricht, 1969). The former
effect results in an increase of the negative after-potential and
the latter in a decrease of the resting membrane potential. De-
pending on the dose and the alkaloid tested, multiple and partly
opposite effects were observed on pre- and postsynaptic events
in sympathetic ganglia (see Haefely, 1972; 1978).

The evoked release of noradrenaline in the isolated perfused cat
spleen was reduced by about 50% by 1 µg/ml protoveratrine
(Kirpekar *et al.*, 1972). This effect was explained by assuming
that, in the concentration used, protoveratrine enhanced the
potassium efflux, which in turn would depress the entry of calcium
during the action potential. The mechanism was thought to be
similar to the situation in which potassium efflux was increased
by raising its concentration in the perfusion fluid (see below).
α-Veratrine or veratrine added to the fluid perfusing the isolated cat heart induced repetitive antidromic firing in cardiac
sympathetic fibres and release of noradrenaline into the perfusate
(Haeusler, unpublished). In the absence of systematic studies of
various concentrations of veratrum alkaloids on the transmitter
output from noradrenergic nerves, it appears likely that both
increases and decreases of the evoked release can be obtained
with varying concentrations of the alkaloid and varying experimental conditions.

D   Tetraethylammonium, Aminopyridines, Barium, Rubidium,
     Nickel and Cesium

These cations have in common the property of prolonging the duration of the action potential of nerve and muscle fibres. The
study of their effect on the evoked release of noradrenaline is,
therefore, of considerable interest.

(a) Tetraethylammonium
Tetraethylammonium depresses the effect of nicotine receptor
stimulants at postganglionic autonomic neurons either by blocking
nicotine receptors or the receptor-regulated sodium channel. At
the squid giant ganglion (Katz & Miledi, 1969) and at the motor
nerve endings (Koketsu, 1958; Collier & Exley, 1963), tetraethylammonium enhances the evoked transmitter release. It is very
probable that this is due to the well-known property of the tetraethylammonium ion to prolong the duration of action potentials.
This prolongation is the result of a specific elimination of the
potassium permeability (see Armstrong, 1969). In the superior
cervical ganglion of the rabbit *in vitro*, tetraethylammonium
(5 mM) prolonged the duration of the antidromic action potential
of single cells up to 6 fold by slowing down the repolarization
phase (Dun *et al.*, 1976).

Bevan (1963) and van Maanen and Wertz (1966) observed an enhancement by tetraethylammonium of the contractile responses of the
pulmonary artery and of the vas deferens, to sympathetic nerve
stimulation. Using the isolated perfused cat spleen, Thoenen,
Haefely and Staehelin (1967) showed that tetraethylammonium increased the amount of noradrenaline recovered in the perfusate
after splenic nerve stimulation; this effect was not due to an
inhibition of the uptake of noradrenaline. In isolated splenic
nerve bundles, tetraethylammonium (30 mM) prolonged the evoked
mass action potential. Although this concentration was about 30
times higher than that required to enhance the noradrenaline output, the authors assumed that the ion may act at lower concentrations in the fine intrasplenic terminals which are better accessible to the quaternary ammonium ion. Support for this view was
their finding that tetraethylammonium blocked antidromic asynchronous firing in the splenic nerves induced by infusing acetylcholine at concentrations reducing the evoked output of noradrenaline.
Moreover, the facilitating effect of tetraethylammonium was absent
when the splenic nerves were stimulated at the maximum frequency
at which these nerves can conduct action potentials.

Kirpekar *et al.* (1972; 1976) confirmed the findings of Thoenen
et al. (1967) and obtained additional evidence for the mode of
action of tetraethylammonium. The ion enhanced the noradrenaline
output in the presence of blockade of uptake and of presynaptic
α-adrenoceptors with phenoxybenzamine. Furthermore, tetraethylammonium partially counteracted the reduction of noradrenaline
release produced by cobalt, which is believed to block calcium
permeability. Tetraethylammonium facilitated the release of noradrenaline at all calcium concentrations in the perfusate, but
the maximum effect was obtained at 2.5 mM Ca^{2+}. Since the
ammonium ion did not enhance the noradrenaline release induced by

high potassium, Kirpekar *et al.* (1972) concluded that it did not
directly facilitate the influx of Ca^{2+} ions; rather, tetraethylammonium produced its effect by inactivating the potassium current,
thereby prolonging the action potential and the time during which
Ca^{2+} ions can enter the noradrenergic nerve terminals. Gillespie
& Tilmisany (1976) studied the effect of tetraethylammonium on
the release of noradrenaline in the isolated rat anococcygeus
muscle when the noradrenergic motor nerves were excited by field
stimulation. In concentrations of 0.125 to 20 mM, the contractile
response of the anococcygeus muscle was potentiated while the
responses to exogenous noradrenaline remained unaltered. Tetraethylammonium also reversed the blocking action of guanethidine.
At higher concentrations, the ion directly released noradrenaline.

The well-documented facilitatory effect of tetraethylammonium is
adequately explained by its retarding effect on the potassium
permeability. This prolongs the duration of action potentials
and, thereby, the time during which Ca^{2+} ions are allowed to move
into the terminal to release noradrenaline. At higher concentrations, the ion induces the release of noradrenaline in the absence
of evoked action potentials; it is not known, whether this effect
is also due to a decreased potassium efflux, a direct increase of
the calcium conductance, or to the ammonium ion acting as a charge
carrier like Ca^{2+}. In addition to increasing the amount of the
evoked release of noradrenaline, tetraethylammonium also potentiates the contractile response of smooth muscles to noradrenaline
and high potassium and produces by itself a calcium-dependent
contraction, effects which have been ascribed to a combination of
reduced potassium permeability and increased calcium permeability
(Haeusler & Thorens, 1975).

(b) Aminopyridines
4-Aminopyridine, a highly ionized molecule, is considerably more
potent than tetraethylammonium in depressing the K^+ current of
the action potential of the squid giant axon (Meves & Pichon,
1975) and of the frog skeletal muscle (Gillespie & Hutter, 1975)
and, thereby, prolonging the repolarization phase of nerve and
muscle action potentials. It potentiates neuromuscular transmission by increasing the evoked output of acetylcholine and is, therefore, used as an anticurare agent (Bowman, Khan & Savage, 1977).

The contractile responses of the isolated rabbit vas deferens to
electrical transmural stimulation, particularly at low frequencies, were markedly potentiated by 4-aminopyridine in concentrations between 0.01 and 1 mM (Johns, Golko, Lauzon & Paton, 1976).
The compound also increased the evoked release of [^{3}H]metaraminol
into the medium, but did not affect to a relevant degree the
accumulation of [^{3}H]noradrenaline by the vas deferens. It is,
therefore, very likely that 4-aminopyridine facilitates the
evoked release of noradrenaline by increasing the duration of the
action potential of noradrenergic nerve terminals, although direct
effects of the compound on the free intracellular Ca^{2+} concentration cannot be excluded (Bowman *et al.*, 1977). Johns *et al.*
(1976) found that the activity of 4-aminopyridine is also present
in pyridine derivatives containing primary amino groups in other
positions.

(c) Barium

The Ba^{2+} ion prolongs the duration of the action potential in nerves (Lorente de Nó & Feng, 1946; Greengard & Straub, 1959; Koketsu et al., 1963) and induces repetitive responses from nerve terminals (Dun & Feng, 1940) and non-terminal axons (Lorente de Nó & Feng, 1946). The permeability of the nodes of Ranvier of peripheral nerves to potassium is reduced more than that to sodium (Lüttgau, 1954). Barium increases the evoked release of acetylcholine from preganglionic cholinergic neurons in the perfused cat superior cervical ganglion (Douglas et al., 1961).

The effect of barium on the evoked release of noradrenaline has been investigated in the isolated perfused cat spleen by Kirpekar et al. (1972). At concentrations between 0.8 and 10 mM, $BaCl_2$ enhanced the spontaneous as well as the stimulation-induced noradrenaline output. This facilitating effect was antagonized by increasing the concentration of potassium in the perfusing medium. The tetraethylammonium-like effect of the Ba^{2+} ion seems to be best explained by the reduction of the potassium efflux. This may enhance the inward movement of calcium during the action potential and possibly also at rest.

(d) Rubidium

The Rb^+ ion inactivates the potassium conductance increase in frog muscle (Adrian, 1964) and markedly prolongs the action potential of the perfused squid axon (Baker et al., 1962).

In the isolated perfused cat spleen, the replacement of K^+ by Rb^+ (5.9 mM) almost doubled the evoked release of noradrenaline (Kirpekar et al., 1972). Adding RbCl (2 mM) to a Krebs solution potentiated the sustained secondary contractile response of the isolated rabbit vas deferens to transmural stimulation and enhanced the evoked release of [3H]metaraminol previously taken up (Johns & Paton, 1976). Although a prolongation of action potentials in noradrenergic neurons has not been demonstrated, such a mechanism may best explain the facilitatory action of the Rb^+ ion.

(e) Nickel

The Ni^{2+} ion produces an enormous prolongation of the action potential of single nodes of toad nerves and makes its membrane highly resistant to depolarization by potassium (Tasaki, 1959). In addition, however, Ni^{2+}, like other transition elements, blocks the late phase of calcium entry during depolarization in giant axons (Baker et al., 1971) and blocks the transmitter release in stellate ganglia of the squid axon (Katz & Miledi, 1969).

In the isolated perfused cat spleen, $NiCl_2$ (2.5 mM) almost completely blocked the stimulation-induced outflow of noradrenaline (Kirpekar et al., 1972). This strong inhibitory effect of nickel strongly suggests that it is not the prolongation of the action potential as such which increases the release of noradrenaline in the case of tetraethylammonium, barium, and rubidium, but rather the increased inflow of calcium; since the Ni^{2+} ions depress the permeability of both potassium and calcium, the net effect on the release of noradrenaline is a depression.

(f) Cesium

Cesium ions prolong nerve action potentials by depressing the
repolarizing K^+-conductance increase (Sjodin, 1966) and facilitate
the evoked transmitter release at mammalian neuromuscular junctions
(Korey & Hamilton, 1974) and sympathetic ganglia (Hancock & Volle,
1969). In noradrenergic ganglion cells of the cat superior cervical ganglion perfused *in situ* with media containing CsCl (5.6 mM)
instead of KCl, both amplitude and duration of orthodromic action
potentials increased (Hancock & Volle, 1969).

In the isolated rabbit vas deferens preparation, the addition of
2-5 mM Cs^+ markedly potentiated the contractile responses to low-
frequency transmural stimulation (Johns & Paton, 1975). This
effect occurred without changes of the muscular responses to exogenous noradrenaline and it was still present after inhibition of
the biosynthesis of prostaglandins by indomethacin. CsCl (2 mM)
enhanced the evoked release of [^{3}H]metaraminol from vasa deferentia previously loaden with this amine. It is resonable to
assume that Cs^+ facilitates the evoked release of noradrenaline
by prolonging the action potential also in noradrenergic nerve
terminals.

E   Potassium

KCl in concentrations above 50 mM induced a short-lasting asynchronous firing of action potentials in noradrenergic nerves of
the isolated perfused cat heart and a concentration-dependent
release of noradrenaline into the perfusate (Haeusler *et al.*,
1968a). In a range of concentrations above normal and below
those that induce the release of noradrenaline, KCl was found to
depress the impulse-induced release of noradrenaline in the isolated perfused cat spleen (Kirpekar *et al.*, 1972) and in the isolated saphenous vein of the dog (Lorenz & Vanhoutte, 1975). These
concentrations are likely to produce a depolarization of noradrenergic nerve terminals and to reduce the amplitude of the action
potentials without blocking their conduction (Furness, 1970).
Kirpekar *et al.* (1972) explained the depression of noradrenaline
release in media with increased concentrations of potassium by a
reduction of the inward movement of calcium during the action potential. Calcium influx is assumed to be decreased by the enhanced outward movement of potassium in the presence of an increased external potassium concentration. The observed reduction
by potassium of the amplitude of the antidromic action potential
in frog sympathetic ganglion cells, which is more marked than the
parallel reduction of the resting membrane potential (Blackman
et al., 1963), might also explain the reduction of the impulse-
induced release of noradrenaline in the presence of increased
potassium.

V   SUMMARY

The compounds and inorganic ions described in this chapter modify
the stimulus-evoked release of noradrenaline in part in opposite

directions and by different molecular mechanisms. Yet, they produce an effect which is common to all of them, i.e., they affect
the initial events in the excitation secretion coupling at noradrenergic nerve terminals. Put in the simplest term, they either
depress or enhance the stimulus-induced influx of Ca^{2+} into the
terminal and, hence, modify the amount of the ion which triggers
the release of the transmitter from intracellular stores. The
inward movement of Ca^{2+} is governed by the Ca^{2+} channel, which is
opened by a depolarization of the neuronal membrane either during
an action potential (electrical stimulus) or in the presence of
high extracellular K^+ or nicotinic stimulants (chemical stimulus).
The stimulus-induced influx of Ca^{2+} can be affected by a direct
action on the Ca^{2+} channel or by primary actions on other membrane
properties that regulate the Ca^{2+} channel.

Classical local anesthetics reduce the influx of Ca^{2+} by a rather
general effect on membranes. Although they have little effect on
resting ionic conductances, they block induced changes of the
conductances for Na^+, K^+, and Ca^{2+} in roughly similar concentrations. Consequently, they depress and eventually block both the
electrical and chemical release of noradrenaline. The effect of
local anesthetics on noradrenergic nerve terminals is not different from that on other excitable membranes.

Tetrodotoxin blocks selectively the electrically controlled Na^+
channel, thereby preventing the conduction and formation of normal action potential spikes in noradrenergic nerve terminals.
Since tetrodotoxin does not affect the depolarization induced by
high potassium or nicotinic stimulants and the resulting influx
of Ca^{2+}, the neurotoxin blocks the electrically-induced but not
the chemically-induced release of noradrenaline.

Adrenergic neuron blocking agents seem to owe their rather selective effect on noradrenergic nerve terminals to a combination of
two properties, namely a moderate membrane stabilizing (local
anesthetic) activity and the high affinity for the amine uptake
mechanism in the noradrenergic neuronal membrane. The latter results in the selective accumulation of adrenergic neuron blockers
in noradrenergic terminals and in the build-up of the high concentration of these agents in the neurolemma required to produce
a stabilization of these terminals. Other effects of some adrenergic neuron blocking agents, such as depletion of noradrenaline,
indirect sympathomimetic effects, inhibition of monoamine uptake
and of the intraneuronal monoamine oxidase, are not essential for
their neuron blocking action, but may modify the latter.

Veratrum alkaloids have complex effects on properties of excitable membranes and, hence, on noradrenergic nerve terminals. By
increasing the resting Na^+- and K^+-conductances of the membrane
and by retarding the inactivation of the Na^+-carrying system,
they initiate a repetitive firing in noradrenergic terminals and
release noradrenaline under certain conditions. Lower concentrations depress the electrical release of noradrenaline, possibly
by increasing the efflux of K^+ and, thereby, reducing the influx
of Ca^{2+}.

The cations tetraethylammonium, Ba^{2+}, and Rb^+ have in common the property of prolonging the action potential by reducing the K^+-conductance increase initiated by the ascending phase of the action potential spike. Prolongation of the spike and reduction of the K^+-efflux augment the amount of Ca^{2+} moving into the terminal and, in consequence, facilitate the stimulus-induced release of noradrenaline.

Nickel, although prolonging the action potential, reduces not only the K^+-conductance, but also the permeability to Ca^{2+}. It depresses the stimulus-induced release of noradrenaline, demonstrating that it is not the depolarization as such which determines the transmitter release, but rather the amount of Ca^{2+} moving into the neuron during depolarization.

Moderate increase of extracellular K^+ depresses the stimulus-induced release of noradrenaline by reducing the influx of trigger-Ca^{2+} either as the consequence of a decreased action potential amplitude or of an enhanced K^+ efflux or of both.

The compounds and inorganic ions described in this chapter can, therefore, be characterized as agents which inhibit the influx of trigger-Ca^{2+} by affecting one or more of the membrane properties that regulate the Ca^{2+} influx. They do not seem to compete directly with Ca^{2+} at its transport sites in the membrane or with its intracellular actions on the transmitter release mechanisms.

VI   REFERENCES

Abbs, E.T. (1966). The release of catecholamines by choline 2,6-xylyl ether, bretylium and guanethidine. *Br. J. Pharmacol.* 26, 162-171.

Abbs, E.T. & Dodd, M.G. (1974). The relation between the adrenergic neurone-blocking and noradrenaline-depleting actions of some guanethidine derivatives. *Br. J. Pharmacol.* 51, 237-247.

Abbs, E.T. & Pycock, C.J. (1973). The effects of bretylium on the subcellular distribution of noradrenaline and on adrenergic nerve function in rat heart. *Br. J. Pharmacol.* 49, 11-22.

Abbs, E.T. & Robertson, M.I. (1970). Selective depletion of noradrenaline: a proposed mechanism of the adrenergic neurone-blocking action of bretylium. *Br. J. Pharmacol.* 38, 776-791.

Abercrombie, G.F. & Davies, B.N. (1963). The action of guanethidine with particular reference to the sympathetic nervous system. *Br. J. Pharmacol.* 20, 171-177.

Adrian, R.H. (1964). The rubidium and potassium permeability of frog muscle membrane. *J. Physiol. (Lond.)* 175, 134-159.

Almgren, O. & Lundberg, D. (1976). Uptake and retention of ^{14}C-bretylium in degenerating postganglionic sympathetic nerves of the rat. *Acta Pharmacol. Toxicol.* 38, 422-432.

Armstrong, C.M. (1969). Inactivation of the potassium conductance and related phenomena caused by quaternary ammonium injection in squid axons. *J. Gen. Physiol.* 54, 553-573.

Athos, W.J., McHugh, B.P., Fineberg, S.E. & Hilton, J.C. (1962). The effects of guanethidine on the adrenal medulla. *J. Pharmacol. Exp. Ther.* 137, 229-234.

Baker, P.F., Blaustein, M.P., Hodgkin, A.L. & Steinhardt, R.A. (1969). The influence of calcium on sodium efflux in squid axons. *J. Physiol. (Lond.)* 200, 431-458.

Baker, P.F., Hodgkin, A.L. & Shaw, T.I. (1962). The effects of changes in internal ionic concentrations on the electrical properties of perfused giant axons. *J. Physiol. (Lond.)* 164, 335-374.

Baker, P.F., Meves, H. & Ridgway, E.B. (1971). Phasic entry of calcium in response to depolarization of giant axons of *Loligo forbesi*. *J. Physiol. (Lond.)* 216, 70P.

Bell, C. (1968). Differential effects of tetrodotoxin on sympathomimetic actions of nicotine and tyramine. *Br. J. Pharmacol.* 32, 96-103.

Bentley, G.A. (1966). The effect of local anaesthetic and anti-adrenaline drugs on the response of sympathetically innervated smooth muscle preparations to electrical stimulation at different frequencies. *Br. J. Pharmacol.* 27, 64-80.

Bevan, J.A. (1963). Action of tetraethylammonium chloride on the sympathetic ganglia-pulmonary artery preparation. *J. Pharmacol. Exp. Ther.* 140, 193-198.

Bigger, J.T. & Jaffe, C.C. (1971). The effect of bretylium tosylate on the elctrophysiologic properties of ventricular muscle and Purkinje fibres. *Amer. J. Cardiol.* 27, 82-92.

Blackman, J.G., Ginsborg, B.L. & Ray, C. (1963). Some effects of changes in ionic concentration on the action potential of sympathetic ganglion cells in the frog. *J. Physiol. (Lond.)* 167, 374-388.

Blaustein, M.P. (1977). Effects of internal and external cations and of ATP on sodium-calcium and calcium-calcium exchange in squid axons. *Biophys. J.* 20, 79-111.

Blaustein, M.P. & Ector, A.C. (1976). Carrier-mediated sodium-dependent and calcium-dependent calcium efflux from pinched-off presynaptic nerve terminals (synaptosomes) *in vitro*. *Biochim. Biophys. Acta* 419, 295-308.

Boullin, D.J., Costa, E. & Brodie, B.B. (1966). Discharge of tritium-labelled guanethidine by sympathetic nerve stimulation as evidence that guanethidine is a false transmitter. *Life Sci.* 5, 803-808.

Boullin, D.J. & O'Brien, R.A. (1969). The accumulation of guanethidine by human blood platelets. *Br. J. Pharmacol.* 35, 90-102.

Boura, A.L.A., Copp, F.C. & Green, A.F. (1959). New antiadrenergic compounds. *Nature (Lond.)* 184, BA70-BA71.

Boura, A.L.A., Copp, F.C., Duncombe, W.G., Green, A.F. & McCoubrey, A. (1960). The selective accumulation of bretylium in sympathetic ganglia and their postganglionic nerves. *Br. J. Pharmacol.* 15, 265-270.

Boura, A.L.A., Duncombe, W.G. & McCoubrey, A. (1961). The distribution of some quaternary ammonium salts in the peripheral nervous system of cats in relation to the adrenergic blocking action of bretylium. *Br. J. Pharmacol.* 17, 92-100.

Boura, A.L.A. & Green, A.F. (1959). The actions of bretylium: adrenergic neurone blocking and other effects. *Br. J. Pharmacol.* 14, 536-348.

Bowman, W.C., Khan, H.H. & Savage, A.O. (1977). Some antagonists of dantrolene sodium on the isolated diaphragm muscle of the rat. *J. Pharm. Pharmacol.* 29, 616-625.

Boyd, H., Chang, V. & Rand, M.J. (1961). The local anaesthetic activity of bretylium in relation to its action in blocking sympathetic responses. *Arch. Int. Pharmacodyn.* 131, 10-23.

Brinley, F.J., Spangler, S.G. & Mullins, L.J. (1975). Calcium and EDTA fluxes in dialyzed squid axons. *J. Gen. Physiol.* 66, 223-250.

Brodie, B.B., Chang, C.C. & Costa, E. (1965). On the mechanism of action of guanethidine and bretylium. *Br. J. Pharmacol.* 25, 171-178.

Burn, J.H. & Welsh, F. (1967). The effect of calcium in removing the blocking action of bretylium and guanethidine. *Br. J. Pharmacol.* 31, 74-81.

Cass, R., Kuntzman, R. & Brodie, B.B. (1960). Norepinephrine depletion as a possible mechanism of action of guanethidine (Su 5864), a new hypotensive agent. *Proc. Soc. Exp. Biol. Med.* 103, 871-872.

Cass, R. & Spriggs, T.L. (1961). Tissue amine levels and sympathetic blockade after guanethidine and bretylium. *Br. J. Pharmacol.* 17, 442-450.

Chang, C.C., Chang, J.C. & Su, C.Y. (1967). Studies on the interactions of guanethidine and bretylium with noradrenaline stores.
Br. J. Pharmacol. 30, 213-223.

Chang, C.C., Costa, E. & Brodie, B.B. (1965). Interactions of
guanethidine with adrenergic neurons. *J. Pharmacol. Exp. Ther.*
147, 303-312.

Chang, C.C., Lai, F.M. & Chiueh, C.C. (1971). Effects of calcium
on smooth muscles and on the adrenergic neuron blocking action
of guanethidine. *Arch. Int. Pharmacodyn.* 190, 34-46.

Clarke, D.E. & Leach, G.D.H. (1968). The influence of bretylium
on the interactions of infused sympathomimetic amines and
tyramine in the reserpine-treated pithed rat. *Br. J.
Pharmacol.* 32, 392-401.

Collier, B. & Exley, K.A. (1963). Mechanism of the antagonism by
tetraethylammonium of neuromuscular block due to d-tubocurarine
or calcium deficiency. *Nature* 199, 702-703.

Davey, M.J., Hayden, M.L. & Scholfield, P.C. (1968). The effects
of bretylium on C fibre excitation and noradrenaline release
by acetylcholine and electrical stimulation. *Br. J. Pharmacol.*
34, 377-387.

Day, M.D. (1962). Effect of sympathomimetic amines on the
blocking action of guanethidine, bretylium and xylocholine.
Br. J. Pharmacol. 18, 421-439.

Day, M.D. & Rand, M.J. (1963). Evidence for a competitive antagonism of guanethidine by dexamphetamine. *Br. J. Pharmacol.*
20, 17-28.

Douglas, W.W. & Gray, J.A.B. (1953). The excitant action of
acetylcholine and other substances on cutaneous sensory pathways and its prevention by hexamethonium and D-tubocurarine.
J. Physiol. (Lond.) 119, 118-128.

Douglas, W.W., Lywood, D.W. & Straub, R.W. (1961). The stimulant
effect of barium on the release of acetylcholine from the superior cervical ganglion. *J. Physiol. (Lond.)* 156, 515-522.

Douglas, W.W. & Ritchie, T.M. (1960). The excitatory action of
acetylcholine on cutaneous non-myelinated fibres. *J. Physiol.
(Lond.)* 150, 501-514.

Dun, F.T. & Feng, T.P. (1940). Studies on the neuro-muscular
junction. XX. The site of origin of the junctional after discharge in muscles treated with guanidine, barium or eserine.
Chin. J. Physiol. 15, 433-444.

Dun, N., Nishi, S. & Karczmar, A.G. (1976). Electrical properties of the membrane of denervated mammalian sympathetic
ganglion cells. *Neuropharmacol.* 15, 219-223.

Eckhardt, S.B., Maxwell, R.A. & Copp, F.C. (1977). Influence of desipramine on the uptake and efflux of radiolabelled brety-lium and bethanidine in the adventitial and media-intimal layers of rabbit aortic strips. *Blood Vessels* 14, 303-317.

Exley, K.A. (1957). The blocking action of choline 2:6-xylyl ether bromide on adrenergic nerves. *Br. J. Pharmacol.* 12, 297-305.

Exley, K.A. (1960). The persistence of adrenergic nerve conduc-tion after TM 10 or bretylium in the cat. In: *Adrenergic Mechanism* (CIBA Foundation), pp. 158-161, Churchill, London.

Feinstein, M.B. & Paimre, M. (1968). Mechanism of cardiovascular action of tetrodotoxin in the cat. *Circulation Res.* 23, 553-565.

Ferry, C.B. (1963). The sympathomimetic effect of acetylcholine on the spleen of the cat. *J. Physiol. (Lond.)* 167, 487-504.

Fielden, R., Roe, A.M. & Willey, G.L. (1964). The adrenergic-neurone blocking action of some coumaran compounds. *Br. J. Pharmacol. Chemother.* 23, 486-507.

Foster, R.W. (1967). The potentiation of the responses to nor-adrenaline and isoprenaline of the guinea-pig isolated tracheal chain preparation by desipramine, cocaine, phentolamine, pheno-xybenzamine, guanethidine, metanephrine and cooling. *Br. J. Pharmacol.* 31, 466-482.

Frazier, D.T., Narahashi, T. & Yamada, M. (1970). The site of action and active form of local anesthetics. II. Experiments with quaternary compounds. *J. Pharmacol. Exp. Ther.* 171, 45-51.

Freis, E.D. (1965). Guanethidine. *Prog. Cardiovasc. Dis.* 8, 183-193.

Furchgott, R.F., Garcia, P.S., Wakade, A.R. & Cervoni, P. (1971). Interactions of bretylium and other drugs on guinea-pig atria: evidence for inhibition of neuronal monoamine oxidase by bre-tylium. *J. Pharmacol. Exp. Ther.* 179, 171-185.

Furness, J.B. (1970). The effect of external potassium ion con-centration on autonomic neuromuscular transmission. *Pflügers Arch. Ges. Physiol.* 317, 310-326.

Gaffney, T.E., Chidsey, C.A. & Braunwald, E. (1963). Study of the relationship between the neurotransmitter store and adren-ergic nerve block induced by reserpine and guanethidine. *Circ. Res.* 12, 264-268.

Gaitondé, B.B. & Nimbkar, A.Y. (1973). Interaction of bretylium and guanethidine on the relaxations of the rat isolated fundal strip preparation, evoked by indirect stimulation. *Br. J. Pharmacol.* 47, 268-271.

Gerkens, J.F., McCulloch, M.W. & Wilson, J. (1969). Mechanism of antagonism between guanethidine and dexamphetamine. *Br. J. Pharmacol*. 35, 563-572.

Giachetti, A. & Hollenbeck, R.A. (1976). Extra-vesicular binding of noradrenaline and guanethidine in the adrenergic neurones of the rat heart: a proposed site of action of adrenergic neurone blocking agents. *Br. J. Pharmacol*. 58, 497-504.

Giachetti, A. & Shore, P.A. (1967). Monoamine oxidase inhibition in the adrenergic neuron by bretylium, debrisoquine, and other adrenergic neuron blocking agents. *Biochem. Pharmacol*. 16, 237-238.

Gillespie, J.I. & Hutter, O.F. (1975). The actions of 4-amino-pyridine on the delayed potassium current in skeletal muscle fibres. *J. Physiol. (Lond.)* 252, 70P-71P.

Gillespie, J.S. & Tilmisany, A.K. (1976). The action of tetra-ethylammonium chloride on the response of the rat anococcygeus muscle to motor and inhibitory nerve stimulation and to some drugs. *Br. J. Pharmacol*. 58, 47-55.

Glitsch, H.G., Reuter, H. & Scholz, H. (1970). The effect of the internal sodium concentration on calcium fluxes in isolated guinea-pig auricles. *J. Physiol*. 209, 25-43.

Greengard, P. & Straub, R.W. (1959). Restoration by barium of action potentials in sodium-deprived mammalian B and C fibres. *J. Physiol. (Lond.)* 145, 562-569.

Gulati, O.D. & Jaykar, S. (1971). Factors affecting the action of guanethidine on adrenergic neurons. *Br. J. Pharmacol*. 42, 352-363.

Haefely, W. (1972). Electrophysiology of the adrenergic neuron. In: *Handbook of Experimental Pharmacology* (eds.) H. Blaschko & E. Muscholl, Vol. 33, pp. 661-725, Springer-Verlag, Berlin.

Haefely, W. (1974). The effects of 1,1-dimethyl-4-phenylpipera-zinium (DMPP) in the cat superior cervical ganglion *in situ*. *Naunyn-Schmiedeberg's Arch. Pharmacol*. 281, 57-91.

Haefely, W. (1978). Non-nicotinic chemical stimulation of auto-nomic ganglia. In: *Handbook of Experimental Pharmacology* (ed.) D.A. Kharkevich, Springer-Verlag, Berlin (in press).

Haeusler, G. (1971). Early pre- and postjunctional effects of 6-hydroxydopamine. *J. Pharmacol. Exp. Ther*. 178, 49-62.

Haeusler, G., Haefely, W. & Huerlimann, A. (1969a). On the mechanism of the adrenergic nerve blocking action of bretylium. *Naunyn-Schmiedebergs Arch. Pharmak*. 265, 260-277.

Haeusler, G., Haefely, W. & Huerlimann, A. (1969b).   Zum Mechanismus der adrenerg blockierenden Wirkung von Bretylium und
   Guanethidin.   *Naunyn-Schmiedebergs Arch. Pharmak.* **264**, 241-243.

Haeusler, G., Lorez, H.P., Bartholini, G., Kettler, R. & Tranzer,
   J.P. (1974).   Absence of degeneration of adrenergic neurons
   after prolonged treatment with debrisoquin.   *J. Pharmacol.
   Exp. Ther.* **189**, 646-658.

Haeusler, G., Thoenen, H., Haefely, W. & Huerlimann, A. (1968a).
   Electrical events in cardiac adrenergic nerves and noradren-
   aline release from the heart induced by acetylcholine and KCl.
   Naunyn-Schmiedebergs Arch. Pharmak. Exp. Path. **261**, 389-411.

Haeusler, G., Thoenen, H., Haefely, W. & Huerlimann, A. (1968b).
   Durch Acetylcholin hervorgerufene antidrome Aktivität im
   kardialen Sympathicus und Noradrenalinfreisetzung unter Guanethidin.   *Helv. Physiol. Pharmacol. Acta* **26**, CR223-CR225.

Haeusler, G. & Thorens, S. (1975).   The effects of tetraethylammonium on contraction, membrane potential and calcium permeability of vascular smooth muscle.   Les Colloques de l'Ins-
   .titut National de la Santé et de la Recherche Médicale,
   INSERM 50, 363-368.

Hanahoe, T.H.P., Ireson, J.D. & Large, B.J. (1969).   Interactions
   between guanethidine and inhibitors of noradrenaline uptake.
   Arch. Int. Pharmacodyn. **182**, 349-353.

Hancock, J.C. & Volle, R.L. (1969).   Enhancement by cesium ions
   of ganglionic hyperpolarization induced by dimethylphenylpiperazinium (DMPP) and repetitive preganglionic stimulation.
   J. Pharmacol. Exp. Ther. **169**, 201-210.

Hertting, G., Axelrod, J. & Patrick, R.W. (1962).   Actions of
   bretylium and guanethidine on the uptake and release of [3]H-
   noradrenaline.   *Br. J. Pharmacol.* **18**, 161-166.

Hey, P. & Willey, G.L. (1954).   Choline 2:6-xylyl ether bromide;
   an active quaternary local anaesthetic.   *Br. J. Pharmacol.* **9**,
   471-475.

Hosotani, T. & Misu, Y. (1977).   Sodium sensitive active transport of bretylium into adrenergic neurons from the development
   of blockade in rabbit ileum.   *Arch. Int. Pharmacodyn.* **226**,
   235-245.

Huston, L.J., Golko, D.S. & Paton, D.M. (1977).   Effect of neuronal uptake inhibitors on the adrenergic neuron blockade produced by guanethidine in rabbit vas deferens.   *Can. J. Physiol.
   Pharmacol.* **55**, 609-614.

Johns, A., Golko, D.S., Lauzon, P.A. & Paton, D.M. (1976). The potentiating effects of 4-aminopyridine on adrenergic transmission in the rabbit vas deferens. *Eur. J. Pharmacol.* 38, 71-78.

Johns, A. & Paton, D.M. (1975). The effect of caesium on adrenergic transmission in rabbit vas deferens. *Can. J. Physiol. Pharmacol.* 53, 410-415.

Johns, A. & Paton, D.M. (1976). Effect of rubidium on responses of rabbit vas deferens to transmural stimulation and to noradrenaline. *Eur. J. Pharmacol.* 35, 145-150.

Katz, B. & Miledi, R. (1969). Tetrodotoxin resistant electric activity in presynaptic terminals. *J. Physiol. (Lond.)* 203, 459-487.

Kirpekar, S.M. & Furchgott, R.F. (1972). Interaction of tyramine and guanethidine in the spleen of the cat. *J. Pharmacol. Exp. Ther.* 180, 38-46.

Kirpekar, S.M., Prat, J.C., Puig, M. & Wakade, A.R. (1972). Modification of the evoked release of noradrenaline from the perfused cat spleen by various ions and agents. *J. Physiol. (Lond.)* 221, 601-615.

Kirpekar, S.M., Wakade, A.R., Dixon, W. & Prat, J.C. (1969). Effect of cocaine, phenoxybenzamine and calcium on the inhibition of norepinephrine output from the cat spleen by guanethidine. *J. Pharmacol. Exp. Ther.* 165, 166-175.

Kirpekar, S.M., Wakade, A.R. & Prat, J.C. (1976). Effect of tetraethylammonium and barium on the release of noradrenaline from the perfused cat spleen by nerve stimulation and potassium. *Naunyn-Schmiedeberg's Arch. Pharmacol.* 294, 23-29.

Koe, B.K. & Constantine, J.W. (1972). Blocking H[3]-norepinephrine uptake and some guanethidine-induced effects with tricyclic psychotherapeutic drugs. *Arch. Int. Pharmacodyn.* 195, 71-80.

Koketsu, K. (1958). Action of tetraethylammonium chloride on neuromuscular transmission in frogs. *Am. J. Physiol.* 193, 213-218.

Koketsu, K., Nishi, S. & Soeda, H. (1963). Effects of calcium ions on prolonged action potentials and hyperpolarizing responses. *Nature* 200, 786-787.

Korey, A. & Hamilton, J.T. (1974). The effect of replacement of potassium by caesium ions on neuromuscular blockade of the rat phrenic nerve-diaphragm preparation *in vitro*. *Can. J. Physiol. Pharmacol.* 52, 61-69.

Kubo, T. & Misu, Y. (1974). Mode of action of guanethidine on adrenergic neurons and its dependence on sodium. *Japan. J. Pharmacol.* 24, 307-318.

Kurahashi, K. & Fujiwara, M. (1976). Adrenergic neuron blocking action of dehydrocorydaline isolated from Corydalis bulbosa. *Can. J. Physiol. Pharmacol.* 54, 287-293.

Lorente de No, R. & Feng, T.P. (1946). Analysis of the effect of barium upon nerve with particular reference to rhythmic activity. *J. Cell. Comp. Physiol.* 28, 397-464.

Lorenz, R.R. & Vanhoutte, P.M. (1975). Inhibition of adrenergic neurotransmission in isolated veins of the dog by potassium ions. *J. Physiol.* 246, 479-500.

Lüttgau, H.-C. (1954). Ueber die Bedingungen zur Auslösung rhythmischer Erregungen an markhaltigen Nervenfasern nach Na^+- und Ba^+-Zusatz, sowie Ca^{++}-Entzug. *Zeitschr. Biol.* 107, 34-46.

Malmfors, T. & Abrams, W.R. (1970). The effects of debrisoquin and bretylium on adrenergic nerves as revealed by fluorescence histochemistry. *J. Pharmacol. Exp. Ther.* 174, 99-110.

Maxwell, R.A. & Eckhardt, S.B. (1975). Concerning the role of the amine pump of the adrenergic innervation of rabbit aorta in sustaining the neuron blockade produced by bethanidine and bretylium. *Blood Vessels* 12, 166-180.

Maxwell, R.A., Plummer, A.J., Schneider, F., Povalski, H. & Daniel, A.I. (1960). Pharmacology of [2-(octahydro-1-azocinyl) -ethyl]-guanidine sulfate (SU-5864). *J. Pharmacol. Exp. Ther.* 128, 22-29.

Meves, H. & Pichon, Y. (1975). Effects of 4-aminopyridine on the potassium current in internally perfused giant axons of the squid. *J. Physiol. (Lond.)* 251, 60P-62P.

Misu, Y. & Kubo, T. (1974). Effect of bretylium on adrenergic neurons and its relation to sodium. *Japan. J. Pharmacol.* 24, 332-334.

Misu, Y. & Nishio, H. (1973). Protective action of guanethidine on atria isolated from reserpinized rabbits during exposure to sodium-deficient media. *Japan. J. Pharmacol.* 23, 740-742.

Mitchell, J.R., Arias, L. & Oates, J.A. (1967). Antagonism of the antihypertensive action of guanethidine sulfate by desipramine hydrochloride. *JAMA* 202, 149-154.

Mitchell, J.R., Cavanaugh, J.H., Arias, L. & Oates, J.A. (1970). Guanethidine and related agents. III. Antagonism by drugs which inhibit the norepinephrine pump in man. *J. Clin. Invest.* 49, 1596-1604.

Mitchell, J.R. & Oates, J.A. (1970). Guanethidine and related
    agents. I. Mechanism of the selective blockade of adrenergic
    neurons and its antagonism by drugs. *J. Pharmacol. Exp. Ther*.
    172, 100-107.

Moe, R.A., Bates, H.M., Palkoski, Z.M. & Banziger, R. (1964).
    Cardiovascular effects of 3,4-dihydro-2(1H)isoquinoline car-
    boxamidine (Declinax $^{T.M.}$). *Current Ther. Res*. 6, 299-318.

Narahashi, T. & Frazier, D.T. (1975). Site of action and active
    form of procaine in squid giant axons. *J. Pharmacol. Exp.
    Ther*. 194, 506-513.

Narahashi, T., Frazier, D.T. & Yamada, M. (1970). The site of
    action and active form of local anesthetics. I. Theroy and pH
    experiments with tertiary compounds. *J. Pharmacol. Exp. Ther*.
    171, 32-44.

Ng, K.K. (1966). Blockade of adrenergic and cholinergic trans-
    missions by emetine. *Br. J. Pharmacol. Chemother*. 28, 228-237.

Ng, K.K. & Ng, Y.T. (1970). Adrenergic neuron blocking action of
    dehydroemetine. *J. Pharm. Pharmacol*. 22, 787.

O'Brien, R.A. & Boullin, D.J. (1972). Accumulation, storage and
    release of adrenergic neuron blocking agents and related drugs
    by human platelets. *Biochem. Pharmacol*. 21, 1817-1827.

Page, I.H. & Dustan, H.P. (1959). A new, potent antihypertensive
    drug. *JAMA* 170, 85/1265-85/1271.

Pettinger, W.A., Korn, A., Spiegel, H., Solomon, H.M., Pocelinko,
    R. & Abrams, W.B. (1969). Debrisoquin, a selective inhibitor
    intraneuronal monoamine oxidase in man. *Clin. Pharmacol. Ther*.
    10, 667-674.

Pluchino, S., Muskus, A.J. & Pluchino, R. (1969). The mechanism
    of action of guanethidine on the isolated mammalian heart. *J.
    Pharmacol. Exp. Ther*. 170, 44-49.

Pocelinko, R. & Solomon, H.M. (1970). Accumulation of debriso-
    quin-^{14}C by the human platelet. *Biochem. Pharmacol*. 19, 697-
    702.

Prasad, C.M., Shah, D.S. & Gulati, O.D. (1973). Some factors
    affecting the neuron blocking action of guanethidine, xylo-
    choline, bretylium and debrisoquin. *Japan. J. Pharmacol*. 23,
    805-811.

Przuntek, H., Guimarães, S. & Philippu, A. (1971). Importance of
    adrenergic neurons of the brain for the rise of blood pressure
    evoked by hypothalamic stimulation. *Naunyn-Schmiedebergs Arch.
    Pharmak*. 271, 311-319.

Rand, M.J. & Wilson, J. (1967). The relationship between adrenergic neurone blocking activity and local anaesthetic activity
in a series of guanidine derivatives. *Eur. J. Pharmacol.* 1,
200-209.

Ross, S.B. & Kelder, D. (1976). Active transport of ^{3}H-bretylium
in the rat vas deferens *in vitro*. *Acta Physiol. Scand.* 97,
209-221.

Shah, D.S., Premanand, N., Jariwala, N.A. & Gulati, O.D. (1974).
Accumulation by rat vas deferens of debrisoquine and guanoxan.
Res. Comm. Chem. Path. Pharmacol. 7, 41-50.

Shand, D.G., Morgan, D.H. & Oates, J.A. (1973). The release of
guanethidine and bethanidine by splenic nerve stimulation: a
quantitative evaluation showing dissociation from adrenergic
blockade. *J. Pharmacol. Exp. Ther.* 184, 73-80.

Sheppard, H. & Zimmermann, J. (1959). Effect of guanethidine
(SU-5864) on tissue catecholamines. *Pharmacologist* 1, 69.

Sjodin, R.A. (1966). Long duration responses in squid axons injected with ^{134}caesium sulphate solutions. *J. Gen. Physiol.*
50, 269-278.

Solomon, H.M., Ashley, C., Spirt, N. & Abrams, W. (1969). The
influence of debrisoquine on the accumulation and metabolism
of biogenic amines by the human platelet, *in vivo* and *in vitro*.
Clin. Pharmacol. Ther. 10, 229-238.

Spriggs, T.L.B. (1966). Peripheral noradrenaline and adrenergic
transmission in the rat. *Br. J. Pharmacol.* 26, 271-281.

Tasaki, I. (1959). Demonstration of two stable states of the
nerve membrane in potassium-rich media. *J. Physiol. (Lond.)*
148, 306-331.

Thoenen, H., Haefely, W. & Staehelin, H. (1967). Potentiation
by tetraethylammonium of the response of the cat spleen of
postganglionic sympathetic nerve stimulation. *J. Pharmacol.
Exp. Ther.* 157, 532-540.

Thoenen, H. & Tranzer, J.P. (1968). Chemical sympathectomy by
selective destruction of adrenergic nerve endings with 6-
hydroxydopamine. *Naunyn-Schmiedebergs Arch. Pharmak. Exp.
Path.* 261, 271-288.

Toda, N. (1972). Interactions of bretylium and drugs that inhibit
the neuronal membrane transport of norepinephrine in isolated
rabbit atria and aortae. *J. Pharmacol. Exp. Ther.* 181, 318-
327.

Ulbricht, W. (1969). The effect of veratridine on excitable membranes of nerve and muscle. *Ergebn. Physiol.* 61, 18-71.

Van Maanen, E.F. & Wertz, A.W. (1966). Vas deferens: potentiation of response by tetraethylammonium. *Fed. Proc.* 25, 228.

Willey, G.L. (1957). Some pharmacological actions of choline 2:5-xylyl ether bromide. *Br. J. Pharmacol.* 12, 128-132.

Wit, A.C., Steiner, C. & Damato, A. (1970). Electrophysiologic effects of bretylium tosylate on single fibers of the canine specialized conducting system and ventricle. *J. Pharmacol. Exp. Ther.* 173, 334-356.

MODIFICATION OF CATECHOLAMINE RELEASE BY NARCOTIC ANALGESICS AND OPIOID PEPTIDES

G. Henderson, J. Hughes and H. W. Kosterlitz

I INTRODUCTION

Elliot (1912) demonstrated that the administration of morphine to the whole animal resulted in a depletion of the adrenaline content of the adrenal medulla. This effect of morphine was mediated by a central action (Stewart & Rogoff, 1916) although a small direct effect may contribute (Yoshizaki, 1973; Anderson & Slotkin, 1976). The first demonstration of a direct effect of narcotic analgesics on adrenergic neurones was made by Trendelenburg (1957). He reported that morphine inhibited the contractions of the cat nictitating membrane to pre- and post-ganglionic sympathetic nerve stimulation. The action of morphine on the nictitating membrane was later shown to be mediated via specific opiate receptors (Cairnie, Kosterlitz & Taylor, 1961). To date there have been many studies on the effects of narcotic analgesics on adrenergic neurones in the peripheral and central nervous systems.

An action of narcotic analgesics is said to be mediated via specific opiate receptors when it satisfies the following criteria: 1) The effect of the narcotic agonist is reversed by a specific antagonist such as naloxone. The antagonist does not mimic the actions of the agonist. 2) The (+)-isomers which are weak or inactive analgesic drugs (Eddy, Halbach & Braenden, 1956) are much less active than the (-)-isomers.

II NORADRENALINE RELEASE

Narcotic analgesic drugs inhibit neuro-effector transmission at some, but not all, adrenergic neuro-effector junctions (Table 1). Why these drugs inhibit transmission at only certain synapses is as yet unclear. In the cat nictitating membrane and mouse (I'O) vas deferens morphine inhibits neuro-muscular transmission at low (< 1 Hz) rather than at high (10-15 Hz) frequencies of nerve stimulation (Henderson, Hughes & Kosterlitz, 1975; Henderson & Hughes, 1976). The site of action of morphine in these tissues is presynaptic since the responses of the muscles to exogenously applied noradrenaline are not reduced. This presynaptic site of action was confirmed by studies on noradrenaline release in which the amount of noradrenaline released from the tissue into the bathing fluid following electrical field stimulation was measured (Henderson *et al.*, 1975; Henderson & Hughes, 1976; Hughes, Kosterlitz & Leslie, 1975a). Morphine depressed the output of

217

TABLE 1   a)   Effect of Narcotic Analgesics on Noradrenaline Release in Various Tissues

Depression of release	No specific effect
Cat nictitating membrane (1)	Cat heart (6)
Guinea-pig jejunum (2)	Cat spleen (6)
Mouse (TO) vas deferens (3)	Rabbit heart (7)
Rat cortex (4)	Rabbit vas deferens (8)
Rat cerebellum (5)	Guinea-pig vas deferens (8)
	Rat vas deferens (8)
	Cat vas deferens (8)
	Hamster vas deferens (8)
	Gerbil vas deferens (8)
	Guinea-pig ileum (9)
	Rabbit portal vein (10)

b)   Tissues Insensitive to Narcotic Analgesics
but Sensitive to Opioid Peptides

Mouse (C57/BL) vas deferens (11)

Rabbit ear artery (12)

(1) Trendelenburg (1957); (2) Szerb (1961); (3) Henderson *et al.*
(1972); (4) Montel *et al.* (1974); (5) Montel *et al.* (1975a);
(6) Cairnie *et al.* (1961); (7) Montel & Starke (1973); (8) Hughes
et al. (1975a); (9) Henderson *et al.* (1975); (10) Hughes, unpublished observations; (11) Henderson & Hughes (1976); (12) Knoll
(1976).

noradrenaline at low (< 1.5 Hz) but not at high (> 15 Hz) frequencies of stimulation. The effect of morphine was present even
after the uptake and metabolism of noradrenaline had been blocked
by pretreatment of the tissues with phentolamine plus cocaine.
The spontaneous release of noradrenaline was unaffected by
morphine in concentrations which markedly inhibited the evoked
release (Henderson, 1976; Hughes *et al.*, 1975a).

The inhibition of neuro-effector transmission in the cat nictitating membrane and mouse (TO) vas deferens was mediated via
specific opiate receptors since (a) it was reversed by naloxone,
and (b) levorphanol was much more potent than its (+)-isomer
dextrorphan. Naloxone itself did not affect the evoked noradrenaline release from the mouse vas deferens. The relative potencies
of narcotic analgesics devoid of any antagonist component to
inhibit contractions of the mouse (TO) vas deferens show a good
correlation with their relative potencies for analgesia in man
(Hughes *et al.*, 1975a). In the vasa from mice rendered tolerant

to morphine by chronic pellet implantation, the ID_{50} value for morphine was much higher than that found in vasa from naive animals (Waterfield, Hughes & Kosterlitz, 1976).

Similar experimental procedures have been used to compare the characteristics of noradrenaline release from tissues in which the noradrenaline output is inhibited by morphine with those from tissues in which the noradrenaline output is not inhibited by morphine (Hughes, 1972; Hughes & Roth, 1974; Henderson *et al.*, 1975; Henderson & Hughes, 1976). Within each group the character-istics of noradrenaline release are very similar. In the morphine-sensitive tissues the noradrenaline output per pulse is constant over a wide range of frequencies (0.2-15 Hz for the nictitating membrane and 0.5-15 Hz for the vas deferens). In these tissues, inhibition of pre- and post-junctional α-adrenoceptors and inhi-bition of neuronal and extraneuronal uptake increased the nor-adrenaline output at each frequency of stimulation but did not greatly alter the relationship between output and frequency of stimulation. Inhibition of prostaglandin synthesis by indometha-cin did not alter this relationship which appears to directly reflect the properties of the noradrenaline release process. In the morphine-insensitive tissues, the noradrenaline output is not constant over such a wide range of frequencies but increases as the frequency of stimulation is increased; for instance, in the rabbit portal vein the output of noradrenaline increases 10-fold between 0.5 and 16 Hz.

In the adrenergic system the major difference between morphine-sensitive and morphine-insensitive tissues is the relatively high noradrenaline output at low (< 1 Hz) frequencies of stimulation observed in morphine-sensitive tissues. A similar relationship between morphine sensitivity and a high transmitter output at low frequencies of stimulation has been observed in the cholinergic system (Greenberg, Kosterlitz & Waterfield, 1970; Lees, Kosterlitz & Waterfield, 1972). It may be significant that in morphine sensitive junctions in both the adrenergic and cholinergic systems the effect of morphine is greatest at low frequencies of stimula-tion.

The release of [^{3}H]noradrenaline following nerve stimulation from slices of rat cortex and cerebellum is reduced by morphine (Montel, Starke & Weber, 1974; Montel, Starke & Taube, 1975a). This effect is stereospecific (Starke, 1977) and reversed by naloxone (Montel *et al.*, 1974). Morphine depressed the release of noradrenaline at frequencies of stimulation below 3 Hz but it did not alter the release due to stimulation at 10 Hz. In rat cortical slices the output of noradrenaline per pulse was greater at 0.3 and 3 Hz than at 10 Hz. In this preparation as in morphine-sensitive neuro-muscular junctions the output of noradrenaline at low frequencies of stimulation is relatively high. Morphine did not depress the spontaneous efflux of [^{3}H]noradrenaline from cor-tical slices.

In cultured hybrid cells which possess specific opiate binding sites (Klee & Nirenberg, 1974) morphine in low concentrations

potentiates and in high concentrations depresses the depolarisation of the cell membrane produced by dopamine (Myers, Livergood
& Shain, 1975). The depression by morphine of the dopamine depolarisation was reversed by equimolar naloxone but stereospecificity of the narcotic analgesics action was not tested.

III   NORADRENALINE UPTAKE

Narcotic analgesics inhibit noradrenaline uptake into various
tissues (Carlsson & Lindqvist, 1969; Carmichael & Israel, 1973;
Ciofalo, 1972; Clouet & Williams, 1974; Dengler & Titus, 1961;
Montel & Starke, 1973). This effect is nonspecific since (1)
high concentrations of the drugs are required, (2) the drugs do
not exhibit any stereospecificity of action, and (3) naloxone
fails to antagonise the effects of the narcotic analgesics and in
some cases mimics them. In the mouse (TO) vas deferens, morphine,
in a concentration sufficient to inhibit the noradrenaline output
by over 50%, has no effect on the active uptake of noradrenaline
(Henderson & Hughes, 1976).

IV   OPIOID PEPTIDES

Hughes *et al*. (1975b) isolated and characterised two pentapeptides
(methionine-enkephalin and leucine-enkephalin) which are endogenous ligands for the opiate receptor. The amino acid sequencies
of these pentapeptides are:

$$\text{Met-enkephalin} \qquad \text{Tyr-gly-gly-phe-met}$$
$$\text{Leu-enkephalin} \qquad \text{Tyr-gly-gly-phe-leu}$$

The met-enkephalin sequence is present at residues 61-65 in the
pituitary peptide β-lipotropin (LPH) and it has been shown that
certain fragments of β-lipotropin whose N terminus is residue 61
(LPH_{61-76}, LPH_{61-77}, LPH_{61-91}) interact specifically with the
opiate receptor (Bradbury, Smyth, Snell, Birdsall & Hulme, 1976;
Cox, Goldstein & Li, 1976; Lazarus, Ling & Guillemin, 1976; Li &
Chung, 1976; Guillemin, Ling & Burgus, 1976). β-Lipotropin itself
is devoid of any opiate activity (Lazarus *et al*., 1976). Met-
and leu-enkephalin produce analgesia when injected into the
cerebral ventricles of the rat (Belluzzi, Grant, Garsky,
Sarantakis, Wise & Stein, 1976). These pentapeptides are much
less potent in producing analgesia than the larger fragments of
β-lipotropin (Graf, Szekely, Ronai, Dunai-Kovacs & Bajusz, 1976;
Feldberg & Smyth, 1977); this is at least in part due to the
greater susceptibility of the pentapeptides to degradation by
peptidases (Hambrook, Morgan, Rance & Smith, 1976).

The enkephalins and LPH_{61-91} inhibit noradrenaline release from
the mouse (TO) vas deferens (Waterfield, Smokcum, Hughes,
Kosterlitz & Henderson, 1977). Naloxone reverses their depression of noradrenaline release. As with the narcotic analgesics
the effect of the opioid peptides is greater at low frequencies
of stimulation. No effect of met-enkephalin could be demonstrated

on the spontaneous release of noradrenaline (Henderson, 1976).
In the vasa from morphine tolerant mice, cross tolerance has been
demonstrated between morphine and met-enkephalin (Waterfield,
Hughes & Kosterlitz, 1976).

There is indirect evidence that in the guinea-pig ileum, endogenous ligands for the opiate receptor released on nerve stimulation act to inhibit the release of acetylcholine (Waterfield &
Kosterlitz, 1975; Puig, Gascon, Graviso & Musacchio, 1977). As
yet there is no evidence for an endogenous ligand exerting a
modulatory role on noradrenaline release from peripheral adrenergic neurones.

Met-enkephalin produces a naloxone-reversible inhibition of the
$[^3H]$noradrenaline output from rat occipital cortex slices evoked
by either electrical field stimulation or high potassium (Taube,
Borowski, Endo & Starke, 1976). Naloxone itself slightly
increases the potassium evoked output of noradrenaline. In rat
striatal slices, morphine, LPH_{61-91} but not met-enkephalin
depressed the potassium evoked output of ^3H-dopamine (Loh, Brase,
Sampath-Khanna, Mar & Way, 1976). Naloxone prevented the effects
of morphine and LPH_{61-91}. Lesions of nigrostriatal pathways
produce a fall in both dopa-decarboxylase activity and enkephalin-
binding sites (Pollard, Llorens-Cortes & Schwartz, 1977) indicating that in the striatum some of the opiate receptors may be
located on dopaminergic nerve terminals.

V   MULTIPLE OPIATE RECEPTORS

In the mouse (TO) vas deferens met-enkephalin is more than 30
times more potent than morphine in inhibiting the contraction to
nerve stimulation at 0.1 Hz (Table 2, Waterfield *et al.*, 1977).

TABLE 2   The Agonist Potencies of the Enkephalins,
          Morphine and Normorphine in the Mouse (TO) Vas
          Deferens and the Guinea-pig Ileum

Compound	Mouse vas deferens ID_{50} (nM)	Guinea-pig Ileum ID_{50} (nM)
Methionine-enkephalin	12.8 ± 1.2 (16)	96.2 ± 8.7 (31)
Leucine-enkephalin	7.8 ± 0.8 (9)	463 ± 59 (10)
Morphine	492 ± 53 (7)	69.2 ± 14.8 (6)
Normorphine	440 ± 42 (9)	72.8 ± 17.7 (6)

The values are the means ± S.E.; the numbers of observations are
given in parentheses.

Reproduced from Waterfield *et al.* (1977).

Leu-enkephalin is slightly more potent than met-enkephalin whilst about 10 times more naloxone is required to reverse the action of the enkephalins than that of morphine. The relative agonist potencies in the vas deferens are markedly different from those found in the guinea-pig ileum. In the guinea-pig preparation there is little difference between the potencies of met-enkephalin and morphine; leu-enkephalin on the other hand is 5 times less potent. Naloxone is equiactive in reversing the actions of the enkephalins and morphine.

From studies on relative potencies and receptor binding assays, it has been postulated that the opiate receptor populations in the mouse vas deferens and guinea-pig ileum are heterogeneous and not identical (Lord, Waterfield, Hughes & Kosterlitz, 1977). Morphine interacts preferentially with μ receptors whereas the enkephalins interact preferentially with δ receptors. It is proposed that the mouse (TO) vas deferens possesses both δ and μ receptors whereas in the guinea-pig ileum there are mainly μ receptors.

In the vasa from C57/BL mice, which are very insensitive to morphine (Henderson & Hughes, 1976), the ID_{50} for met-enkephalin is similar to that found in vasa from TO mice (Waterfield, Gillan, Hughes & Kosterlitz, unpublished results). Thus the vasa from C57/BL mice may possess mainly δ receptors. The vasoconstrictor nerves of the rabbit ear artery are inhibited by the enkephalins (naloxone reversible) but not by morphine (Knoll, 1976); this tissue may also possess only δ receptors. The actions of opioid peptides mediated via δ receptors do not appear to be confined to neurones which possess a high output of noradrenaline at low frequencies of stimulation.

Studies in brain homogenates (Lord *et al.*, 1977) indicate that the opiate receptors present in the central nervous system are also heterogeneous. The evidence available at present is insufficient to attempt to allocate different receptors to different physiological functions.

VI   MECHANISM OF ACTION

The action of narcotic analgesic drugs and opioid peptides to inhibit noradrenaline release is <u>not</u> mediated via the following mechanisms:

1)   Stimulation of noradrenaline uptake. An inhibition of noradrenaline release by narcotic analgesics is apparent in the presence of high concentrations of phentolamine plus cocaine (Henderson & Hughes, 1976).

2)   Stimulation of presynaptic muscarinic receptors or α-adrenoceptors. Atropine and phentolamine do not prevent the inhibition of noradrenaline release by narcotic analgesics (Henderson & Hughes, 1976; Starke, 1977).

3) Stimulation of prostaglandin release. In the CNS inhibition
    of prostaglandin biosynthesis does not prevent the depression
    of noradrenaline release (Montel, Starke & Taube, 1975b).

At the concentrations used to inhibit noradrenaline release the
narcotic analgesics are devoid of any local anaesthetic action
(Kosterlitz & Wallis, 1964). In the cat nictitating membrane and
mouse vas deferens the inhibition of noradrenaline release is not
due to an inhibition of ganglionic transmission. There are few
if any ganglion cells in the nictitating membrane (Gardiner,
Hellmann & Thompson, 1962) and in the vas deferens the contractions to nerve stimulation are not reduced by hexamethonium
(Henderson, Hughes & Kosterlitz, 1972). Stripping the outer coat
of the vas deferens does not alter the inhibition produced by
morphine (Henderson & Hughes, unpublished observations). Thus
the site of action of the narcotic analgesics and opioid peptides
must be on the postganglionic nerve fibre. No effect of the
narcotic analgesics has been observed on adrenergic storage vesicles from rat brain or adrenal medulla (Anderson & Slotkin, 1975;
Blosser & Catravas, 1974).

It has been postulated (Henderson & Hughes, 1974) that the high
output of noradrenaline at low frequencies of stimulation in
morphine-sensitive tissues may reflect some property of the
mechanisms involved in calcium utilization by the stimulus-
secretion process. Narcotic analgesics and opioid peptides may
act by inhibiting the availability of calcium (see Starke, 1977).
At present no direct experimental evidence is available to support
this view.

In the guinea-pig ileum myenteric plexus ganglion, narcotic analgesics and opioid peptides produce a stereospecific and naloxone
reversible reduction in cell excitability by hyperpolarising the
cell membrane (North & Tonini, 1976; North & Williams, 1976;
North, personal communication). An hyperpolarisation of adrenergic nerve fibres by the narcotic analgesics and opioid peptides
could reduce noradrenaline release by preventing the action
potentials invading the sites of release.

Why specific opiate receptors have been observed on only certain
adrenergic neurones (Table 1) is unknown. This apparently random
distribution of opiate receptors in the peripheral nervous system
may be resolved by the following considerations. Opiate receptors
are present in the peripheral nervous system to mediate the
actions of endogenous opioid peptides. The enkephalins are found
in many parts of the peripheral nervous system, e.g. vagus and
sympathetic ganglia (Hughes *et al.*, 1977). The genetic coding
for enkephalin synthesis may be paralleled by coding for opiate
binding sites. This does not indicate a physiological function.
Since there is a relationship between frequency-output and opiate
action at μ receptors it may be that these opiate binding sites
are widely distributed but they are only detected by pharmacological means at those sites showing certain release characteristics. This hypothesis could be resolved by a series of binding
studies in peripheral tissues but at present such experiments are

fraught with difficulties.

VII   REFERENCES

Anderson, T.R. & Slotkin, T.A. (1975). Effects of morphine on rat adrenal medulla. *Biochem. Pharmacol.* 24, 671-679.

Anderson, T.R. & Slotkin, T.A. (1976). The role of neural input in the effects of morphine on the rat adrenal medulla. *Biochem. Pharmacol.* 25, 1071-1074.

Belluzzi, J.D., Grant, N., Garsky, V., Sarantakis, D., Wise, C.D. & Stein, L. (1976). Analgesia induced *in vivo* by central administration of enkephalin in rat. *Nature (Lond.)* 260, 625-626.

Blosser, J.C. & Catravas, G.N. (1974). Action of reserpine in morphine-tolerant rats: Absence of antagonism of catecholamine depletion. *J. Pharmacol. Exp. Ther.* 191, 284-289.

Bradbury, A.F., Smyth, C.R., Snell, N.J., Birdsall, N.J.M. & Hulme, E.C. (1976). C-fragment of lipotropin has a high affinity for brain opiate receptors. *Nature (Lond.)* 260, 793-795.

Cairnie, A.B., Kosterlitz, H.W. & Taylor, D.W. (1961). Effect of morphine on some sympathetically innervated effectors. *Br. J. Pharmacol.* 17, 539-551.

Carlsson, A. & Lindqvist, M. (1969). Central and peripheral monoaminergic membrane-pump blockade by some addictive analgesics and antihistamines. *J. Pharm. Pharmacol.* 21, 460-464.

Carmichael, F.J. & Israel, Y. (1973). *In vitro* inhibitory effects of narcotic analgesics and other psychotropic drugs on the active uptake of norepinephrine in mouse brain tissue. *J. Pharmacol. Exp. Ther.* 186, 253-260.

Ciofalo, F.R. (1972). Effects of some narcotics and antagonists on synaptosomal ^{3}H-norepinephrine uptake. *Life Science*, 11, 573-580.

Clouet, D.H. & Williams, N. (1974). The effect of narcotic analgesic drugs on the uptake and release of neurotransmitters in isolated synaptosomes. *J. Pharmacol. Exp. Ther.* 188, 419-428.

Cox, B.M., Goldstein, A. & Li, C.H. (1976). Opioid activity of a peptide, β-lipotropin-(61-91) derived from β-lipotropin. *Proc. Natl. Acad. Sci. USA* 73, 1821-1823.

Dengler, H.J. & Titus, E.O. (1961). Die Aufnahme von ^{3}H-Noradrenalin in Gewebeschnitte und deren Beeinflussung durch Pharmaka. *N.S. Arch. Exp. Pathol. Pharmacol.* 241, 523.

Eddy, N.B., Halbach, H. & Braenden, O.J. (1956). Synthetic
    substances with morphine-like effect. *Bull. WHO* 14, 353-402.

Elliot, T.R. (1912). The control of the suprarenal glands by the
    splanchnic nerves. *J. Physiol. (Lond.)* 44, 374-409.

Feldberg, W. & Smyth, D.G. (1977). C-fragment of lipotropin - an
    endogenous potent analgesic peptide. *Br. J. Pharmacol.* 60,
    445-454.

Gardiner, J.E., Hellmann, K. & Thompson, J.W. (1962). The nature
    of the innervation of the smooth muscle, Harderian gland and
    blood vessels of the cat's nictitating membrane. *J. Physiol.*
    (Lond.) 163, 436-456.

Graf, L., Szekely, J.I., Ronai, A.Z., Dunia-Kovacs, Z. & Bajusz,
    S. (1976). Comparative study on analgesic effect of met-
    enkephalin and related lipotropin fragments. *Nature (Lond.)*
    263, 240-241.

Greenberg, R., Kosterlitz, H.W. & Waterfield, A.A. (1970). The
    effects of hexamethonium, morphine and adrenaline on the out-
    put of acetylcholine from the myenteric plexus-longitudinal
    muscle preparation of the ileum. *Br. J. Pharmacol.* 40, 553P.

Guillemin, R., Ling, N. & Burgus, R. (1976). Endorphines, pep-
    tides d'origine hypothalamique et neurohypophysaire à activité
    morphinomimétique. Isolement et structure moléculaire d'α
    endorphine. *C.R. Hebd. Seances Acad. Sci. (Paris)* 282, 783-
    785.

Hambrook, J.M., Morgan, B.A., Rance, M.J. & Smith, C.F.C. (1976).
    Mode of deactivation of the enkephalins by rat and human
    plasma and rat brain homogenates. *Nature (Lond.)* 262, 782-
    783.

Henderson, G. (1976). Effect of normorphine and enkephalin on
    spontaneous potentials in the vas deferens. *Eur. J. Pharmacol.*
    39, 409-412.

Henderson, G. & Hughes, J. (1974). Modulation of frequency-
    dependent noradrenaline release by calcium, angiotensin and
    morphine. *Br. J. Pharmacol.* 52, 455P.

Henderson, G. & Hughes, J. (1976). The effects of morphine on
    the release of noradrenaline from the mouse vas deferens.
    Br. J. Pharmacol. 57, 551-557.

Henderson, G., Hughes, J. & Kosterlitz, H.W. (1972). A new
    example of a morphine-sensitive neuro-effector junction:
    adrenergic transmission in the mouse vas deferens. *Br. J.*
    Pharmacol. 46, 764-766.

Henderson, G., Hughes, J. & Kosterlitz, H.W. (1975). The effects of morphine on the release of noradrenaline from the cat isolated nictitating membrane and the guinea-pig ileum myenteric plexus-longitudinal muscle preparation. *Br. J. Pharmacol.* 53, 505-512.

Hughes, J. (1972). Evaluation of mechanisms controlling the release and inactivation of the adrenergic transmitter in the rabbit portal vein and vas deferens. *Br. J. Pharmacol.* 44, 472-491.

Hughes, J. & Roth, R.H. (1974). Variation in noradrenaline output with changes in stimulus frequency and train length: Role of different noradrenaline pools. *Br. J. Pharmacol.* 51, 373-381.

Hughes, J., Kosterlitz, H.W. & Leslie, F.M. (1975a). Effect of morphine on adrenergic transmission in the mouse vas deferens. Assessment of agonist and antagonist potencies of narcotic analgesics. *Br. J. Pharmacol.* 53, 371-381.

Hughes, J., Kosterlitz, H.W. & Smith, T.W. (1977). The distribution of methionine-enkephalin and leucine-enkephalin in the brain and peripheral tissues. *Br. J. Pharmacol.* 61, 639-648.

Hughes, J., Smith, T.W., Kosterlitz, H.W., Fothergill, L.A., Morgan, B.A. & Morris, H.R. (1975b). Identification of two related pentapeptides from the brain with potent opiate agonist activity. *Nature (Lond.)* 258, 577-579.

Klee, W. & Nirenberg, M. (1974). A neuroblastoma x glioma hybrid cell line with morphine receptors. *Proc. Natl. Acad. Sci. USA* 71, 3474-3477.

Knoll, J. (1976). Neuronal peptide (enkephalin) receptors in the ear artery of the rabbit. *Eur. J. Pharmacol.* 39, 403-407.

Kosterlitz, H.W. & Wallis, D.I. (1964). The action of morphine-like drugs on impulse transmission in mammalian nerve fibres. *Br. J. Pharmacol.* 22, 499-510.

Lazarus, L.H., Ling, N. & Guillemin, R. (1976). β-Lipotropin as a prohormone for the morphinomimetic peptides endorphins and enkephalins. *Proc. Natl. Acad. Sci. USA* 73, 2156-2159.

Lees, G.M., Kosterlitz, H.W. & Waterfield, A.A. (1972). Characteristics of morphine-sensitive release of neurotransmitter substances. In: *Agonist and Antagonist Actions of Narcotic Analgesic Drugs* (eds.) H.W. Kosterlitz, H.O.J. Collier & J.E. Villarreal, Macmillan, London, pp. 142-152.

Li, C.H. & Chung, D. (1976). Isolation of an untriakontapeptide with opiate activity from camel pituitary glands. *Proc. Natl. Acad. Sci. USA* 73, 1145-1148.

Loh, H.H., Brase, D.A., Sampath-Khanna, S., Mar, J.B. & Way, E.L. (1976). β-Endorphin *in vitro* inhibition of striatal dopamine release. *Nature (Lond.)* 264, 567-568.

Lord, J.A.H., Waterfield, A.A., Hughes, J. & Kosterlitz, H.W. (1977). Endogenous opioid peptides: Multiple angonists and receptors. *Nature (Lond.)* 267, 495-499.

Montel, H. & Starke, K. (1973). Effects of narcotic analgesics and their antagonists on the rabbit isolated heart and its adrenergic nerves. *Br. J. Pharmacol.* 49, 628-641.

Montel, H., Starke, K. & Taube, H.D. (1975a). Influence of morphine and naloxone on the release of noradrenaline from rat cerebellar cortex slices. *N.S. Arch. Pharmacol.* 288, 427-433.

Montel, H., Starke, K. & Taube, H.D. (1975b). Narcotic analgesics and central noradrenaline neurones. An *in vitro* study. In: *Abstracts of the Symposium Acute Effects of Narcotic Analgesics*, Nokkala, Finland, pp. 45-47.

Montel, H., Starke, K. & Weber, F. (1974). Influence of morphine and naloxone on the release of noradrenaline from rat brain cortex slices. *N.S. Arch. Pharmacol.* 283, 357-369.

Myers, P.R., Livergood, D.R. & Shain, W. (1975). Effect of morphine on a depolarising dopamine response. *Nature (Lond.)* 257, 238-240.

North, R.A. & Tonini, M. (1976). Hyperpolarization by morphine of myenteric neurones. In: *Opiates and Endogenous Opioid Peptides*, Elsevier North, Holland, pp. 205-212.

North, R.A. & Williams, J.T. (1976). Enkephalin inhibits firing of myenteric neurones. *Nature (Lond.)* 264, 460-461.

Pollard, H., Llorens-Cortez, C. & Schwartz, J.C. (1977). Enkephalin receptors on dopaminergic neurones in rat striatum. *Nature (Lond.)* 268, 745-746.

Puig, M.M., Gascon, P., Graviso, G.L. & Musacchio, J.M. (1977). Endogenous opiate receptor ligand: Electrically induced release in the guinea-pig ileum. *Science* 195, 419-420.

Starke, K. (1977). Regulation of noradrenaline release by pre-synaptic receptor systems. *Rev. Physiol. Biochem. Pharmacol.* 77, 1-124.

Stewart, G.N. & Rogoff, J.M. (1916). The influence of certain factors, especially emotional disturbances, on the epinephrin content of the adrenals. *J. Exp. Med.* 24, 709-738.

Szerb, J.C. (1961). The effect of morphine on adrenergic nerves of the isolated guinea-pig ileum. *Br. J. Pharmacol.* 16, 23-31.

Taube, H.D., Borowski, E., Endo, T. & Starke, K. (1976). Enke-
    phalin: A potential modulator of noradrenaline release in rat
    brain. *Eur. J. Pharmacol.* 38, 377-380.

Trendelenburg, U. (1957). The action of morphine on the superior
    cervical ganglion and the nictitating membrane. *Br. J.
    Pharmacol.* 12, 79-85.

Waterfield, A.A., Hughes, J. & Kosterlitz, H.W. (1976). Cross
    tolerance between morphine and methionine-enkephalin. *Nature
    (Lond.)* 260, 624-625.

Waterfield, A.A. & Kosterlitz, H.W. (1975). Stereospecific
    increase by narcotic antagonists of evoked acetylcholine out-
    put in guinea-pig ileum. *Life Science* 16, 1787-1792.

Waterfield, A.A., Smokcum, R.W.J., Hughes, J., Kosterlitz, H.W. &
    Henderson, G. (1977). *In vitro* pharmacology of the opioid
    peptides, enkephalins and endorphins. *Eur. J. Pharmacol.* 43,
    107-116.

Yoshizaka, T. (1973). Effect of histamine, bradykinin and mor-
    phine on adrenaline release from rat adrenal gland. *Jap. J.
    Pharmacol.* 23, 695-699.

MODIFICATION OF RELEASE BY LYSERGIC ACID DIETHYLAMIDE

J. C. McGrath

I   INTRODUCTION

Although lysergic acid diethylamide (LSD) has recently been shown to be a powerful sympatholytic and a sympathomimetic agent in peripheral tissues (Ambache, Dunk, Verney & Zar, 1973; Hughes, 1973; Ambache, Killick, Sprinivasan & Zar, 1975, Gillespie & McGrath, 1975) these effects must be viewed against the background of its earlier known actions.

The diethylamide of lysergic acid was synthesised in 1938 with the hope, based on the similarity of the molecule to that of niketha- mide, of finding a new analeptic. Initial screening demonstrated that it possessed a powerful uterotonic action similar to that of ergometrine but the therapeutic uses of the compound became limited when Hofmann discovered its powerful hallucinogenic properties in 1943 (Hofmann, 1975).

New interest in the pharmacological properties of lysergic acid diethylamide (LSD) was aroused when Gaddum and his co-workers found that it was a potent and relatively specific inhibitor of certain of the effects of 5-hydroxytryptamine on isolated tissues (Gaddum, 1953; Gaddum & Hameed, 1954; Gaddum & Picarelli, 1957). At the same time the presence of 5-hydroxytryptamine in the brain and in peripheral tissues was exciting considerable interest in regard to its possible physiological role as a neurotransmitter (Rapport, 1948; Rand & Reid, 1951; Erspamer & Asero, 1952; Amin, Crawford & Gaddum, 1954). 5-Hydroxytryptamine subsequently became more firmly established as a putative transmitter substance in the central nervous system than in the periphery (Anden, Carlsson, Hillarp & Magnusson, 1964; Haigler & Aghajanian, 1974). Interest in LSD as a tool for the study of neurotransmission mechanisms has, therefore, until recently been confined to the C.N.S., with its use on peripheral tissue limited to that of one of a number of antagonists of the pharmacological actions of 5-hydroxytryptamine (Gyermek, 1966).

More recently attention has also been focused on an agonist action of LSD at central dopamine receptors (von Hungen, Roberts & Hill, 1974; Kelly & Iversen, 1975; Da Prada, Saner, Burkard, Bartholini & Pletscher, 1975). Just as other actions of LSD have been related to similarities of the molecule to ergot or to 5-hydroxytryptamine, a structural correlation between LSD and apomorphine, a dopamine receptor agonist, has been implicated in this latter action of LSD (Nichols, 1976).

Nevertheless, in the course of investigating, in peripheral
tissues, phenomena which were or might have been related to an
action of 5-hydroxytryptamine, a number of effects of LSD have
come to light which may owe as much to its relationship with other
ergot derivatives as with 5-hydroxytryptamine.

II   CONTRACTILE EFFECTS OF LSD

LSD produces contraction of smooth muscle in several isolated
tissues including the cat nictitating membrane (Thomson, 1958),
the rat or cat anococcygeus (McGrath, 1973; Ambache et al., 1975;
Gillespie & McGrath, 1975) and rat vas deferens (Gillespie &
McGrath, 1975) and raises the blood pressure of the pithed rat
(Salmoiraghi, McCubbin & Page, 1957; McGrath, 1973). In each of
these cases the agonist effect of LSD can be reduced by α-adrenoceptor blocking agents and has been ascribed to a mixture of
direct effects on post-junctional α-adrenoceptors and indirect
sympathomimetic effects via the release of noradrenaline from
sympathetic nerve varicosities.

In the case of the rat vas deferens and rat or cat anococcygeus
the motor effect of LSD is abolished by prior treatment with 6-
hydroxydopamine (Gillespie & McGrath, 1975). In rat anococcygeus
LSD releases ^{3}H from tissues whose adrenergic nerves have been
previously loaded with [^{3}H]noradrenaline (McGrath & Olverman,
1977). LSD is not, however, an indirect sympathomimetic in all
tissues, e.g. it does not increase the rate of beating of isolated
mammalian atria (Trendelenburg, 1960) nor produce tachycardia in
pithed rats (McGrath, 1973).

Direct stimulation of smooth muscle by LSD has been demonstrated
on the non-innervated smooth muscle of umbilical blood vessels
(Dyer & Gant, 1973) and, after reserpinisation of the animals,
Ambache et al. (1975) found that LSD contracted rat anococcygeus.
The contractile effect of LSD may therefore be a mixture of direct
and indirect actions as is the case with 5-hydroxytryptamine
(Innes, 1962; Pluchino, 1972).

The nature and location of the receptors for LSD and 5-hydroxy-
tryptamine contraction has not been clarified due to the multiple
properties of both the agonists and antagonists involved in such
a study. For example, using "specific" antagonists on cat splenic
strips and nictitating membrane, Innes (1962) and Pluchino (1972)
both concluded that 5-hydroxytryptamine has a combination of
direct and indirect actions but could not finally define whether
the direct effects of 5-hydroxytryptamine and catecholamines were
exerted against the "same" receptor since both 2-bromo-lysergic
acid diethylamide, and dihyroergotamine inhibited the net effects
of adrenaline or of 5-hydroxytryptamine (Innes, 1962) but the
"direct" effect of 5-hydroxytryptamine was not blocked by phentolamine (Pluchino, 1972). Similarly in rat or cat anococcygeus LSD
and 5-hydroxytryptamine seem to act on the same receptors in producing contraction. In sub-contractile concentrations LSD or
methysergide antagonised the contractile effect of 5-hydroxytryp-
tamine but not of noradrenaline suggesting that LSD may be acting

as a partial agonist at the receptors activated by 5-hydroxytryp-
tamine in these tissues (McGrath, 1973; Gillespie & McGrath, 1974,
1975). Due to the presence of the indirect component due to noradrenaline released by LSD (Gillespie & McGrath, 1975; McGrath &
Olverman, 1977) or by 5-hydroxytryptamine (McGrath, 1973), however,
phentolamine or other α-adrenoceptor blockers always produce some
inhibition of the contractile response rendering "absolute" separation of receptors impossible without resort to a polypharmaceuti-
cal milieu.

III   INHIBITION OF NERVE-INDUCED CONTRACTION BY LSD

An action of ergot-derivatives at the post-ganglionic sympathetic
junction was first demonstrated by Dale (1906) who found motor
effects on various tissues and antagonism of the effects of sympathetic nerve stimulation. Gaddum and Hameed (1954) reported
that LSD did not antagonise the contractile effects of adrenaline
on rabbit ear artery. The effects of LSD on sympathetic neurotransmission did not receive much further attention until Ambache
et al. (1973) demonstrated that contractile responses of the isolated guinea-pig vas deferens to motor nerve stimulation were
inhibited by LSD. This inhibition was reduced by the α-adrenoceptor blocker phentolamine while contractile responses to noradrenaline were not reduced by LSD suggesting a pre-junctional,
phentolamine-sensitive site of action. Since the motor nerve
response itself was not abolished by phentolamine or by prior
reserpinisation of the animals, it was concluded that the nerves
involved in this pre-junctional effect of LSD were not adrenergic
(Ambache & Zar, 1971; Ambache et al., 1973).

It was subsequently found that LSD could also inhibit contractions
to sympathetic nerve stimulation, but not to noradrenaline, in
tissues where the relevant transmission was undoubtedly noradrenergic such as rat or cat anococcygeus (Gillespie & McGrath, 1974,
1975; Ambache et al., 1975), dog retractor penis (Ambache et al.,
1975), rat heart (Drew, 1976) and the vasopressor fibres in the
pithed rat (Clanachan & McGrath, unpublished observations). This
effect was a relatively specific one since the non-adrenergic
inhibitory nerve responses of the anococcygeus and of the dog
retractor penis were not reduced by LSD at concentrations larger
than were necessary to abolish the adrenergic nerve responses
(Gillespie & McGrath, 1974, 1975; Ambache et al., 1975).

In the tissues which have so far been examined most closely, the
response of the post-junctional tissue is a particularly unreliable
guide to the inhibitory properties of a drug such as LSD for two
main reasons:

(1)   In tissues where LSD itself exerts a motor action the net
effect seen may be a balance between pre-junctional inhibition
and post-junctional facilitation. This particularly applies to
the vas deferens where the contractile effect of LSD is quantitatively small compared with the effects of nerve stimulation
(Gillespie & McGrath, 1975) but where facilitation of nerve-
mediated responses may still be considerable as has been found

with a variety of other smooth muscle stimulants including 5-hydroxytryptamine (Sjostrand & Swedin, 1968; Sjostrand, 1973). In the anococcygeus LSD produces a contraction whose onset is often delayed until several minutes after addition to the bath, whose maximum is usually attained within 5-15 min and which thereafter gradually declines to baseline after a further 15-30 min (Gillespie & McGrath, 1975). This delayed onset is often found with other indirect sympathomimetics e.g. tyramine, amphetamine, guanethidine and 5-hydroxytryptamine, and while the decline of the response is not associated with any desensitisation to the direct contractile effects of noradrenaline, some cross-tachyphylaxis with tyramine is found (McGrath, 1973). As a consequence of this early contractile effect of LSD, during which equilibrium conditions have not been established, the degree of inhibition of nerve responses is difficult to determine. When assessing this latter effect, therefore, it is necessary to wait at least until the contractile effect has subsided at which time the inhibitory effect will have approached its maximum (Gillespie & McGrath, 1975). This time factor is highly critical when assessing any pharmacodynamic study with LSD on peripheral tissues, e.g. Gaddum, Hameed, Hathaway and Stephens (1955) found that the magnitude of the inhibition by LSD of the contractile effect of 5-hydroxytryptamine in rat uterus increased steadily with time.

(2) The presence of another set of nerve fibres in addition to the adrenergic ones will also make interpretation of the net effect difficult. In the anococcygeus and retractor penis the influence of the non-adrenergic, non-cholinergic inhibitory nerve fibres present within the tissue (Luduena & Grigas, 1966; Gillespie, 1972) cannot be removed when the tissues are field stimulated *in vitro* since no selective blocker of their effects is yet known. This can be partly surmounted by studying the anococcygeus *in situ* in the pithed rat, selectively stimulating the sympathetic outflow at L1-2 and thus avoiding stimulation of the sacral inhibitory outflow (Gillespie & McGrath, 1973). This manoeuvre can be used to confirm the selective nature of the inhibition by LSD (McGrath, unpublished observations) but carries with it the disadvantages of the vascular effects of LSD and the introduction of the ganglion synapse. In vas deferens the situation is even more complex since the response to field stimulation consists of two motor components (Swedin, 1971; McGrath, 1977) which cannot even be separated *in situ* since they share a common vertebral origin (Duncan & McGrath, 1976; Anton, Duncan & McGrath, 1977). In this case one of the components is clearly adrenergic since it can be blocked by α-adrenoceptor blockers and potentiated by blockade of the neuronal re-uptake of noradrenaline (Swedin, 1971; McGrath, 1977) while another, which is resistant to α-adrenoceptor blockade may involve either a resistant type of noradrenergic transmission (Swedin, 1971; Furness, 1974) or non-adrenergic transmission (Ambache & Zar, 1971).

In the face of these complications it would thus appear that measurement of the nerve-induced overflow of noradrenaline or [3H]noradrenaline would be a more reliable guide to the pre-junctional inhibitory effect of LSD (e.g. Hughes, 1973; McGrath & Olverman, 1977) especially if the contractile effects of nerve

stimulation are also monitored. However, this approach also
carries with it some drawbacks especially in the case of the vas
deferens. First, if a transmitter affected by LSD is not noradrenaline, as postulated in guinea-pig vas deferens by Ambache
et al. (1973), then assessing the output of noradrenaline will
shed no light on this aspect of the drug's action. Secondly,
the nerve induced overflow of noradrenaline from guinea-pig vas
deferens bears little relationship to the corresponding contraction of the tissue (Stjarne, 1973). This is partly due to the
transience of the initial "twitch" response and also due to the
"desensitisation" of the tissue to prolonged stimulation by an
agonist drug or transmitter substance (Hotta, 1969; Wadsworth,
1974). Thirdly, the inhibitory effect of LSD in the vas deferens
seems to be exerted to a relatively greater extent against the
contractile response to the first few pulses in a train (Ambache
et al., 1973; Gillespie & McGrath, 1975). The reason for this is
not yet fully understood but may be related to the post-junctional
stimulant effect of LSD overcoming the reduction in transmitter
output (Booth & McGrath, unpublished observations). Nevertheless,
it must be considered that due to the limited sensitivity of
overflow studies in the absence of further pharmacological interference (e.g. blockade of noradrenaline uptake), such experiments
only give an indication of the average output of noradrenaline
over a relatively long train of pulses.

IV   COMPARISON OF THE EFFECTS OF LSD ON THE NERVE-INDUCED
      OVERFLOW OF [^{3}H]NORADRENALINE AND ON THE ACCOMPANYING
      CONTRACTILE RESPONSES

Two studies have been carried out to assess the effect of LSD
against the nerve induced release of [^{3}H]noradrenaline from pre-
labelled isolated tissues. Both confirm that LSD can reduce the
release of noradrenaline from the adrenergic nerves.

Hughes (1973) demonstrated that in guinea-pig vas deferens, LSD
inhibited the overflow of labelled noradrenaline into the organ
bath during intramural nerve stimulation and caused a reduction
in the corresponding contraction of the smooth muscle. In the
presence of phentolamine both the nerve-induced overflow of labelled noradrenaline and the nerve-induced contractions were increased compared with controls, but LSD no longer reduced either
parameter. It was concluded that LSD inhibits the release of
noradrenaline from the intramural nerves. Since the contractile
response was also reduced, this could be taken to support the
classical concept that noradrenaline is the motor transmitter in
the vas deferens contrary to the view of Ambache and Zar (1971)
and Ambache *et al*. (1973). If, however, the nerve-induced contractile response consists of both adrenergic and hypothetically
"non-adrenergic" components even at low frequencies or with single
pulses (McGrath, 1977) and if in guinea-pig vas deferens this
"non-adrenergic" response is inhibited by LSD (Ambache *et al*.,
1973), then the hypothesis that part of the contractile response
is not adrenergic is not contradicted by these overflow experiments.

The abolition by phentolamine of the inhibitory effect of LSD suggests that LSD may be acting as an agonist on pre-junctional inhibitory α-adrenoceptors located on the motor nerves and that phentolamine is antagonising this action. This might also explain why the inhibitory effect of LSD against nerve-induced contractions was more effective against low frequencies and short trains of stimuli (Hughes, 1973) since the intrinsic feedback control of release by endogenous transmitter might be less under these conditions leaving more scope for inhibition by extraneous agents. An alternative explanation proposed by Hughes (1973) is that the antagonism of the effects of LSD by phentolamine is not a direct pharmacological antagonism but a physiological antagonism consequent on the increased efflux of noradrenaline produced by the phentolamine. Whatever is the nature of the antagonism between α-adrenoceptor blockers and the sympatholytic action of LSD, Drew (1976) has shown in rat heart that such antagonism by a range of α-adrenoceptor blocking agents is associated with those which are relatively selective for pre-junctional rather than post-junctional α-adrenoceptors. It is interesting that yohimbine and phentolamine, two of the agents which were found to be most effective against the sympatholytic effect of LSD and clonidine on rat heart, (Drew, 1976), were among the earliest known antagonists of the peripheral actions of 5-hydroxytryptamine (Reid & Rand, 1951; Wooley & Shaw, 1953; Meier, Tripod & Wirz, 1957).

Selectivity of the agonists and antagonists for the "receptors" involved in pre-junctional inhibition by drugs is vital in identifying any physiological or pathological significance of such phenomena. For example, the reversal of the sympatholytic effect of LSD by α-adrenoceptor antagonists, in the tissues where all or part of the post-junctional effect is not due to α-adrenoceptor stimulation (Hughes, 1973; Drew, 1976) can be explained simply by considering LSD as a relatively selective agonist at pre-junctional α-adrenoceptors analogous to clonidine or oxymetazoline. Other observations, however, suggest a more complex picture. Ambache *et al*. (1973) noted that although LSD could completely inhibit the contractile response to nerve stimulation in the guinea-pig vas deferens, in rat vas deferens the response to even a single pulse could not be abolished by LSD. If this single pulse response is analysed in transversely bisected portions of rat vas deferens, the α-adrenoceptor sensitive "noradrenergic" and resistant "non-adrenergic" components can be distinguished by their different time courses (McGrath, 1977). When the effect of LSD was assessed against these responses it was found that the "adrenergic" component was susceptible while the "non-adrenergic" component was resistant to the inhibitory effect of LSD. In contrast, clonidine inhibited both components while yohimbine reversed the effect of both LSD and clonidine (Booth, McGrath & Summers, unpublished observations). This suggests that if LSD exerts its inhibitory effect via pre-junctional α-adrenoceptors, it does not activate all such receptors. It was also found that methysergide and 5-hydroxytryptamine had a qualitatively similar effect to LSD but that higher doses were required. Dopamine and apomorphine, which also inhibit nerve-induced contraction of the rat vas deferens (Simon & Van Maanen, 1976; Tayo, 1977), presumably via pre-junctional "dopamine receptors", had a contrasting

effect, inhibiting the "non-adrenergic" but not the "adrenergic"
component. A wide range of pre-junctional receptors therefore
appear to be present in this tissue. The peripheral inhibitory
effect of LSD, however, seems to be more closely related to α-
adrenoceptor or "tryptamine" receptors than to dopamine receptors
in contrast to the situation in the central nervous system where
both "tryptamine" and dopamine receptors are involved in certain
actions of LSD (see introduction).

In the isolated, superfused, rat anococcygeus, when the sympathetic
terminals were pre-labelled with [^{3}H]noradrenaline, LSD produced
two effects on the efflux of ^{3}H (McGrath & Olverman, 1977). First
LSD produced an increase in the background efflux of ^{3}H, accompanied by contraction of the tissue. These effects were reproduced by tyramine but not by carbachol or barium chloride. LSD
did not produce contraction after treatment with 6-hydroxydopamine
(Gillespie & McGrath, 1975). These results confirm that LSD can
act as an indirect sympathomimetic in this tissue. However,
since a wide range of drugs which do not necessarily produce the
release of noradrenaline in all tissues e.g. guanethidine, cocaine,
ascorbic acid, can act as powerful indirect sympathomimetics in
the anococcygeus (McGrath, 1973), this may not be an ubiquitous
action of LSD. Nevertheless, it indicates that LSD may enter the
neurone and displace noradrenaline from stores within the nerve
terminal. Since LSD can also alter the release and reuptake of
noradrenaline in isolated bovine splenic nerve granules (Euler,
1970), an action at an intracellular site may also be involved
in the sympatholytic action of LSD.

The second action of LSD on the superfused anococcygeus was a
reduction in both the nerve-induced efflux of ^{3}H and in the
accompanying contractile response. This occurred despite the
relatively high stimulation frequencies of 5-20 Hz that were employed (McGrath & Olverman, 1977). A frequency of 0.2 Hz was employed in the similar study in guinea-pig vas deferens (Hughes,
1973). Although the contractile responses in vas deferens are
relatively less inhibited or even potentiated at high frequencies
(Hughes, 1973; Ambache et al., 1973; Gillespie & McGrath, 1975),
it would be interesting to know whether the efflux of noradrenaline is similarly resistant to inhibition by LSD or whether the
presence of another nerve response unrelated to noradrenaline
efflux levels had complicated the contractile response. Such a
complication is present with the anococcygeus but can be more
easily interpreted since the second set of nerves produce an inhibitory response. When the percentage inhibition by LSD of contractile responses to field stimulation was plotted against inhibition of nerve-induced efflux of [^{3}H]noradrenaline, it was found
that the adrenergic contractile response was apparently completely
extinguished when the efflux of [^{3}H]noradrenaline was still
approximately 50% of control values (McGrath & Olverman, unpublished observations). This can be readily explained by the continuous unaltered presence of the inhibitiry nerve response and
indicates the increased accuracy of noradrenaline efflux over
contractile responses in circumstances where only effects on
adrenergic nerves are of interest.

In conclusion, LSD produces considerable effects on release of transmitter from adrenergic nerves which deserve closer investigation. Although the concentrations required are high compared for example to hallucinogenic doses in humans, in certain tissues, on a molar basis, it is a more potent sympathomimetic than tyramine and a more potent sympatholytic than guanethidine (Gillespie & McGrath, 1975; McGrath & Olverman, 1977).

V   REFERENCES

Ambache, N., Dunk, L.P., Verney, J. & Zar, M.A. (1973). An inhibition of postganglionic motor transmission in the mammalian vas deferens by D-Lysergic acid diethylamide. *J. Physiol.* 231, 251-270.

Ambache, N., Killick, S.W., Srinivasan, V. & Zar, M.A. (1975). Effects of lysergic acid diethylamide on autonomic post-ganglionic transmission. *J. Physiol.* 246, 571-593.

Ambache, N. & Zar, M.A. (1971). Evidence against adrenergic motor transmission in the guinea-pig vas deferens. *J. Physiol.* 216, 359-389.

Amin, A.H., Crawford, T.B.B. & Gaddum, J.H. (1954). The distribution of substance P and 5-hydroxytryptamine in the central nervous system of the dog. *J. Physiol.* 126, 596-618.

Anden, N.-E., Carlsson, A., Hillarp, N.-A. & Magnusson, T. (1964). 5-hydroxytryptamine release by nerve stimulation of the spinal cord. *Life Sci.* 3, 473-478.

Anton, P.G., Duncan, M.E. & McGrath, J.C. (1977). An analysis of the anatomical basis for the mechanical response to motor nerve stimulation of the rat vas deferens. *J. Physiol.*, 273, 23-43.

Dale, H.H. (1906). On some physiological actions of ergot. *J. Physiol.* 34, 163-206.

Da Prada, M., Saner, A., Burkard, W.P., Bartholini, G. & Pletscher, A. (1975). Lysergic acid diethylamide: Evidence for stimulation of cerebral dopamine receptors. *Brain Res.* 94, 67-73.

Drew, G.M. (1976). Effects of α-adrenoceptor agonists and antagonists on pre- and post-synaptically located α-adrenoceptors. *Eur. J. Pharmacol.* 36, 313-320.

Duncan, M.E. & McGrath, J.C. (1976). Observations on the origin of the complex mechanical response to motor nerve stimulation of the rat vas deferens. *J. Physiol.* 259, 54P-55P.

Dyer, D.C. & Gant, D.W. (1973). Vasoconstriction produced by hallucinogens on isolated human and sheep umbilical vasculature. *J. Pharm. Exp. Ther.* 184, 366-375.

Erspamer, V. & Asero, B. (1952). Identification of enteramine, the specific hormone of the enterochromaffin cell system, as 5-hydroxytryptamine. *Nature (Lond.)* 169, 800-801.

Euler, U.S. von (1970). Effect of some metabolic factors and drugs on uptake and release of catecholamines *in vitro* and *in vivo*. In: *New Aspects of Storage and Release Mechanisms of Catecholamines*, (eds.) H.J. Schumann & G. Kroneberg, Springer-Verlag, Berlin, pp. 144-158.

Furness, J.B. (1974). Transmission to the longitudinal muscle of the guinea-pig vas deferens: The effect of pretreatment with guanethidine. *Br. J. Pharmacol.* 50, 63-68.

Gaddum, J.H. (1953). Antagonism between lysergic acid diethyl-amide and 5-hydroxytryptamine. *J. Physiol.* 121, 15P.

Gaddum, J.H. & Hameed, K.A. (1954). Drugs which antagonise 5-hydroxytryptamine. *Br. J. Pharmacol.* 9, 240-248.

Gaddum, J.H., Hameed, K.A., Hathaway, D.E. & Stephens, F.F. (1955). Quantitative studies of antagonists for 5-hydroxy-tryptamine. *Q. J. Exp. Physiol.* 40, 49-74.

Gaddum, J.H. & Picarelli, Z.P. (1957). Two kinds of tryptamine receptors. *Br. J. Pharmacol. Chemother.* 12, 323-328.

Gillespie, J.S. (1972). The rat anococcygeus muscle and its response to nerve stimulation and to some drugs. *Br. J. Pharmacol.* 45, 404-416.

Gillespie, J.S. & McGrath, J.C. (1973). The spinal origin of the motor and inhibitory innervation of the rat anococcygeus muscles. *J. Physiol.* 230, 659-672.

Gillespie, J.S. & McGrath, J.C. (1974). The response of the cat anococcygeus muscle to nerve and drug stimulation and a comparison with the rat anococcygeus. *Br. J. Pharmacol.* 50, 109-118.

Gillespie, J.S. & McGrath, J.C. (1975). The effects of lysergic acid diethylamide on the response to field stimulation of the rat vas deferens and the rat and cat anococcygeus muscles. *Br. J. Pharmacol.* 54, 481-488.

Gyermek, L. (1966). Drugs which antagonise 5-hydroxytryptamine and related indolealkylamines. In: *Handbook of Experimental Pharmacology*, Vol. XIX, *5-Hydroxytryptamine and Related indole-alkylamines*, (eds.) O. Erchler & A. Farah, Springer-Verlag, Berlin, pp. 469-528.

Haigler, H.J. & Aghajanian, G.K. (1974). Lysergic acid diethyl-amide and serotonin: A comparison of effects on serotonergic neurons and neurons receiving a serotonergic input. *J. Pharmacol. Exp. Ther.* 188, 688-699.

238   J. C. McGrath

Hofmann, A. (1975). The chemistry of LSD and its modification.
    In: *LSD a Total Study* (ed.) Siva D.V. Sankar, P.J.D. Publi-
    cations, N.Y.

Hotta, Y. (1969). Some properties of the junctional and extra-
    junctional receptors in the vas deferens of the guinea-pig.
    Agents and Actions 1, 13-21.

Hughes, J. (1973). Inhibition of noradrenaline release by lyser-
    gic acid diethylamide. *Br. J. Pharmacol*. 49, 706-708.

von Hungen, K., Roberts, S. & Hill, D.F. (1974). LSD as an agon-
    ist and antagonist at central dopamine receptors. *Nature* 252,
    588-589.

Innes, I.R. (1962). An action of 5-hydroxytryptamine on adren-
    aline receptors. *Br. J. Pharmacol*. 19, 427-441.

Kelly, P.H. & Iversen, L.L. (1975). LSD is an agonist at meso-
    limbic dopamine receptors. *Psychopharmacologia (Berl.)* 45,
    221-224.

Luduena, F.P. & Grigas, E.D. (1966). Pharmacological study of
    autonomic innervation of dog retractor penis. *Am. J. Physiol*.
    210, 435-444.

McGrath, J.C. (1973). In: *The Inhibitory and Motor Innervation
    of the Anococcygeus Muscle*, Ph.D. Thesis, University of Glasgow.

McGrath, J.C. (1977). Adrenergic motor responses to single pulse
    stimulation in the rat vas deferens. *J. Physiol*. 270, 52P-53P.

McGrath, J.C. & Olverman, H.J. (1977). Release of (^{3}H)-noradren-
    aline by field stimulation and by drugs from the anococcygeus
    muscle. *Br. J. Pharmacol*. 60, 305-306P.

Meir, R., Tripod, J. & Wirz, E. (1957). Classification d'une
    serie d'antagonistes de la serotonine et analyse de ses points
    d'attaque vasculaires periferiques. *Arch. Int. Pharmacodyn.
    Ther*. 114, 55-77.

Nichols, D.E. (1976). Structural correlation between apomorphine
    and LSD: Involvement of dopamine as well as serotonin in the
    actions of hallucinogens. *J. Theor. Biol*. 59, 167-177.

Pluchino, S. (1972). Direct and indirect effects of 5HT and tyr-
    amine on cat smooth muscle. *Naunyn-Schmiedeberg's Arch.
    Pharmacol*. 272, 189-224.

Rand, M. & Reid, G. (1951). Source of "serotonin" in serum.
    Nature (Lond.) 168, 385.

Rapport, M.M. (1948). Serum vasoconstrictor (serotonin) V. Pre-
    sence of creatinine in complex. Proposed structure of vasocon-
    strictor principle. *J. Biol. Chem*. 180, 961-969.

Reid, G. & Rand, M. (1951). Physiological actions of the partially purified serum vasoconstrictor (Serotonin). *Aust. J. Exp.
Biol. Med. Sci.* 29, 401-415.

Salmoiraghi, G.C., McCubbin, J.W. & Page, I.H. (1957). Effects
of d-lysergic acid diethylamide and its brom derivative on
cardiovascular responses to serotonin and on arterial pressure.
J. Pharmacol. Exp. Ther. 119, 240-247.

Simon, A. & Van Maanen, E.F. (1976). Dopamine receptors and dopaminergic nerves in the vas deferens of the rat. *Arch. Int.
Pharmacodyn. Ther.* 222, 4-15.

Sjostrand, N.O. (1973). Effects of acetylcholine and some other
smooth muscle stimulants on the electrical and mechanical responses of the guinea-pig vas deferens to nerve stimulation.
Acta Physiol. Scand. 89, 1-9.

Sjostrand, N.O. & Swedin, G. (1968). Potentiation by smooth muscle stimulants of the hypogastric nerve - vas deferens preparation from normal and castrated guinea-pigs. *Acta Physiol.
Scand.* 74, 472-479.

Stjärne, L. (1973). Lack of correlation between profiles of transmitter efflux and of muscular contraction in response to nerve
stimulation in isolated guinea-pig vas deferens. *Acta Physiol.
Scand.* 88, 137-144.

Swedin, G. (1971). Studies on neurotransmission mechanisms in
the rat and guinea-pig vas deferens. *Acta Physiol. Scand.*
Suppl. 369.

Tayo, F.M. (1977). Further evidence for dopaminoceptors in the
vas deferens. *Br. J. Pharmacol.* 59, 511P-512P.

Thomson, J.W. (1958). Studies on the response of the isolated
nictitating membrane of the cat. *J. Physiol.* 141, 46-72.

Trendelenburg, U. (1960). The action of histamine and 5-hydroxy-
tryptamine on isolated mammalian atria. *J. Pharmacol. Exp.
Ther.* 130, 450-460.

Wadsworth, R.M. (1974). Excitatory and inhibitory effects of noradrenaline on the isolated guinea-pig vas deferens. *Clin. Exp.
Pharmacol. Physiol.* 1, 135-145.

Wooley, D.W. & Shaw, E. (1953). Yohimbine and ergotoxin as natu-
rally occurring antimetabolites of serotonin. *Fed. Proc.* 12,
293.

MODIFICATION OF CATECHOLAMINE RELEASE BY ANAESTHETICS AND ALCOHOLS

M. Göthert

I   INTRODUCTION

Evidence has been accumulating in recent years that alcohols and anaesthetics influence catecholamine pathways both in the central nervous system and in the periphery. It appears that anaesthetic-induced alterations of noradrenaline release from peripheral sympathetic nerves are clinically significant (Ngai, 1974), since they may contribute to various side effects of these drugs, in particular those involving the cardiovascular system. It has been suggested that an inhibition of the function of catecholamine neurons in the brain may be involved in the mechanism of action of anaesthetics. This suggestion is based on investigations with drugs which alter the concentrations of catecholamines in the brain or which cause monoamine release. After treatment with these drugs, the anaesthetic concentration or dose that is necessary for the induction of anaesthesia has been found to be modified (Miller, Way & Eger, 1968; Johnston, Way & Miller, 1972; Hatch, 1973; Stoelting, Creasser & Martz, 1975). For example, the action of anaesthetics is potentiated by pretreatment with reserpine or α-methyldopa (Miller et $al.$, 1968); in contrast, acute injection of amphetamine (Johnston et $al.$, 1972) or pretreatment with an inhibitor of monoamine oxidase (Miller et $al.$, 1968) or cocaine (Stoelting et $al.$, 1975) increases anaesthetic requirements. Changes in the activity of catecholamine neurons also seem to play a role in ethanol physical dependence, since drugs which interfere with catecholamine pathways, including α-methyl-p-tyrosine, α- and β-adrenoceptor blocking drugs and reserpine, increase the severity of alcohol withdrawal reactions (Goldstein, 1973; Griffiths, Littleton & Ortiz, 1974).

More direct evidence for the ability of anaesthetics and alcohols to modify catecholamine release comes from studies of the transmitter output from isolated brain tissues or peripheral tissues and from in $vivo$ studies of the turnover of the catecholamines in the central nervous system and in peripheral organs. This review will concentrate on such studies performed with aliphatic alcohols and drugs used for the induction of general anaesthesia. However, it must be remembered that not only these compounds but also a variety of other lipid soluble drugs exert anaesthetic actions, including neuroleptics, anticonvulsants, and sedatives (Seeman, 1972). In the final section, dealing with the possible site and mechanism of action of the anaesthetics and alcohols, an anticonvulsant and a few neuroleptics will also be considered and the effects of general anaesthetics will be compared to that of local

241

anaesthetics.

Many attempts have been made to study the influence of anaesthetics and alcohols on noradrenaline release from peripheral sympathetic nerves by measuring the noradrenaline concentration in the
blood. Most of these estimations were made using spectrofluorimetric assays. These, however, do not appear to be sensitive
enough to disclose inhibitory effects of the drugs. (More
detailed discussion of this problem appears in the section about
inhalation anaesthetics). Moreover, since determinations of
noradrenaline in blood and urine do not allow one to determine
whether the changes observed are due to alterations of the release
from sympathetic nerves or from the adrenal medulla, such studies
will be mentioned only briefly.

II   EFFECTS OF ALCOHOLS

Turnover Studies. Studies have been made of the effects of relatively large acute doses of ethanol on the turnover of dopamine
and noradrenaline in the brains of rats. Ethanol administration
decreased the brain levels of noradrenaline but not of dopamine
to a greater extent than in controls, when the synthesis of the
amines was blocked by pretreatment with the inhibitor of tyrosine
hydroxylase, α-methyl-p-tyrosine (Corrodi, Fuxe & Hökfelt, 1966b;
Hunt & Majchrowicz, 1974). The disappearance of dopamine and
noradrenaline after treatment with α-methyl-p-tyrosine provides
indirect information on large modifications in monoamine release
from nerve terminals and is probably dependent on nerve impulses,
since the disappearance was almost completely inhibited by an
acute axotomy (Andén, Corrodi, Dahlström, Fuxe & Hökfelt, 1966;
Andén, Corrodi, Fuxe & Ungerstedt, 1971). Hence, the acceleration of α-methyl-p-tyrosine-induced disappearance of noradrenaline by ethanol suggests that the alcohol caused an increase in
noradrenaline release. However, an alternative explanation must
be considered, i.e., that the re-uptake of noradrenaline is
inhibited by ethanol (Israel, Carmichael & Macdonald, 1973).

In contrast to these results, Pohorecky (1974) determined the
contents of [^{3}H]noradrenaline and its metabolites in various
tissues after [^{3}H]tyrosine injection and found that a relatively
large acute dose of ethanol (4 g/kg) decreased noradrenaline
turnover in the hypothalamus, brainstem, telencephalon, and in
the heart and spleen. However, 30-60 min after injection of a
moderate dose of ethanol (1 g/kg) the noradrenaline turnover in
the brain was increased (Pohorecky & Jaffe, 1975); interestingly,
behavioural studies have shown that this dose has a brief stimulant effect on locomotor activity in rats (Carlsson, Engel &
Svensson, 1972).

After chronic ethanol intake, there was an acceleration of noradrenaline turnover in the brain and heart (Thadani & Truit,
1973; Pohorecky, 1974; Hunt & Majchrowicz, 1974). The turnover
of brain and peripheral noradrenaline was also increased in
alcohol-dependent rats withdrawn from ethanol (Pohorecky, 1974;

Hunt & Majchrowicz, 1974). These effects were found either using
the α-methyltyrosine technique or by determination of [3H]nor-
adrenaline and its metabolites after injection of [3H]tyrosine.
The noradrenaline concentration in the blood of human alcoholics
was also increased during ethanol withdrawal (Carlsson &
Häggendal, 1967). In rats withdrawn from ethanol, the acceleration of noradrenaline turnover was antagonized by re-introduction
of ethanol (Pohorecky, Jaffe & Berkeley, 1974).

Contradictory results have been reported regarding the effect of
ethanol withdrawal on the turnover rate of dopamine in the brain
of ethanol-dependent rats: Hunt and Majchrowicz (1974) determined
a decrease, whereas Ahtee and Svartström-Fraser (1975) found no
alteration. In both investigations, the turnover was determined
from the rate of depletion of brain dopamine after administration
of α-methyltyrosine.

Conclusions. Only the findings of studies concerning the effects
of chronic ethanol administration and of ethanol withdrawal on
noradrenaline turnover are consistent: The acceleration of noradrenaline turnover appears to reflect an increase in noradrenaline release. However, it cannot be evaluated whether the
changes observed result from direct actions of ethanol on catecholamine neurons or whether they represent a secondary effect
caused by an action on other neurons which then influence noradrenergic neurons.

Studies in Synaptosomes and Isolated Tissues. Determination of
the influence of alcohols on the catecholamine release from
synaptosomes, brain slices or isolated tissues with adrenergic
innervation provides more direct information on the site and
mechanism of action of the compounds. In synaptosomes prepared
from rat caudate nuclei and loaded with [3H]dopamine *in vitro*,
ethanol enhanced the spontaneous release of dopamine by a direct
action on the nerve endings (Seeman & Lee, 1974). The threshold
concentration for the dopamine-releasing effect was 50 mM and is
equivalent to the plasma concentration at which ethanol produces
general anaesthesia (Dundee, 1970). However, very high concentrations of ethanol (0.44-0.66 M) were necessary to cause a
slight increase in nonstimulated release of dopamine from superfused rat brain cortex slices preloaded *in vitro* with tritiated
catecholamines (Carmichael & Israel, 1975); the spontaneous
release of noradrenaline was not affected by ethanol (0.01-0.66 M).
In synaptosomes of mouse brain loaded with [3H]noradrenaline by
intraventricular injection, ethanol induced a biphasic effect on
spontaneous noradrenaline release: Concentrations of 20-100 mM
were inhibitory, whereas higher concentrations (0.2-1.3 M)
enhanced noradrenaline release (Sun, 1976).

Ethanol (1.37 M) and 1-pentanol (3.8 μM) also increased the spontaneous release of endogenous noradrenaline from the terminal
sympathetic nerves of the isolated rabbit heart (Göthert &
Thielecke, 1976; Göthert, Kennerknecht & Thielecke, 1976b); lower
ethanol concentrations had no effect. It has been suggested that
the increase in spontaneous noradrenaline release by lethal

concentrations of the alcohols may be due to a non-specific impairment of the cell membrane of the varicosities and/or of the membrane of the storage vesicles (Göthert & Thielecke, 1976; Göthert *et al.*, 1976b), since the compounds possess the ability to accumulate in the membranes and to destroy them (Seeman, 1966, 1972). The depolarizing effect of high concentrations of alcohols that has been shown in various nerve and muscle cells (Knutsson, 1961; Houck, 1969) may be an alternative explanation for the enhanced release. However, this possibility seems to be impro-bable, since the depolarization is rather small.

In concentrations up to 0.22 M, ethanol did not affect the elec-trically stimulated release of [^{3}H]noradrenaline from incubated brain cortical slices of guinea-pigs (Israel *et al.*, 1973) or from superfused rat cortical slices (Carmichael & Israel, 1975). Higher concentrations inhibited the electrically stimulated release of both noradrenaline and dopamine from rat brain corti-cal slices (Carmichael & Israel, 1975); the concentrations of ethanol that caused 50% inhibition (IC$_{50}$) were 0.42 and 0.41 M, respectively. In addition, the effects of l-butanol and l-hexanol on noradrenaline release were compared to that of ethanol. There was an increasing inhibitory potency with an increasing chain length of the alcohols; the inhibitory potency was found to correlate with the lipid solubility of the alcohols.

Noradrenaline release in response to electrical stimulation was also studied in isolated rabbit hearts with an intact post-ganglionic sympathetic nerve supply (Göthert & Thielecke, 1976); higher concentrations of ethanol than those which decreased the release from central noradrenergic neurons were required to inhibit release from peripheral nerves (for IC$_{50}$, see Table 1). Ethanol, l-propanol, l-butanol, and l-pentanol also inhibited noradrenaline release from cardiac sympathetic nerves produced by 80 mM KCl or by nicotinic agonists (Göthert & Thielecke, 1976; Göthert *et al.*, 1976b). The release evoked by nicotinic agonists was most sensitive to the alcohols, whereas the opposite holds true for electrically stimulated release. The inhibitory potency was correlated with the membrane/buffer partition coefficients of the compounds (Fig. 1). The noradrenaline release produced by activation of the tryptamine receptors on the terminal sympathetic nerves of the rabbit heart (Fozard & Mwaluko, 1976; Fozard & Mobarok Ali, 1976; Göthert & Klupp, in press) was also inhibited by ethanol at a slightly higher concentration than that which decreased the acetylcholine-induced release (see Table 1; Dührsen & Göthert, unpublished).

Conclusions. Direct studies of catecholamine release from adre-nergic neurons have clearly shown that acute administration of alcohols decreases release in response to various methods of stimulation, whereas the spontaneous output is increased. At present it is difficult to correlate these results with those obtained in turnover studies after the administration of a single, large dose of ethanol, since the latter findings are contradic-tory.

TABLE 1

Inhibitory Effects of Various Drugs on the Stimulated Release of Noradrenaline from the Sympathetic Nerves of the Isolated Rabbit Heart; the Concentrations (M) of the Drugs which caused 50% Inhibition are given.

	Method of Stimulation Used			
	Acetylcholine, 180 μM (in the presence of 3.5 μM atropine)	5-Hydroxytryptamine, 500 nmoles (bolus injection)	80 mM KCl	Electrical stimulation (5 Hz)
Ethanol	1.5×10^{-1}*	2.0×10^{-1}§	8.3×10^{-1}∇	1.2×10^{0}∇
1-Propanol	1.9×10^{-2}*			
1-Butanol	6.0×10^{-3}*			
1-Pentanol	1.2×10^{-3}*			
Diethyl ether	5.1×10^{-3}*	6.0×10^{-3}§	7.1×10^{-2}¶	
Halothane	3.0×10^{-4}*	7.9×10^{-4}§	4.6×10^{-3}¶	**
Enflurane	2.9×10^{-4}*		4.4×10^{-3}¶	**
Chloroform	2.6×10^{-4}*			
Methoxyflurane	3.8×10^{-5}*			
Phenobarbital	1.7×10^{-4}+			10^{-3}+
Pentobarbital	3.5×10^{-5}△		1.9×10^{-4}△	4.4×10^{-4}△
Thiopental	7.1×10^{-6}+	2.1×10^{-5}§		8.9×10^{-4}¶
Ketamine	2.5×10^{-6}+			

* Göthert et al., 1976b. + Göthert & Rieckesmann, unpublished. △ Göthert & Rieckesmann, 1976. § Dührsen & Göthert, unpublished. ∇ Göthert & Thielecke, 1976. ¶ Göthert, unpublished. ** No inhibition by halothane (Göthert, 1974) and enflurane (Göthert & Kennerknecht, 1976) at concentrations up to 1.1×10^{-3} and 1.2×10^{-3}M, respectively.

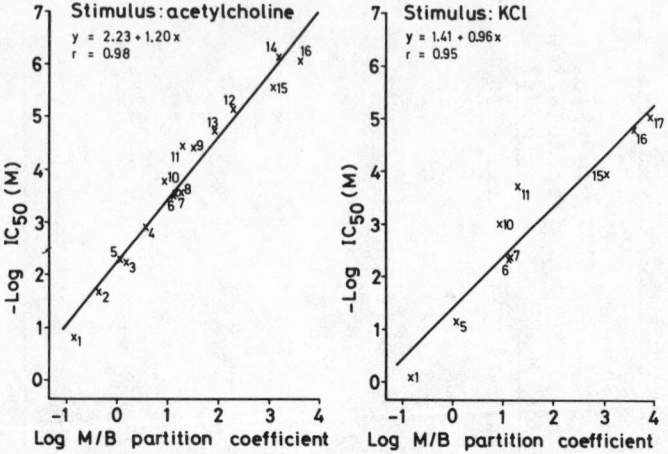

Fig. 1   Correlation between the inhibitory potencies of
various compounds on the noradrenaline output
from the isolated rabbit heart evoked by 80 mM
KCl or 180 μM acetylcholine (3.5 μM atropine
present throughout the experiments) and their
membrane/buffer (M/B) partition coefficients.
Abscissa: Logarithms of the membrane/buffer
partition coefficients (from Seeman, 1972;
Staiman & Seeman, 1974; some of the coefficients
were calculated from the olive oil/water or
octanol/water partition coefficients by the use
of the relations between the coefficients; these
relations were determined by Seeman, 1972).
Ordinate: Negative logarithms of the concentrations of the compounds causing 50% inhibition of
the noradrenaline output (IC_{50}). 1, ethanol;
2, 1-propanol; 3, 1-butanol; 4, 1-pentanol; 5,
diethyl ether (IC_{50} from Göthert *et al.*, 1976b);
6, halothane (IC_{50} from Göthert, 1974); 7, enflurane; 8, chloroform; 9, methoxyflurane (IC_{50} from
Göthert *et al.*, 1976b); 10, phenobarbital (IC_{50}
from Göthert & Rieckesmann, unpublished). 11;
pentobarbital (IC_{50} from Göthert & Rieckesmann,
1976); 12, thiopental; 13, phenytoin; 14, chlorpromazine (IC_{50} from Göthert & Rieckesmann,
unpublished); 15, droperidol; 16, haloperidol;
17, trifluperidol (IC_{50} from Göthert, Lox &
Rieckesmann, 1977).

III   EFFECTS OF INHALATION ANAESTHETICS

Turnover Studies and Catecholamine Determinations in Brain and
Blood. Halothane anaesthesia in rats did not affect the disappearances of brain dopamine and noradrenaline caused by pretreatment with α-methyl-p-tyrosine (Andén, Magnusson & Stock,
1974), or the haloperidol-induced acceleration of the α-methyl-

dopamine-evoked disappearance of dopamine (Andén *et al.*, 1974).

Recently, microdissection techniques and radioisotopic-enzymatic assays were used to measure the catecholamine concentrations in 20 different nuclei, fiber tracts or nerve terminal regions in brain of rats anaesthetized with halothane or cyclopropane (Roizen, Kopin, Thoa, Zivin, Muth & Jacobowitz, 1976a). Both anaesthetics increased the dopamine level in the nucleus accumbens and the noradrenaline content in the locus coeruleus, nucleus accumbens and central gray catecholamine areas. The elevated catecholamine concentrations may reflect a decrease in release, but could also be caused by increased synthesis or re-uptake.

The effects of halothane anaesthesia on catecholamine concentrations in plasma were first estimated using spectrofluorimetric techniques. Contradictory results have been obtained. Whereas Price, Linde, Jones, Black and Price (1959) did not find significant changes during anaesthesia with halothane, others have reported slightly increased concentrations (Anton, Gravenstein & Wheat, 1964; Ahnefeld & Frey, 1965). Hamelberg, Sprouse, Mahaffey and Richardson (1960) found slightly increased concentrations of serum catecholamines during light halothane anaesthesia, but no alterations during deep anaesthesia. Roizen, Moss, Henry and Kopin (1974) called attention to the relative insensitivity of the fluorimetric techniques which probably is the reason for the inconclusive results. Using radioisotopic enzymatic techniques which provide the required sensitivity, they found striking decreases in plasma catecholamines in both normal and adrenalectomized rats anaesthetized with halothane. Planz, Yilmaz and Palm (1973) reported a decrease in activity of dopamine-β-hydroxylase in the plasma during halothane anaesthesia in children, suggesting that the anaesthetic decreased exocytotic release from the sympathetic nerves, since the dopamine-β-hydroxylase in plasma arises mainly from sympathetic nerve endings and not from the adrenal medulla (Weinshilboum & Axelrod, 1971; Weinshilboum, Kvetnansky, Axelrod & Kopin, 1971). The inhibition of release from the terminal sympathetic nerves can partly be explained by central inhibition of the sympathetic nervous system, indicated by a decrease in preganglionic cervical sympathetic activity in cats during halothane anaesthesia (Millar, Warden, Cooperman & Price, 1969; Skovsted, Price & Price, 1969; Tauberger, Schulte am Esch & Steinringer, 1975). The ganglionic blocking effect of halothane (reviewed by Alper & Flacke, 1968; Gardier, 1972) probably also contributes to the decreased noradrenaline release *in vivo*.

Studies of Effects on Sympathetic Nerve Terminals in Tissues with Noradrenergic Innervation. Halothane, enflurane, methoxyflurane, chloroform, and diethyl ether did not affect the spontaneous noradrenaline release from isolated rabbit hearts (Göthert *et al.*, 1976b). Contradictory results have been reported regarding the influence of halothane on the electrically stimulated release of noradrenaline. Both in the dog heart *in vivo* (Price, Warden, Cooperman & Price, 1968) and in the isolated rabbit heart (Göthert, 1974; Göthert & Guth, 1975), halothane did not affect

noradrenaline release evoked by stimulation of the postganglionic
sympathetic nerve axons. Indirect determination of the noradrenaline release from the dog heart *in vivo* also revealed that halothane had no effect on the release induced by nerve impulses
(Gersh, Prys-Roberts & Baker, 1972); neither the positive chronotropic effect of sympathetic nerve stimulation nor that of exogenous isoprenaline was altered by the anaesthetic. Similarly,
in isolated, sympathetically innervated cat atria, halothane did
not alter the positive chronotropic response to either exogenous
noradrenaline or electrical stimulation of the sympathetic nerves
(Naito & Gillis, 1968). In contrast, another indirect study in
which the isolated saphenous vein of dogs was used, indicated
that halothane inhibited the electrically stimulated release of
noradrenaline (Muldoon & Vanhoutte, 1975): Halothane considerably
depressed the increase in tension of the vein strips induced by
electrical field stimulation, but did not alter that in response
to noradrenaline.

Direct evidence for a decrease in noradrenaline release evoked by
nerve impulses was obtained in an investigation by Roizen, Thoa,
Moss and Kopin (1975) using the isolated guinea-pig vas deferens-
hypogastric nerve preparation; halothane inhibited the release of
endogenous noradrenaline evoked by electrical nerve stimulation,
but it did not decrease the stimulation-induced release of
dopamine-β-hydroxylase. It is difficult to explain this dissociation between catecholamine and enzyme release. Since the ratio
of noradrenaline to dopamine-β-hydroxylase released is normally
constant and approximates that of noradrenaline to soluble enzyme
in tissue, it has been concluded that exocytosis is the mechanism
by which noradrenaline secretion occurs from electrically stimulated sympathetic nerves (Weinshilboum, Thoa, Johnson, Kopin &
Axelrod, 1971) and that dopamine-β-hydroxylase release is an
index of exocytosis. Roizen *et al.* (1975) have suggested that
halothane may enhance the binding of noradrenaline to the vesicular membrane, thus impairing noradrenaline release during exocytosis.

The discrepancies concerning the effect of halothane on electrically stimulated release of noradrenaline cannot be accounted
for by differences in the concentrations of the anaesthetic used,
since all investigations were carried out in a similar concentration range. Moreover, since contradictory results were obtained
in the same species (dog), they cannot be attributed to species
differences. Hence, the most plausible explanation appears to be
that the discrepancies are due to tissue differences.

Similarly, cyclopropane inhibited the electrically stimulated
release of noradrenaline but not that of dopamine-β-hydroxylase
from the guinea-pig vas deferens (Roizen, Thoa, Moss & Kopin,
1976b), but did not alter the nerve-mediated noradrenaline
release from the cardiac sympathetic nerves of dogs (Price *et al.*,
1968). Enflurane also did not affect the electrically stimulated
release of noradrenaline from the sympathetic nerves of the
isolated rabbit heart (Göthert & Kennerknecht, 1976).

Interestingly, it has been shown (Göthert, 1974; Göthert & Kennerknecht, 1976; Göthert *et al.*, 1976b) that halothane, enflurane, methoxyflurane, chloroform, and diethyl ether in a concentration range compatible with surgical anaesthesia inhibit the noradrenaline release from the sympathetic nerves of the isolated rabbit heart evoked by dimethylphenylpiperazinium or acetylcholine in the presence of atropine; at considerably higher concentrations the compounds also decreased the release in response to 80 mM KCl (see Table 1). The inhibitory potency of the compounds was proportional to their membrane/buffer partition coefficients (see Fig. 1). Diethyl ether and halothane at concentrations slightly higher than those which decreased the release evoked by acetylcholine also inhibited the release induced by 5-hydroxytryptamine (see Table 1; Dührsen & Göthert, unpublished).

Conclusions. In peripheral neurons, inhalation anaesthetics inhibit the noradrenaline release evoked by KCl or by activation of the nicotinic receptors on the nerve terminals (the latter at concentrations equivalent to those measured during anaesthesia). The decrease in noradrenaline concentration and in activity of dopamine-β-hydroxylase in plasma during halothane anaesthesia suggest an inhibition of noradrenaline release from the sympathetic nerves *in vivo*. This effect is probably mainly due to a decreased rate of impulse flow in the postganglionic sympathetic nerve fibers. The inhibition of the release per impulse found in the sympathetic nerves of the saphenous vein and of the vas deferens (but not of the heart) may also contribute to a minor extent to the inhibition of noradrenaline release found *in vivo*.

IV   EFFECTS OF INTRAVENOUS ANAESTHETICS

Turnover Studies. In the whole brain (Corrodi, Fuxe & Hökfelt, 1966a; Andén *et al.*, 1974) and in the neocortex (Lidbrink, Corrodi, Fuxe & Olson, 1972) of rats pentobarbital decelerates the α-methyl-p-tyrosine-induced disappearance of noradrenaline. The disappearance of whole brain dopamine after pretreatment of rats with α-methyl-p-tyrosine was also inhibited by pentobarbital (Corrodi *et al.*, 1966a; Andén *et al.*, 1974). Moreover, pentobarbital decreased the disappearance of noradrenaline in the whole brain after treatment with an inhibitor of dopamine-β-hydroxylase (Persson & Waldeck, 1971). The acceleration of the α-methyl-p-tyrosine-induced disappearances of dopamine and of noradrenaline after administration of haloperidol, in the brain of rats, was significantly reduced by pentobarbital, whereas it did not affect the acceleration of the α-methyl-p-tyrosine-induced disappearance of dopamine from the rat forebrain caused by injection of 25% KCl into the neostriatum (Andén *et al.*, 1974).

Studies in Synaptosomes and Isolated Tissues. In rat cerebral cortical slices preloaded with [³H]noradrenaline, pentobarbital and phenobarbital did not alter the spontaneous release of noradrenaline (Lidbrink & Farnebo, 1973; Carmichael & Israel, 1975). These barbiturates also did not affect the spontaneous release

from cardiac sympathetic nerves of the isolated rabbit heart
(Göthert & Rieckesmann, unpublished).

The release of [^{3}H]noradrenaline from rat cerebral cortical
slices evoked by electrical field stimulation was unaffected by
phenobarbital and pentobarbital in a concentration range compatible with general anaesthesia (Lidbrink & Farnebo, 1973).
However, high concentrations of pentobarbital and phenobarbital
(300 μM - 10 mM) inhibited the electrically stimulated release of
noradrenaline in rat cerebral cortical slices preincubated with
[^{3}H]noradrenaline (Carmichael & Israel, 1975). In mouse forebrain
synaptosomes depolarized with 50 mM KCl or veratridine, pentobarbital at a rather low concentration (200 μM) decreased the
efflux of [^{3}H]noradrenaline when Ca^{2+} was present in the incubation medium (Haycock, Levy & Cotman, 1977). In contrast, the
efflux found during incubation with a solution containing 50 mM
KCl but no Ca^{2+} was unaffected by pentobarbital. Interestingly,
this drug also failed to affect the Ca^{2+}-dependent release of
noradrenaline evoked by the Ca^{2+} ionophore A 23187 which is
known to increase Ca^{2+} permeability of the cell membrane without
causing a depolarization.

Pentobarbital at very high concentrations also decreased the noradrenaline release from the sympathetic nerves of the isolated
rabbit heart evoked by electrical stimulation of nerves (see
Table 1; Göthert & Rieckesmann, 1976). Moreover, in this preparation, pentobarbital, phenobarbital, and thiopental inhibited the
noradrenaline release in response to 80 mM KCl and to acetylcholine in the presence of atropine (see Table 1; Göthert &
Rieckesmann, 1976; Göthert & Rieckesmann, unpublished). The concentration range in which the inhibition of the acetylcholine-
induced release occurred corresponds to concentrations that were
measured in the blood during general anaesthesia, while the inhibition of the KCl-induced release was found at higher concentrations. The inhibitory potency of the compounds was proportional
to their membrane/buffer partition coefficient (see Fig. 1). The
5-hydroxytryptamine-induced release from the sympathetic nerves
of the rabbit heart was also inhibited by thiopental (Dührsen &
Göthert, unpublished).

At first sight, the results obtained with ketamine and phencyclidine are contradictory to those obtained with the other intravenous anaesthetics, since in slices of the rat occipital cortex
preloaded with [^{3}H]noradrenaline, these drugs enhanced both the
spontaneous outflow of tritium and that evoked by electrical field
stimulation (Taube, Montel, Hau & Starke, 1975); however, these
effects were mainly due to an inhibition of the re-uptake of
released [^{3}H]noradrenaline (but not to an increase in the release
from the nerve terminals), since the drugs inhibited the accumulation of tritium during incubation of the slices with [^{3}H]nor-
adrenaline (Taube *et al.*, 1975; Smith, Azzaro, Turndorf & Abbott,
1975). Very high concentrations of ketamine and phencyclidine
(10 and 1 mM, respectively) abolished the electrically stimulated
outflow of tritium from the slices (Taube *et al.*, 1975), indicating that the release from the nerve endings was decreased. In the

isolated rabbit heart, ketamine in a concentration range of 10 -
320 μM also increased the electrically stimulated outflow of
endogenous noradrenaline (Montel, Starke, Görlitz & Schümann,
1973). This was not due to an increase in noradrenaline release
from the nerve terminals, but also reflected an inhibition of the
uptake of noradrenaline into the peripheral sympathetic nerve
endings (Montel *et al.*, 1973; Nedergaard, 1973; Miletich,
Ivankovic, Albrecht, Zahed & Ihali, 1973). Ketamine also inhibited
the noradrenaline release from the sympathetic nerves of the isolated rabbit heart evoked by KCl and acetylcholine in the presence
of atropine (see Table 1; Göthert & Rieckesmann, unpublished).

In man, ketamine anaesthesia increases the plasma concentration
of noradrenaline (determined by a radiometric technique) and the
activity of dopamine-β-hydroxylase (Appel, Simrock, Palm, Wnuk &
Dudziak, 1977), suggesting that the neuronal uptake of noradrenaline is decreased (see above) or that noradrenaline release is
stimulated probably by a central mechanism of action. The latter
possibility appears to be more likely, since evidence has been
presented in the pithed rat that ketamine in doses used clinically
does not potentiate the effects of noradrenaline (Clanachan &
McGrath, 1976) and since the serum concentrations measured during
ketamine anaesthesia in man (Wieber, Gugler, Hengstmann & Dengler,
1975) are lower than those which have been shown to cause an
inhibition of neuronal uptake *in vitro*.

Conclusions. Direct studies of noradrenaline release from central
and peripheral neurons have shown that all intravenous anaesthetics
investigated can cause an inhibition of stimulated noradrenaline
release, at least when KCl and acetylcholine are used for stimulation. However, since pentobarbital inhibits the electrically
stimulated release of noradrenaline from brain tissue only at
lethal concentrations, the inhibition of noradrenaline release
found in *in vivo* turnover studies does not appear to be due to a
direct effect of the drug on the nerve terminals (i.e., to an
inhibition of the per pulse release), but rather results from a
decreased rate of impulse flow.

V   POSSIBLE SITE AND MECHANISM OF ACTION UNDERLYING THE
INHIBITION OF STIMULATED RELEASE

As outlined in the previous sections, it is a common property of
all alcohols and anaesthetics investigated that they inhibit the
stimulated noradrenaline release from central and peripheral
noradrenaline neurons. However, considerably different concentrations of a drug were necessary for the inhibition of release
evoked by the various methods of stimulation used, indicating
that different sites of action appear to exist. Evidence has
been accumulating that, in principle, the cell membrane is the
site of action of the anaesthetics and alcohols (reviewed by
Seeman, 1972). In particular, it has been shown that these drugs
are capable of decreasing the Na^+ and Ca^{2+} permeability of the
membrane (Seeman, 1972; Andersen & Amaranath, 1973; Blaustein &
Christie Ector, 1975).

As a rule, lethal concentrations of anaesthetics and alcohols were necessary to cause inhibition of the noradrenaline release induced by nerve impulses or by KCl. The failure of halothane, enflurane, and cyclopropane to decrease electrically stimulated release from cardiac sympathetic nerves (see Section III; Table 1) probably does not indicate that there is a fundamental difference between these anaesthetics and the other compounds, but rather is due to the fact that the concentrations investigated to date were not large enough to cause inhibition. The noradrenaline release from peripheral sympathetic nerves evoked by KCl and electrical stimulation has been shown to be Ca^{2+}-dependent, but only the nerve impulse-induced depolarization of the nerve terminals is dependent on an increase in Na^+ permeability of the membrane (reviewed by Smith & Winkler, 1972). It has been suggested (Göthert & Thielecke, 1976; Göthert & Rieckesmann, 1976) that ethanol and anaesthetics (at high concentrations which inhibit the release by both methods of stimulation) produce this effect mainly by decreasing the Ca^{2+} permeability of the membrane; blockade of Na^+ conductance may be an additional factor contributing to the inhibition of release evoked by nerve impulses.

The effects of local anaesthetics on the peripheral sympathetic nerves are different from those of the general anaesthetics, since tetracaine at concentrations up to 100 μM did not alter KCl-induced noradrenaline release (Göthert, 1974), whereas electrically stimulated release was inhibited by this drug (Huković & Muscholl, 1962; Starke, Wagner & Schümann, 1972: IC_{50} = 8 μM). It was concluded that in the terminal and/or preterminal parts of the nerves, tetracaine does not inhibit the permeability of the membrane to Ca^{2+} ions but only that to Na^+ ions (Göthert, 1974).

The decrease in stimulated noradrenaline release (by KCl or impulses) from central noradrenaline neurons caused by alcohols and barbiturates has also been suggested to be due to an inhibition of ion conductance of the cell membrane (Carmichael & Israel, 1975; Haycock et al., 1977). In particular, evidence has been presented that pentobarbital impairs Ca^{2+} influx into the nerve terminals, since the compound selectively inhibited the depolarization-induced calcium-dependent release, leaving the Ca^{2+}-independent release unaffected (Haycock et al., 1977). The possibility that the compound depresses one of the steps in transmitter secretion subsequent to Ca^{2+} influx was excluded by experiments with the Ca^{2+} ionophore A 23187: The A 23187-facilitated Ca^{2+}-dependent release was unaffected by pentobarbital.

It has been shown both in central (Carmichael & Israel, 1975) and in peripheral (see Fig. 1) noradrenaline neurons that the interaction between the anaesthetics and alcohols and the membrane constituents essential to the inhibition of noradrenaline release is hydrophobic in nature, since a correlation was found between the inhibitory potencies of a great number of drugs and their hydrophobic properties; this finding is consistent with the classical rule of anaesthesia of Meyer (1899; 1901) and Overton (1901). According to the definition of an anaesthetic given by

Seeman (1972), phenytoin and neuroleptics also belong to this group of drugs. Hence, phenytoin and various neuroleptics were included in the study in peripheral sympathetic nerves (see Fig. 1); this appeared to be of interest because of their very high lipid solubility.

The intercepts and the slopes of the regression lines calculated for the inhibition of acetylcholine and KCl-induced release are different from each other (see Fig. 1), suggesting that the sites of action underlying the inhibition of acetylcholine and KCl-induced release are different from each other. The chain of events initiated by activation of the nicotine receptors on the nerve terminals is identical to that initiated by electrical stimulation: Activation of these receptors also induces depolarization and Ca^{2+} influx which in turn causes noradrenaline release by exocytosis (reviewed by Smith & Winkler, 1972). It has been concluded that the selective inhibition of acetylcholine-induced noradrenaline release caused by alcohols and anaesthetics in low concentrations is neither due to an impairment of the exocytotic release mechanism, nor to an inhibition of depolarization, nor to a decrease in Ca^{2+} inward current, but that the site of action underlying the inhibition is the nicotine receptor (Göthert, 1974; Göthert & Thielecke, 1976) which may be a highly hydrophobic protein (De Robertis, 1975). This suggestion was also based on the finding that alcohols and anaesthetics interact with hydrophobic regions of membrane and enzyme proteins which undergo conformational change on binding the compounds (Seeman, 1972; Ueda & Kamaya, 1973; Eyring, Woodbury & D'Arrigo, 1973; Seeman, 1974). A conformational change of the nicotine receptor may prevent agonist-receptor interaction or inhibit an event subsequent to the binding of the agonist to the receptor. Similar alterations of tryptamine receptors may account for the inhibition of the 5-hydroxytryptamine-induced release caused by low concentrations of ethanol and anaesthetics (see Table 1).

The suggestion that the nicotine receptor is the site of action of alcohols and anaesthetics is further supported by two findings: (1) Administration of diethyl ether, pentobarbital, or chloralose to cats *in vivo* reversibly reduced the ability of acetylcholine (injected into the left atrial appendage) to set up antidromic nerve impulses in thoracic postganglionic sympathetic fibres (Cabrera, Torrance & Viveros, 1966); and, (2) The response to activation of nicotine receptors was also selectively inhibited by halothane in cardiac sympathetic ganglia of dogs (Alper, Fleisch & Flacke, 1969) and in isolated bovine adrenals (Göthert, Dorn & Loewenstein, 1976a).

In conclusion, there is evidence that ethanol in concentrations compatible with moderate intoxication and anaesthetics at concentrations equivalent to those measured during clinical anaesthesia may affect receptors in the membrane of noradrenaline neurons. Since nicotine receptors mediating noradrenaline release have been shown to be located on neurons of different brain areas (Westfall, 1974), a similar action on these receptors may contribute to the effects of the drugs on the central nervous system.

VI   REFERENCES

Ahnefeld, F.W. & Frey, R. (1965). Untersuchungen über den Plasma-Katecholaminspiegel nach Operationen und Traumen. *Anaesthesist* 14, 36-38.

Ahtee, L. & Svartström-Fraser, M. (1975). Effect of ethanol dependence and withdrawal on the catecholamines in rat brain and heart. *Acta Pharmacol. Toxicol.* 36, 289-298.

Alper, M.H. & Flacke, W. (1969). The peripheral effects of anaesthetics. *Annu. Rev. Pharmacol.* 9, 273-296.

Alper, M.H., Fleisch, J.H. & Flacke, W. (1969). The effects of halothane on the responses of cardiac sympathetic ganglia to various stimulants. *Anesthesiology* 31, 429-436.

Anden, N.E., Corrodi, H., Dahlström, A., Fuxe, K. & Hökfelt, T. (1966). Effects of tyrosine hydroxylase inhibition on the amine levels of central monoamine neurons. *Life Sci.* 5, 605-611.

Andén, N.E., Corrodi, H., Fuxe, K. & Ungerstedt, U. (1971). Importance of nervous impulse flow for the neuroleptic-induced increase in amine turnover in central dopamine neurons. *Eur. J. Pharmacol.* 15, 193-199.

Andén, N.E., Magnusson, T. & Stock, G. (1974). Effect of anaesthetic agents on the synthesis and disappearance of brain dopamine normally and after haloperidol, KCl or axotomy. *Naunyn-Schmiedeberg's Arch. Pharmacol.* 283, 409-418.

Andersen, N.B. & Amaranath, L. (1973). Anesthetic effects on transport across cell membranes. *Anesthesiology* 39, 126-152.

Anton, A.H., Gravenstein, J.S. & Wheat, Jr., M.W. (1964). Extracorporeal circulation and endogenous epinephrine and norepinephrine in plasma, atrium and urine in man. *Anesthesiology* 25, 262-269.

Appel, E., Simrock, R., Palm, D., Wnuk, A. & Dudziak, R. (1977). Enhancement of sympathoneuronal and sympathoadrenal activity during ketamine anaesthesia. *Naunyn-Schmiedeberg's Arch. Pharmacol.*, Suppl. to Vol. 297, R59.

Blaustein, M.P. & Christie Ector, A. (1975). Barbiturate inhibition of calcium uptake by depolarized nerve terminals *in vitro*. *Mol. Pharmacol.* 11, 369-378.

Cabrera, R., Torrance, R.W. & Viveros, H. (1966). The action of acetyl choline and other drugs upon the terminal parts of the postganglionic sympathetic fibre. *Br. J. Pharmacol.* 27, 51-63.

Carlsson, A., Engel, J. & Svensson, T.H. (1972). Inhibition of
    ethanol-induced excitation in mice and rats by alpha-methyl-
    p-tyrosine. *Psychopharmacologia* 26, 307-312.

Carlsson, C. & Häggendal, J. (1967). Arterial noradrenaline
    levels after ethanol withdrawal. *Lancet* 2, 889.

Carmichael, F.J. & Israel, Y. (1975). Effects of ethanol on
    neurotransmitter release by rat brain cortical slices. *J.
    Pharmacol. Exp. Ther.* 193, 824-834.

Clanachan, A.S. & McGrath, J.C. (1976). Effects of ketamine on
    the peripheral autonomic nervous system of the rat. *Br. J.
    Pharmacol.* 58, 247-252.

Corrodi, H., Fuxe, K. & Hökfelt, T. (1966a). The effects of
    barbiturates on the activity of the catecholamine neurones in
    the rat brain. *J. Pharm. Pharmacol.* 18, 556-558.

Corrodi, H., Fuxe, K. & Hökfelt, T. (1966b). The effect of
    ethanol on the activity of central cetacholamine neurons in
    rat brain. *J. Pharm. Pharmacol.* 18, 821-823.

DeRobertis, E. (1975). Synaptic receptor proteins. Isolation
    and reconstitution in artificial membranes. *Rev. Physiol.
    Biochem. Pharmacol.* 73, 9-38.

Dundee, J.W. (1970). Intravenous ethanol anaesthesia: A study
    of dosage and blood levels. *Anesth. Analg. Curr. Res.* 49,
    467-475.

Eyring, H., Woodbury, J.W. & D'Arrigo, J.S. (1973). A molecular
    mechanism of general anaesthesia. *Anesthesiology* 38, 415-424.

Fozard, J. & Mwaluko, G. (1976). Mechanism of the indirect
    sympathomimetic effect of 5-hydroxytryptamine on the isolated
    heart of the rabbit. *Br. J. Pharmacol.* 57, 115-125.

Fozard, J.R. & Mobarok Ali, A.T.M. (1976). Inhibition of the
    stimulant effect of 5-hydroxytryptamine on cardiac sympathetic
    nerves by 5-hydroxytryptamine and related compounds. *Br. J.
    Pharmacol.* 58, 416P-417P.

Gardier, R.W. (1972). Autonomic nervous system. In: *Handbook of
    Experimental Pharmacology* (ed.) M.B. Chenoweth, Vol. 30, pp.
    123-148, Springer, Berlin, Heidelberg, New York.

Gersh, B.J., Prys-Roberts, C. & Baker, A.B. (1972). The effects
    of halothane on the interactions between myocardial contrac-
    tility, aortic impedance and left ventricular performance.
    III. Influence of stimulation of sympathetic nerves, beta
    adrenergic receptors, and myocardial fibres. *Br. J. Anaesth.*
    44, 997-1005.

Goldstein, D.B. (1973). Alcohol withdrawal reactions in mice: Effects of drugs that modify neurotransmission. *J. Pharmacol. Exp. Ther.* 186, 1-9.

Göthert, M. (1974). Effects of halothane on the sympathetic nerve terminals of the rabbit heart. Differences in membrane actions of halothane and tetracaine. *Naunyn-Schmiedeberg's Arch. Pharmacol.* 286, 125-143.

Göthert, M. & Guth, M. (1975). Zum Einfluß von Halothan auf die Wirkungen von endogenem und exogenem Noradrenalin am isolierten druckkonstant perfundierten Kaninchenherzen. *Anaesthesist* 24, 27-31.

Göthert, M. & Kennerknecht, E. (1976). Effects of general anaesthetics on the cell membrane of sympathetic nerve terminals: An investigation of the mechanism of action of anaesthetics. *Excerpta Medica International Congress Series No. 387.* 6th World Congress of Anaesthesiology, Mexico City, April 24-30. Abstract No. 145 (F5-1/2). Amsterdam: Excerpta Medica.

Göthert, M. & Klupp, N. (1978). Cardiovascular effects of neurotoxic indolethylamines. *Ann. NY Acad. Sci.*, in press.

Göthert, M. & Rieckesmann, J.M. (1976). Effects of intravenous anaesthetics and hypnotics on the sympathetic nerves of the isolated rabbit heart. *Naunyn-Schmiedeberg's Arch. Pharmacol.* Suppl. 294, R1.

Göthert, M. & Thielecke, G. (1976). Inhibition by ethanol of noradrenaline output from peripheral sympathetic nerves: Possible interaction of ethanol with neuronal receptors. *Eur. J. Pharmacol.* 37, 321-328.

Göthert, M., Dorn, W. & Loewenstein, I. (1976a). Inhibition of catecholamine release from the adrenal medulla by halothane. Site and mechanism of action. *Naunyn-Schmiedeberg's Arch. Pharmacol.* 294, 239-249.

Göthert, M., Kennerknecht, E. & Thielecke, G. (1976b). Inhibition of receptor-mediated noradrenaline release from the sympathetic nerves of the isolated rabbit heart by anaesthetics and alcohols in proportion to their hydrophobic property. *Naunyn-Schmiedeberg's Arch. Pharmacol.* 292, 145-152.

Göthert, M., Lox, H.-J. & Rieckesmann, J.-M. (1977). Effects of butyrophenones on the sympathetic nerves of the isolated rabbit heart and on the postsynaptic α-adrenoceptors of the isolated rabbit aorta. *Naunyn-Schmiedeberg's Arch. Pharmacol.* 300, 255-265.

Griffiths, P.J., Littleton, J.M. & Ortiz, A. (1974). Changes in monoamine concentrations in mouse brain associated with ethanol dependence and withdrawal. *Br. J. Pharmacol.* 50, 489-498.

Hamelberg, W., Sprouse, J.H., Mahaffey, J.E. & Richardson, J.A. (1960). Catecholamine levels during light and deep anesthesia. *Anesthesiology* 21, 297-301.

Hatch, R.C. (1973). Experiments on antagonism of barbiturate anesthesia with adrenergic, serotonergic, and cholinergic stimulants given alone and in combination. *Am. J. Vet. Res.* 34, 1321-1331.

Haycock, J.W., Levy, W.B. & Cotman, C.W. (1977). Pentobarbital depression of stimulus-secretion coupling in brain. Selective inhibition of depolarization-induced calcium-dependent release. *Biochem. Pharmacol.* 26, 159-161.

Houck, D.J. (1969). Effect of alcohols on potentials of lobster axons. *Am. J. Physiol.* 216, 364-367.

Huković, S. & Muscholl, E. (1962). Die Noradrenalin-Abgabe aus dem isolierten Kaninchenherzen bei sympathischer Nervenreizung und ihre pharmakologische Beeinflussung. *Naunyn-Schmiedeberg's Arch. Exp. Pathol. Pharmacol.* 244, 81-96.

Hunt, W.A. & Majchrowicz, E. (1974). Alterations in the turnover of brain norepinephrine and dopamine in alcohol-dependent rats. *J. Neurochem.* 23, 549-552.

Israel, Y., Carmichael, F.J. & Macdonald, J.A. (1973). Effects of ethanol on norepinephrine uptake and electrically stimulated release in brain tissue. *Ann. NY Acad. Sci.* 215, 38-48.

Johnston, R.R., Way, W.L. & Miller, R.D. (1972). Alteration of anesthetic requirement by amphetamine. *Anesthesiology* 36, 357-363.

Knutsson, E. (1961). Effects of ethanol on the membrane potential and membrane resistance of frog muscle fibres. *Acta Physiol. Scand.* 52, 242-253.

Lidbrink, P. & Farnebo, L.-O. (1973). Uptake and release of noradrenaline in rat cerebral cortex *in vitro:* No effect of benzodiazepines and barbiturates. *Neuropharmacology* 12, 1087-1095.

Lidbrink, P., Corrodi, H., Fuxe, K. & Olson, L. (1972). Barbiturates and meprobamate: Decreases in catecholamine turnover of central dopamine and noradrenaline neuronal systems and the influence of immobilization stress. *Brain Res.* 45, 507-524.

Meyer, H. (1899). Zur Theorie der Alkoholnarkose. Erste Mittheilung. Welche Eigenschaft der Anästhetica bedingt ihre narkotische Wirkung? *Arch. Exp. Pathol. Pharmacol.* 42, 109-118.

Meyer, H. (1901). Zur Theorie der Alkoholnarkose. 3. Mittheilung
    Der Einfluß wechselnder Temperatur auf Wirkungsstärke und
    Theilungscoefficient der Narcotica. *Arch. Exp. Pathol.*
    Pharmacol. 46, 338-346.

Miletich, D.J., Ivankovic, A.D., Albrecht, R.F., Zahed, B. &
    Ihali, A.A. (1973). The effect of ketamine on catecholamine
    metabolism in the isolated perfused rat heart. *Anesthesiology*
    39, 271-277.

Millar, R.A., Warden, J.C., Cooperman, L.H. & Price, L.H. (1969).
    Central sympathetic discharge and mean arterial pressure during
    halothane anaesthesia. *Br. J. Anaesth*. 41, 918-928.

Miller, R.D., Way, W.L. & Eger, E.I. (1968). The effects of
    alpha-methyldopa, reserpine, guanethidine and iproniazid on
    minimum alveolar anesthetic requirement (MAC). *Anesthesiology*
    29, 1153-1158.

Montel, H., Starke, K., Görlitz, B.-D. & Schümann, H.J. (1973).
    Tierexperimentelle Untersuchungen zur Wirkung des Ketamins auf
    periphere sympathische Nerven. *Anaesthesist* 22, 111-116.

Muldoon, S. & Vanhoutte, P. (1975). Venous relaxation by halo-
    thane acting on the sympathetic nerves. *Arch. Int. Pharmacodyn*.
    213, 330-331.

Naito, H. & Gillis, C.N. (1968). Anesthetics and response of
    atria to sympathetic nerve stimulation. *Anesthesiology* 29,
    259-266.

Nedergaard, O.A. (1973). Cocaine-like effect of ketamine on
    vascular adrenergic neurons. *Eur. J. Pharmacol*. 23, 153-161.

Ngai, S.H. (1974). Plasma catecholamines - their significance in
    anesthesia. *Anesthesiology* 41, 429-431.

Overton, E. (1901). *Studien über die Narkose* (ed.) E. Overton,
    Jena: G. Fischer.

Persson, T. & Waldeck, B. (1971). A reduced rate of turnover of
    brain noradrenaline during pentobarbitone anaesthesia. *J.*
    Pharm. Pharmacol. 23, 377-378.

Planz, G., Yilmaz, E. & Palm, D. (1973). Plasma dopamine - β -
    hydroxylase activity as a measure of sympathetic activity
    during halothane anaesthesia in children. *Eur. J. Clin.*
    Pharmacol. 6, 228-233.

Pohorecki, L.A. (1974). Effects of ethanol on central and peri-
    pheral noradrenergic neurons. *J. Pharmacol. Exp. Ther*. 189,
    380-391.

Pohorecky, L.A. & Jaffe, L.S. (1975). Noradrenergic involvement in the acute effects of ethanol. *Res. Commun. Chem. Pathol. Pharmacol.* 12, 433-448.

Pohorecky, L.A., Jaffe, L.S. & Berkeley, H.A. (1974). Ethanol withdrawal in the rat: Involvement of noradrenergic neurons. *Life Sci.* 15, 427-437.

Price, H.L., Linde, H.W., Jones, R.E., Black, G.W. & Price, M.L. (1959). Sympathoadrenal responses to general anesthesia in man and their relation to hemodynamics. *Anesthesiology* 20, 563-575.

Price, H.L., Warden, J.C., Cooperman, L.H. & Price, M.L. (1968). Enhancement by cyclopropane and halothane of heart rate responses to sympathetic stimulation. *Anesthesiology* 29, 478-483.

Roizen, M.F., Moss, J., Henry, D.P. & Kopin, I.J. (1974). Effects of halothane on plasma catecholamines. *Anesthesiology* 41, 432-439.

Roizen, M.F., Thoa, N.B., Moss, J. & Kopin, I.J. (1975). Inhibition by halothane of release of norepinephrine, but not of dopamine - β - hydroxylase, from guinea pig vas deferens. *Eur. J. Pharmacol.* 31, 313-318.

Roizen, M.F., Kopin, I.J., Thoa, N.B., Zivin, J., Muth, E.A. & Jacobowitz, D.M. (1976a). The effect of two anesthetic agents on norepinephrine and dopamine in discrete brain nuclei, fiber tracts, and terminal regions of the rat. *Brain Res.* 110, 515-522.

Roizen, M.F., Thoa, N.B., Moss, J. & Kopin, I.J. (1976b). Inhibition by cyclopropane of release of norepinephrine, but not dopamine - β - hydroxylase from the guinea-pig vas deferens. *Anesthesiology* 44, 54-56.

Seeman, P. (1966). Membrane stabilization by drugs: Tranquilizers, steroids and anesthetics. *Int. Rev. Neurobiol.* 9, 145-221.

Seeman, P. (1972). The membrane actions of anesthetics and tranquilizers. *Pharmacol. Rev.* 24, 583-655.

Seeman, P. (1974). The membrane expansion theory of anesthesia: Direct evidence using ethanol and a high-precision density meter. *Experientia* 30, 759-760.

Seeman, P. & Lee, T. (1974). The dopamine-releasing actions of neuroleptics and ethanol. *J. Pharmacol. Exp. Ther.* 190, 131-140.

Skovsted, P., Price, M.L. & Price, H.L. (1969). The effects of
halothane on arterial pressure, preganglionic sympathetic
activity and barostatic reflexes. *Anesthesiology* 31, 507-514.

Smith, A.D. & Winkler, H. (1972). Fundamental mechanisms in the
release of catecholamines. In: *Handbook of Experimental
Pharmacology* (eds.) H. Blaschko and E. Muscholl, Vol. 33, pp.
538-617, Springer: Berlin-Heidelberg-New York.

Smith, D.J., Azzaro, A.J., Turndorf, H. & Abbott, S.B. (1975).
The effect of ketamine HCl on the *in vitro* metabolism of
norepinephrine in rat cerebral cortex tissue. *Neuropharmacology*
14, 473-481.

Staiman, A. & Seeman, P. (1975). The impulse-blocking concentrations of anesthetics, alcohols, anticonvulsants, barbiturates,
and narcotics on phrenic and sciatic nerves. *Can. J. Physiol.
Pharmacol.* 52, 535-550.

Starke, K., Wagner, J. & Schümann, H.J. (1972). Adrenergic neuron
blockade by clonidine: Comparison with guanethidine and local
anaesthetics. *Arch. Int. Pharmacodyn.* 195, 291-308.

Stoelting, R.K., Creasser, C.W. & Martz, R.C. (1975). Effect of
cocaine administration on halothane MAC in dogs. *Anesth.
Analg. Curr. Res.* 54, 422-424.

Sun, A.Y. (1976). Alcohol-membrane interaction in the brain:
Norepinephrine release. *Res. Commun. Chem. Pathol. Pharmacol.*
15, 705-720.

Taube, H.D., Montel, H., Hau, G. & Starke, K. (1975). Phencyclidine
and ketamine: Comparison with the effect of cocaine on the
noradrenergic neurones of the rat brain cortex. *Naunyn-
Schmiedeberg's Arch. Pharmacol.* 291, 47-54.

Tauberger, G., Schulte am Esch, J. & Steinringer, W. (1975). Der
Einfluß kombinierter Narkosen mit Halothan und Neuroleptanal-
gesie auf die praeganglionäre Sympathicusaktivität des Atem-
zentrums und den Kreislauf. *Anaesthesist* 24, 491-495.

Thadani, P.V. & Truitt, E.G. (1973). Norepinephrine turnover
effects of ethanol and acetaldehyde in rat brain. *Fed. Proc.*
32, 697.

Ueda, I. & Kamaya, H. (1973). Kinetic and thermodynamic aspects
of the mechanism of general anesthetics in a model system of
firefly luminescence *in vitro*. *Anesthesiology* 38, 425-436.

Weinshilboum, R.M. & Axelrod, J. (1971). Serum dopamine - β -
hydroxylase: Decrease after chemical sympathectomy. *Science*
173, 931-934.

Weinshilboum, R.M., Kvetnansky, R., Axelrod, J. & Kopin, I.J. (1971). Elevation of serum dopamine - β - hydroxylase activity with forced immobilization. *Nature (New Biol.)* 230, 287-288.

Weinshilboum, R.W., Thoa, N.B., Johnson, D.G., Kopin, I.J. & Axelrod, J. (1971). Proportional release of norepinephrine and dopamine - β - hydroxylase from sympathetic nerves. *Science* 174, 1349-1351.

Westfall, T.C. (1974). Effect of nicotine and other drugs on the release of ^{3}H-norepinephrine and ^{3}H-dopamine from rat brain slices. *Neuropharmacology* 13, 693-700.

Wieber, J., Gugler, R., Hengstmann, J.H. & Dengler, H.J. (1975). Pharmacokinetics of ketamine in man. *Anaesthesist* 24, 260-263.

MODIFICATION OF RELEASE BY ADENOSINE AND ADENINE NUCLEOTIDES

A. S. Clanachan

I   INTRODUCTION

It is now well established that the release of noradrenaline from
noradrenergic neurons can be influenced via receptor systems
located on the outer surface of the nerve ending (see Section A;
this volume). Stimulation of these presynaptic receptors may
either inhibit (α adrenoceptor; dopamine, prostaglandin, opiate
and muscarine receptors) or facilitate (β adrenoceptor; angiotensin and nicotine receptors) noradrenaline release. Experimental investigations intent on elucidating the role of cyclic
adenosine 3',5'-monophosphate (cAMP) in the process of neurotransmitter release uncovered the finding that agents which increased intracellular levels of cAMP (e.g., adrenaline or dibutyryl cyclic 3',5'-monophosphate) increased acetylcholine release
at the neuromuscular junction (Goldberg & Singer, 1969). In contrast, adenosine, in doses which increased intracellular cAMP in
brain slices (Sattin & Rall, 1970) inhibited neuromuscular transmission by decreasing acetylcholine release (Ginsborg & Hirst,
1972; Ribeiro & Walker, 1975). Such studies, then, uncovered
this hitherto unknown property of adenosine. Similar presynaptic
inhibitory effects of adenine nucleotides and adenosine on parasympathetic neurotransmission have been observed in intestinal
smooth muscle (Takagi & Takayanagi, 1972; Sawynok & Jhamandas,
1976; Vizi & Knoll, 1976). The effects of adenine nucleotides
and adenosine on noradrenergic neurotransmission have been investigated only recently (Hedqvist & Fredholm, 1976; Clanachan &
Paton, 1977; Clanachan, Johns & Paton, 1977; Enero & Saidman,
1977; Verhaeghe, Vanhoutte & Shepherd, 1977). This chapter is
intended as a review of the experimental evidence which suggests
that presynaptic 'purinergic' (adenine nucleotide and/or adenosine)
receptors may exist on noradrenergic neurones.

II   EFFECTS OF ADENINE NUCLEOTIDES AND ADENOSINE ON
        NORADRENALINE RELEASE

   A.   Indirect Studies

Isometric contractions of isolated rat vas deferens elicited by
field stimulation are inhibited by ATP, ADP, AMP and adenosine
whereas those to exogenous noradrenaline are unaffected (Clanachan
& Paton, 1977; Clanachan et al., 1977). The inhibition is rapid
in onset and is readily reversed by washing. In canine blood
vessels, ATP, ADP, and adenosine produce a greater inhibition of

the mechanical responses produced by electrical stimulation than those produced by exogenous noradrenaline (Verhaeghe *et al.*, 1977). In addition, these authors demonstrated that adenosine possesses a similar activity *in vivo*. These results provide indirect evidence that adenine nucleotides and adenosine inhibit neurotransmission at a presynaptic site by inhibiting noradrenaline release.

B.   Direct Studies

The presynaptic effects of adenine nucleotides and adenosine have been investigated directly by measuring the basal and stimulus-induced efflux of $(-)-[^3H]$noradrenaline. Adenosine inhibits the nerve stimulated release of noradrenaline in perfused adipose tissue and perfused kidney *in vitro* and *in vivo* (Hedqvist & Fredholm, 1976), in guinea pig (Hedqvist & Fredholm, 1976) and rat vas deferens (Clanachan *et al.*, 1977), in rat portal vein (Enero & Saidman, 1977) and in canine blood vessels (Verhaeghe *et al.*, 1977). Similarly, ATP has been shown to reduce noradrenaline release in perfused adipose tissue (Fredholm, 1974), in blood vessels (Verhaeghe *et al.*, 1977; Enero & Saidman, 1977) and in rat vas deferens (Clanachan *et al.*, 1977). Thus, although the postsynaptic effects of adenine nucleotides are variable (e.g., noradrenaline-induced responses are potentiated in kidney, unchanged in rat vas deferens and reduced in isolated blood vessels) the predominant presynaptic effect is inhibition of noradrenaline release.

III   SITE OF ACTION

The possibility existed that adenosine-induced inhibition of noradrenaline release was mediated via an indirect action on other, previously reported presynaptic receptor systems. For example, it is well established that prostaglandins can act at a presynaptic site to inhibit noradrenaline release (Hedqvist, 1974). As adenine nucleotides and adenosine can stimulate the biosynthesis of endogenous prostaglandins (Needleman, Minkes & Douglas, 1974; Kamikawa & Shimo, 1976), the presynaptic inhibitory effects of the purines may be prostaglandin mediated. However, this is unlikely as indomethacin, an inhibitor of prostaglandin synthetase (Flower & Vane, 1974) did not change their inhibitory actions in vas deferens (Hedqvist & Fredholm, 1976; Clanachan *et al.*, 1977). In addition, the inhibition is not caused by the stimulation of presynaptic muscarine receptors which would also inhibit transmitter release (Löffelholz & Muscholl, 1969) as atropine did not antagonise ATP and adenosine-induced inhibition (Clanachan *et al.*, 1977). Similarly, stimulation of presynaptic *a*-adrenoceptors which would also inhibit noradrenaline release (Langer, 1974; 1977) was discounted as phenoxybenzamine did not change the inhibitory actions of ATP or adenosine (Hedqvist & Fredholm, 1976; Clanachan *et al.*, 1977).

Theophylline, a commonly used postsynaptic antagonist of ATP and adenosine (Burnstock, 1975) can antagonise their presynaptic

effect in vas deferens (Clanachan *et al.*, 1977) and in blood
vessels (Verhaeghe *et al.*, 1977). However, theophylline, in
addition to its antagonist properties on adenosine receptors,
also produces mobilisation of intracellular calcium pools
(Isaacson & Sandow, 1967; Johnson & Inesi, 1969) and phosphodiesterase inhibition (Berthet, Sutherland & Rall, 1957). It
should be noted, however, that the antagonism by theophylline is
specific for the purine compounds. For example, the inhibition
of nerve stimulated responses of vas deferens by the presynaptic
α adrenoceptor agonist, clonidine (Starke & Altman, 1973) is not
affected (Clanachan & Paton, unpublished observations). Similarly, dopamine-induced inhibition of parasympathetic neurotransmission was unchanged by theophylline (Sawynok & Jhamandas, 1976).
The specific antagonism of the presynaptic actions of adenosine
and ATP indicates that a presynaptic purinergic receptor system
(see Burnstock, 1972) may be involved.

Dipyridamole and 2-amino-6[2-hydroxy-5-nitro-benzylthio]-9-β-D-
ribofuranosylpurine (HNBTG), which potentiate the postsynaptic
effects of adenosine by inhibiting its uptake and hence its inactivation (Stafford, 1966; Paterson, Kim, Bernard & Cass, 1975;
Baer, Frew & Burnstock, 1977), also potentiated the presynaptic
action of adenosine in the rat vas (Clanachan *et al.*, 1977).
This effect is, at first, surprising since adenine nucleotides,
unlike adenosine, do not readily traverse cell membranes (Hattori,
Miyazaki & Nakamura, 1969). A plausible explanation is that the
nucleotides must be first hydrolysed by extracellular phospha-
tases to adenosine in order to cause presynaptic inhibition.
Rapid hydrolysis of ATP to adenosine is known to occur in heart
(Bär & Drummond, 1968), intestine (Burnstock, 1972) and trachea
(Coleman, 1976). This theory is also supported by the finding
that 2-2'-pyridylisatogen tosylate (PIT), an antagonist which has
been claimed to inhibit selectively the postsynaptic actions of
ATP and ADP without affecting those of AMP and adenosine
(Spedding & Weetman, 1976), does not antagonise the presynaptic
inhibitory effects of these compounds in the rat vas (Clanachan
et al., 1977).

A relationship between presynaptic opiate (Hughes, Kosterlitz &
Leslie, 1976) and presynaptic purinergic actions on parasympathetic nerves have been found in studies on acetylcholine release in intestinal smooth muscle (Sawynok & Jhamandas, 1976).
However, these authors also found that naloxone, a specific
opiate receptor antagonist (Hughes *et al.*, 1975), did not antagonise ATP or adenosine-induced inhibition and suggested that
morphine may be releasing an "adenosine-like" substance. This is
unlikely to be a widespread phenomenon as opiates do not inhibit
noradrenaline release from all noradrenergic nerve endings, e.g.,
those in rat vas deferens, a tissue where presynaptic purinergic
inhibition has been demonstrated (Clanachan *et al.*, 1977).
Nevertheless, a specific opiate-purinergic interaction on noradrenergic neurones has not, as yet, been investigated.

IV   MECHANISM OF ACTION

The mechanism responsible for the purine-mediated inhibition of noradrenaline release appears to be similar in nature to that of other presynaptic receptor systems. For example, a greater inhibition of noradrenaline release at low frequencies of stimulation is seen with both presynaptic α-adrenoceptor (Langer, 1977) and presynaptic purinergic receptor agonists (Verhaeghe et al., 1977). Verhaeghe et al.(1977) examined the effect of adenosine on (-)-[^{3}H]noradrenaline release from canine saphenous vein strips induced by electrical field stimulation and by nerve depolarisation with an elevated potassium ion concentration (30 mM). These are calcium-dependent processes. Noradrenaline release was also induced by tyramine, a calcium independent process (Thoa, Wollen, Axelrod & Kopin, 1975). Release by nerve stimulation and potassium were inhibited whereas that caused by tyramine was not. Thus, adenosine, like other presynaptic agonists (Langer, 1977) only interferes with calcium dependent processes. However, whether adenosine acts by hyperpolarising the neuronal membrane, by directly inhibiting calcium influx, or by interfering with a further step in excitation-secretion coupling remains to be answered. An inhibitory effect on calcium permeability has, however, been reported to be involved in adenosine action postsynaptically in cardiac muscle (Schrader, Rubio & Berne, 1975) and in vascular smooth muscle (Herlihy, Bockman, Berne & Rubio, 1976).

Pre- and postsynaptic α 'adrenoceptors are not necessarily identical entities as they differ in their ability to be stimulated by α adrenoceptor agonists and to be blocked by α adrenoceptor antagonists. This has led to the suggestion that postsynaptic α adrenoceptors be termed α1 while the presynaptic α adrenoceptors should be termed α2 (Langer, 1974). No such difference between pre- and postsynaptic 'purinergic' receptors has been suggested. Extensive structure-activity data is available for presynaptic purinergic receptor agonists in rat vas deferens (Paton, Bär, Clanachan & Lauzon, 1977) and for purinergic receptor-induced relaxation of intestinal smooth muscle (McKenzie, Frew & Bär, 1977a) which presumably is mediated postsynaptically. Comparisons of these data indicate no marked differences in the structure-activity relationships (Paton et al., 1977). The common structural requirements for activity include a primary or secondary amine function at C6 of the purine ring. For example, omission of the amino group, as in inosine, the natural deamination metabolite of adenosine, results in an inactive compound. Furthermore, there is little tolerance for steric changes or substitutions on the sugar moiety, indicating that the sugar plays a key role in receptor activation.

Postsynaptic actions of purine compounds have been linked to stimulation of the adenylate cyclase-cAMP system (Sattin & Rall, 1970; Huang & Drummond, 1976) although more recent evidence tends to dispute this finding (Herlihy et al., 1976; McKenzie, Frew & Bär, 1977b; Verhaeghe, 1977). No such relationship is likely to occur presynaptically. As mentioned above, an increase in intraneuronal cAMP is associated with an increase in the release of

acetylcholine (Goldberg & Singer, 1969). A similar conclusion
has been reached from studies on noradrenaline release irrespective of whether cAMP levels were elevated by β adrenoceptor
agonists (see Langer, 1977), by phosphodiesterase inhibition or
by exogenous cyclic nucleotide analogues (Cubeddu, Barnes &
Weiner, 1975).

In addition, a comparison of the structure activity data obtained
in rat vas (Paton *et al.*, 1977) with those for cAMP formation in
brain slices (Mah & Daly, 1976), heart slices (Huang & Drummond,
1976) and in smooth muscle of the rabbit intestine (McKenzie *et
al.*, 1977b) indicates several noteworthy discrepancies. Mah &
Daly (1976) reported that adenosine analogues with modifications
to the ribose moiety antagonised the stimulant effect of adenosine on cAMP in brain tissue. These compounds (2'- and 3'-deoxy-
adenosine) showed no antagonist activity on adenosine-induced inhibition of noradrenergic neurotransmission (Paton *et al.*, 1977).
Similarly, the depression of electrical activity in central neurons by adenosine is also unaffected by these analogues (Phyllis
& Edstrom, 1976). These results indicate distinct differences
between adenosine actions on the adenylate cyclase-cAMP system
and those on adenosine receptors located either pre- or post-
synaptically.

High concentrations of adenosine (0.4 mM), but not ATP, can increase the basal (unstimulated) efflux of $(-)$-[^{3}H]noradrenaline
and deaminated metabolites from vascular preparations (Verhaeghe
et al., 1977). This suggests that at higher concentrations,
adenosine acts intracellularly, perhaps via changes in cAMP
levels, to increase the intraneuronal leakage of noradrenaline
out of storage vesicles (Verhaeghe *et al.*, 1977).

V   SIGNIFICANCE OF PRESYNAPTIC 'PURINERGIC' RECEPTORS

It should be pointed out that inhibition of noradrenaline release
can only be demonstrated in the presence of relatively high concentrations (> 10^{-5}M) of ATP and adenosine. This raises doubts
about assigning a role to these compounds in the physiological
regulation of noradrenaline release. However, great care should
be taken when trying to compare concentrations of drugs *in vitro*
with those which may occur in the 'biophase' in the synaptic
cleft. There are several possible sources of ATP and adenosine
which could act presynaptically (Fig. 1). ATP is released with
catecholamines from the adrenal medulla (Smith & Winkler, 1972)
and probably also with noradrenaline from noradrenergic nerve
endings (see Burnstock, 1976). It has been suggested that ATP
released in this manner may be responsible for the residual non-
cholinergic, non-adrenergic responses of the nictitating membrane
to nerve stimulation following reserpine pretreatment (Langer &
Pinto, 1976). It is interesting to consider that ATP released
from noradrenergic nerves is metabolised to adenosine which may
'feedback' and influence noradrenaline release.

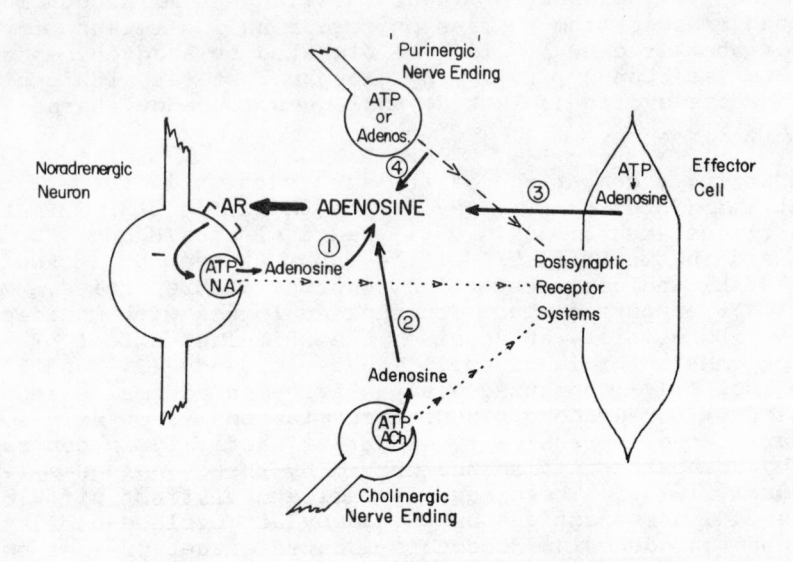

Fig. 1.   Diagrammatic representation of possible sources
          of adenosine which could stimulate presynaptic
          adenosine (adenine riboside, AR) receptors to
          inhibit the release of noradrenaline. (1) and
          (2) represent ATP, which may be released by ex-
          ocytosis with noradrenaline and acetylcholine
          from noradrenergic and cholinergic nerves res-
          pectively. ATP is rapidly degraded to adenosine
          by extracellular phosphatases. (3) adenosine
          released from postsynaptic sites and (4) adeno-
          sine released from 'purinergic nerves'.

Vesicles in cholinergic nerve terminals contain, in addition to
acetylcholine, considerable amounts of nucleotides (Whittaker,
Dowdall & Boyne, 1972). It has been suggested that following release, ATP, or its metabolites ADP, AMP and adenosine may 'feedback' to inhibit acetylcholine release (Vizi & Knoll, 1977).
Thus, they may also act on surrounding noradrenergic neurones and
inhibit noradrenaline release. Another possible source of ATP or
adenosine is from the so-called 'purinergic nerves' (see Burnstock,
1972) which are claimed to exist in some tissues. Enero & Saidman
(1977) have shown that in rat portal vein, a tissue in which a
purinergic innervation has been postulated (Hughes & Vane, 1970;
Su, 1975), inhibition of adenosine uptake and metabolism (with
dilazep and erythro-9-(2 hydroxy-3-monyl) adenine respectively)
significantly reduced the stimulation-induced overflow of noradrenaline. However, the drugs used to decrease adenosine inactivation may have produced a direct depression of noradrenaline release. Adenosine may also be released from postsynaptic sites.
Degradation of adenine nucleotides to adenosine has been demon-

strated in anoxic slices of myocardium (Imai, Riley & Berne, 1964), ischemic myocardium (Scheuer & Steyoski, 1968) and the arrested heart (Parker, Smith & Jones, 1976). It is possible that adenosine produced during such conditions may exhibit profound effects on cardiac neurotransmission. Adenosine has also been shown to be released from the cortex by stimulation (McIlwain, 1972; Pull & McIlwain, 1972) and so may be continuously controlling transmitter release in the central nervous system.

VI   CONCLUSION

Adenine nucleotides and adenosine have been shown to inhibit noradrenergic neurotransmission in a variety of preparations *in vitro* and *in vivo*. This inhibition occurs at a presynaptic site by reducing noradrenaline release and is mediated by a 'purinergic' receptor system which is probably not linked to adenylate cyclase.

A regulating role of ATP or adenosine is difficult to show experimentally. Theophylline antagonises the effects of exogenous purine compounds (Verhaeghe *et al.*, 1977; Clanachan *et al.*, 1977). If endogenous purines produce presynaptic inhibition it would be expected that theophylline would increase transmitter release. This has been confirmed for acetylcholine release in intestinal smooth muscle (Vizi & Knoll, 1976). Although theophylline is commonly used as an antagonist of adenosine, it is relatively weak and, due to its effects on calcium and phosphodiesterase, it may be non-specific. Before any conclusions can be made regarding the role of endogenous purines in the regulation of transmitter release, a more potent and specific adenosine receptor antagonist is required.

Acknowledgements

The author wishes to acknowledge the financial support of a Research Fellowship from the Canadian Heart Foundation.

VII   REFERENCES

Bär, H.-P. & Drummond, G.I. (1968). Catabolism of adenine nucleotides by the isolated perfused rat heart. *Proc. Soc. Exp. Biol. Med.* 127, 33-36.

Baer, H.-P., Frew, R. & Burnstock, G. (1977). Effect of dipyridamole and 6-(2-nydroxy-5-nitro)-benzylthioguanosine on low-frequency-stimulated relaxation in the guinea-pig taenia coli. *Can. J. Physiol. Pharmacol.* 55, 394-398.

Berthet, J., Sutherland, E.W. & Rall, T.W. (1957). The assay of glucagon and epinephrine with use of liver homogenates. *J. Biol. Chem.* 229, 351-361.

Burnstock, G. (1972). Purinergic nerves. *Pharmacol. Rev.* 24, 509-581.

Burnstock, G. (1975). Purinergic transmission. In: *Handbook of Psychopharmacology* (eds.) L.I. Iversen, S.D. Iversen & S.H. Snyder, Vol. 5, pp. 131-194, Plenum Press, New York.

Burnstock, G. (1976). Do some nerve cells release more than one transmitter? *Neuroscience* 1, 239-248.

Clanachan, A.S. & Paton, D.M. (1977). Inhibitory actions of adenine nucleotides and adenosine on transmission in rat vas deferens. *Br. J. Pharmacol.* 59, 53P.

Clanachan, A.S., Johns, A. & Paton, D.M. (1977). Presynaptic inhibitory actions of adenine nucleotides and adenosine on neurotransmission in rat vas deferens. *Neuroscience* 2, 597-602.

Coleman, R.A. (1976). Effects of some purine derivatives on the guinea-pig trachea and their interaction with drugs that block adenosine uptake. *Br. J. Pharmacol.* 57, 51-57.

Cubeddu, L., Barnes, X.E. & Weiner, N. (1975). Release of norepinephrine and dopamine-β-hydroxylase by nerve stimulation. IV. An evaluation of a role for cyclic adenosine monophosphate. *J. Pharmacol. Exp. Ther.* 193, 105-127.

Enero, M.A. & Saidman, B.Q. (1977). Possible feed-back inhibition of noradrenaline release by purine compounds. *Naunyn Schmiedeberg's Arch. Pharmacol.* 297, 39-46.

Flower, R.J. & Vane, J.R. (1974). Inhibition of prostaglandin biosynthesis. *Biochem. Pharmacol.* 23, 1439-1450.

Fredholm, B.B. (1974). Vascular and metabolic effects of theophylline, dibutyryl cyclic AMP and dibutyryl cyclic GMP in canine subcutaneous adipose tissues *in situ*. *Acta Physiol. Scand.* 90, 226-236.

Ginsborg, B.L. & Hirst, G.I.S. (1972). The effect of adenosine on the release of the transmitter from the phrenic nerve of the rat. *J. Physiol.* 224, 629-645.

Goldberg, A.L. & Singer, J.J. (1969). Evidence for a role of cyclic AMP in neuromuscular transmission. *Proc. Natn. Acad. Sci., U.S.A.* 64, 134-141.

Hattori, E., Miyazaki, T. & Nakamura, M. (1969). Incorporation of adenosine and adenosine triphosphate into rat myocardium. *Jap. Heart J.* 10, 47-52.

Hedqvist, P. (1974). Prostaglandin action on noradrenaline release and mechanical responses in the stimulated guinea-pig vas deferens. *Acta Physiol. Scand.* 90, 86-93.

Hedqvist, P. & Fredholm, B.B. (1976). Effects of adenosine on adrenergic transmission; prejunctional inhibition and postjunctional enhancement. *Naunyn Schmiedeberg's Arch. Exp. Path. Pharmak.* 293, 217-223.

Herlihy, J.T., Bockman, E.L., Berne, R.M. & Rubio, R. (1976).
Adenosine relaxation of isolated vascular smooth muscle. *Am. J. Physiol*. 230, 1239-1243.

Huang, M. & Drummond, G.I. (1976). Effect of adenosine on cyclic AMP accumulation in ventricular myocardium. *Biochem. Pharmacol*. 25, 2713-2719.

Hughes, J. & Vane, J.R. (1970). Relaxations of the isolated portal vein of the rabbit induced by nicotine and electrical stimulation. *Br. J. Pharmacol*. 39, 476-489.

Hughes, J., Kosterlitz, H.W. & Leslie, F.M. (1975). Effect of morphine on adrenergic transmission in the mouse vas deferens. Assessment of agonist and antagonist potencies of narcotic analgesics. *Br. J. Pharmacol*. 53, 371-381.

Imai, S., Riley, A.L. & Berne, R.M. (1964). Effect of ischemia on adenine nucleotides in cardiac and skeletal muscle. *Circ. Res*. 15, 443-450.

Isaacson, A. & Sandow, A. (1967). Quinine and caffeine effects on calcium movements in frog sartorius muscle. *J. Gen. Physiol*. 50, 2109-2128.

Johnson, P.N. & Inesi, A. (1969). The effects of methylxanthines and local anaesthetics on fragmented sarcoplasmic reticulum. *J. Pharmacol. Exp. Ther*. 169, 308-314.

Kamikawa, Y. & Shimo, Y. (1976). Mediation of prostaglandin E_2 in the biphasic response to ATP of the isolated tracheal muscle of guinea-pigs. *J. Pharm. Pharmacol*. 38, 294-297.

Langer, S.Z. (1974). Presynaptic regulation of catecholamine release. *Biochem. Pharmacol*. 23, 1793-1800.

Langer, S.Z. (1977). Presynaptic receptors and their role in the regulation of transmitter release. *Br. J. Pharmacol*. 60, 481-497.

Langer, S.Z. & Pinto, J.E.B. (1976). Possible involvement of a transmitter different from norepinephrine in the residual responses to nerve stimulation of the cat nictitating membrane after pretreatment with reserpine. *J. Pharmacol. Exp. Ther*. 196, 697-713.

Löffelholz, K. & Muscholl, E. (1969). A muscarinic inhibition of the noradrenaline release evoked by postganglionic sympathetic nerve stimulation. *Naunyn Schmiedeberg's Arch. Exp. Path. Pharmak*. 265, 1-15.

Mah, H.D. & Daly, J.W. (1976). Adenosine-dependent formation of cyclic AMP in brain slices. *Pharmacol. Res. Commun*. 8, 65-79.

McIlwain, H. (1972). Regulatory significance of the release and
    action of adenine derivatives in cerebral system. *Biochem.*
    Soc. Symp. 36, 69-85.

McKenzie, S.G., Frew, R. & Bär, H.-P. (1977a). Characteristics
    of the relaxant response of adenosine and its analogs in in-
    testinal smooth muscle. *Eur. J. Pharmacol.* 41, 183-192.

McKenzie, S.G., Frew, R. & Bär, H.-P. (1977b). Effects of adeno-
    sine and related compounds on adenylate cyclase and cyclic AMP
    levels in smooth muscle. *Eur. J. Pharmacol.* 41, 193-203.

Needleman, P., Minkes, M.S. & Douglas, J.R. (1974). Stimulation
    of prostaglandin biosynthesis by adenine nucleotides. *Circ.*
    Res. 34, 455-460.

Parker, J.C., Smith, E.E. & Jones, C.E. (1976). The role of nuc-
    leoside and nucleobase metabolism in myocardial adenine nucleo-
    tide regeneration after cardiac arrest. *Circ. Shock* 3, 11-20.

Paterson, A.R.P., Kim, S.C., Bernard, O. & Cass, C.E. (1975).
    Transport of nucleosides. *Ann. N.Y. Acad. Sci.* 255, 402-411.

Paton, D.M., Bär, H.-P., Clanachan, A.S. & Lauzon, P. (1977).
    Structure activity relations for inhibition of neurotrans-
    mission in rat vas deferens by adenosine. *Neuroscience,* in
    press.

Phyllis, J.W. & Edstrom, J.P. (1976). Effects of adenosine ana-
    logs on rat cerebral cortical neurons. *Life Science* 19, 1041-
    1054.

Pull, L. & McIlwain, H. (1972). Metabolism of [^{14}C] adenosine and
    derivatives by cerebral tissues superfused and electrically
    stimulated. *Biochem. J.* 126, 965-972.

Ribeiro, J.A. & Walker, J. (1975). The effects of adenosine tri-
    phosphate and adenosine diphosphate on transmission at the rat
    and frog neuromuscular junctions. *Br. J. Pharmacol.* 54, 213-
    218.

Sattin, A. & Rall, T.W. (1970). The effect of adenosine and ad-
    enine nucleotides on the cyclic adenosine 3',5'-phosphate con-
    tent of guinea-pig cerebral cortex slices. *Mol. Pharmacol.* 6,
    13-23.

Sawynok, J. & Jhamandas, K.H. (1976). Inhibition of acetylcholine
    release from cholinergic nerves by adenosine, adenine nucleo-
    tides and morphine: antagonism by theophylline. *J. Pharmacol.*
    Exp. Ther. 197, 379-390.

Scheuer, J. & Steyoski, S.W. (1968). Effects of high-energy phos-
    phate depletion and repletion on the dynamics and electro-
    cardiogram of isolated rat hearts. *Circ. Res.* 23, 519-522.

Schrader, J., Rubio, R. & Berne, R.M. (1975). Inhibition of slow
    action potentials of guinea-pig atria by adenosine. *J. Mol.
    Cell. Cardiol.* 7, 427-433.

Smith, A.D. & Winkler, H. (1972). Fundamental mechanisms in the
    release of catecholamines. In: *Catecholamines, Handbook of
    Experimental Pharmacology* (eds.) H. Blaschko & E. Muscholl,
    Vol. 33, pp. 538-617, Springer-Verlag, Berlin.

Spedding, M. & Weetman, D.F. (1976). Identification of separate
    receptors for adenosine and adenosine 5'-triphosphate in
    causing relaxations of the isolated taenia of the guinea-pig
    caecum. *Br. J. Pharmacol.* 57, 305-310.

Stafford, A. (1966). Potentiation of adenosine and the adenine
    nucleotides by dipyridamole. *Br. J. Pharmacol. Chemother.* 28,
    218-227.

Starke, K. & Altman, K.P. (1973). Inhibition of adrenergic neuro-
    transmission by clonidine: An action of prejunctional α recep-
    tors. *Neuropharmacology* 12, 339-347.

Su, C. (1975). Neurogenic release of purine compounds in blood
    vessels. *J. Pharmacol. Exp. Ther.* 195, 159-166.

Takagi, K. & Takayanagi, I. (1972). Effect of N^6,2'-O-dibutryl
    3',5'-cyclic adenosine monophosphate, 3',5'-cyclic adenosine
    monophosphate and adenosine triphosphate on acetylcholine out-
    put from cholinergic nerves in guinea-pig ileum. *Jap. J.
    Pharmacol.* 22, 33-36.

Thoa, N.B., Wosten, G.F., Axelrod, J. & Kopin, I.S. (1975). On
    the mechanism of release of norepinephrine from sympathetic
    nerves induced by depolarizing agents and sympathomimetic
    drugs. *Mol. Pharmacol.* 11, 10-18.

Verhaeghe, R.H. (1977). Action of adenosine and adenine nucleo-
    tides on dogs' isolated veins. *Am. J. Physiol.* 233, 114-121.

Verhaeghe, R.H., Vanhoutte, P.M. & Shepard, J.T. (1977). Inhibi-
    tion of sympathetic neurotransmission in canine blood vessels
    by adenosine and adenine nucleotides. *Circ. Res.* 40, 208-215.

Vizi, E.S. & Knoll, J. (1976). The inhibitory effect of adeno-
    sine and related nucleotides on the release of acetylcholine.
    Neuroscience 1, 391-398.

Whittaker, U.P., Dowdall, M.J. & Boyne, A.F. (1972). The storage
    and release of acetylcholine by cholinergic nerve terminals:
    recent results with non-mammalian preparations. *Biochem. Soc.
    Sym.* 36, 48-79.

RELEASE INDUCED BY NICOTONIC AGONISTS

K. Löffelholz

I   INTRODUCTION

Chronic administration of nicotine to rats caused an increase in
urinary catecholamine excretion (Westfall, 1965). Since the rise
in blood pressure produced by the intravenous administration of
nicotine or of 1,1-dimethyl-4-phenylpiperazine (DMPP) was blocked
after adrenalectomy (Franko, Ward & Alphin, 1963; Jones, Gomez
Alonso De La Sierra & Trendelenburg, 1963), the pressor response
to nicotinic drugs was assumed to be evoked by the release of
catecholamines from the adrenal medulla. The actions of nicotine
in vivo on the adrenal medulla may be mediated by three distinct
mechanisms (reviewed by Seidler & Slotkin, 1976):   (1) by indirect
stimulation via central firing of the splanchnic nerve (Patrick &
Kirshner, 1971), (2) by direct stimulation of chromaffin cells
via nicotine receptors (Wilson & Kirshner, 1977), and (3) by
indirect stimulation via increased steroidogenesis in the adrenal
cortex (Rubin & Warner, 1975). Denervation of the rat adrenal
gland unmasked the contribution of the increased central input to
the effects of chronic administration (Seidler & Slotkin, 1976).
As will be shown in section VII, the cardiovascular effects of
nicotine in small doses administered intravenously or by inhalation of tobacco smoke are mediated by stimulation of afferent
nerves.

Acetylcholine is the physiological substance that stimulates postsynaptic nicotine receptors. Inhibition of cholinesterase activity, e.g. by organophosphates, caused the release of catecholamines
from adrenergic neurons and from chromaffin cells (see section
VII) as a result of a marked increase in the acetylcholine concentration in the blood plasma of animals (Stewart, 1952) and man
(Okonek, 1975).

It is difficult to confine the actions of nicotine *in vivo* to one
site of attack because of the widespread distribution of nicotine
receptors among central and peripheral, afferent and efferent
nerves. The distribution even extends to extrasynaptic areas of
the nerves (see sections V and VI).

The present chapter reviews our knowledge about the neuronal
release of catecholamines directly evoked by nicotinic agonists,
i.e. where stimulation of the nicotine receptor and transmitter
release are events confined to the same nerve cell. Except in a
few rare cases (see below) the ganglionic nicotine receptor has

been studied after separation from the terminal parts of the nerve
(reviewed by Nishi, 1976), while the postganglionic nicotine
receptor has been characterized after separation from the cell
body. The ganglionic receptor was investigated by measuring
ganglionic responses such as changes in the membrane potential or
the activities of the enzymes involved in transmitter synthesis
(Otten & Thoenen, 1976). On the other hand, the release of noradrenaline has been used as a tool for studying the postganglionic
nicotine receptor.

Knowledge of the release of catecholamines evoked by nicotinic
agonists is essentially based on experiments using stimulation of
postganglionic receptors. However, Chinn and Hilton (1976) have
elegantly demonstrated that stimulation of the cardiac sympathetic
nerves of the dog heart by intra-arterial application of a nicotinic drug into the left stellate and caudal ganglia may be advan-
tageous for the solution of certain problems. One such problem
is the unequal distribution of ganglionic receptors (Chinn &
Hilton, 1976) and of postganglionic (presynaptic) receptors
(Endo, Starke, Bangerter & Taube, 1977). In other words, a nerve
or a group of nerves may be characterized by a certain pattern of
(post)-ganglionic receptors. A good example is the results
obtained from the cardiac sympathetic ganglia of the dog:
Impulses travelling via the third thoracic ramus or above it
mediate myocardial contractile responses through stimulation of
predominantly nicotine receptors whereas the muscarine type
receptors dominate the cardiac responses elicited by impulses
travelling via the fourth thoracic ramus or below it (Chinn &
Hilton, 1976).

Several reviews on the release of the adrenergic transmitter by
nicotinic drugs are available (Muscholl, 1970; Kosterlitz & Lees,
1972; Baldessarini, 1975; Starke, 1977), and have been employed
in the preparation of this chapter. These reviews will be cited
in the sections which have not been reviewed in detail because
of the limited space available.

    II   BASIC EVIDENCE

Heart. One year before von Euler (1946; reviewed by Iversen,
1967) identified the adrenergic transmitter of mammalian sympathetic nerves as being predominantly noradrenaline, the cardio-
stimulant effect of acetylcholine (in the presence of atropine)
in various mammalian hearts had been interpreted to result from
the release of an "epinephrine-like" substance (Hoffmann,
Hoffmann, Middleton & Talesnik, 1945) which according to von
Euler's discovery appeared to be noradrenaline (Richardson &
Woods, 1959).

Although the ability of nicotinic drugs to cause the release of
catecholamines from the isolated heart (for reviews see section
I) is beyond doubt, the discussion about whether the positive
chronotropic and inotropic effects of these drugs are caused by
stimulation of neurons or myocardial cells is still active.

Stimulation of the isolated cat, rabbit or rat heart preparations
by nicotine has been observed after surgical denervation (Ginzel
& Kottegoda, 1953, 1954) or after pretreatment with reserpine
(Basset, Wiggins, Danilo, Nilsson & Gelbard, 1974; Chiang &
Leaders, 1968). However, these latter effects did not show
tachyphylaxis (Bassett *et al.*, 1974), required high concentrations
of nicotine (> 10^{-4}M) and were possibly evoked by a non-specific
membrane effect rather than by an interaction with a nicotine
receptor (Buccino, Sonnenblick, Cooper & Braunwald, 1966). In
the rat left atrium (electrically driven), nicotine increased the
force of contraction only at concentrations above 10^{-4}M, an effect
which was not antagonized by 10^{-7}M propranolol (Löffelholz,
unpublished). Experiments on hearts of anaesthetized dogs using
constant rate and isovolumic contractions cast some doubt on the
existence of a positive postsynaptic cardiac action of nicotine,
since intracoronary injection of nicotine over the entire dose
range used (25 to 200 µg) failed to cause positive effects after
denervation (Priola, Spurgeon & Geis, 1977). Moreover, 2 x 10^{-4}M
nicotine (in the presence of 2.9 x 10^{-6}M atropine) had no effect
on the force of contraction of spontaneously beating right atria,
electrically driven left atria or strips from the right ventricle
of the isolated chicken heart; the cardiac sympathetic nerves of
this species lack presynaptic nicotine receptors (Engel &
Löffelholz, 1976).

The dose of nicotine used to produce cardiostimulation by intracoronary injection in the anaesthetized dog ranged between 10 and
200 µg (Chiba, Tamura, Kubota & Hashimoto, 1972; Ross, 1973;
Priola *et al.*, 1977). The isolated dog heart was found to be 5-
10 times more sensitive to nicotine than the heart of the monkey
(Nishikawa & Tsujimoto, 1975). The concentration of nicotine
used by the latter authors to stimulate the monkey's heart (0.5 -
5 x 10^{-5}M) corresponded well with those used for the hearts of
other mammals (cat: Basset *et al.*, 1974; rabbit: Löffelholz,
1970a; guinea-pig: Lindmar, 1962; Bhagat, 1966). However, it was
found that nicotine ($\leq$ 2 x 10^{-4}M) failed to cause positive effects
in rat atria (Lindmar, 1962; Löffelholz, unpublished observation,
see above) and in chicken atria and perfused heart (Engel &
Löffelholz, 1976). In the isolated rabbit heart, the bell-shaped
concentration-response curves showing nicotine-evoked increases
in rate and amplitude of contraction were nearly identical with
that showing the overflow of noradrenaline into the perfusate
(Löffelholz, 1970a). It is concluded from pharmacological
analysis and from the arguments presented above that the cardio-
stimulant effects of nicotine are essentially or even exclusively
(at concentrations $\leq$ 2 x 10^{-4}M) caused via the release of the
adrenergic transmitter.

The nicotine-evoked release of the adrenergic transmitter has been
demonstrated by measuring the appearance of catecholamines in the
perfusate ("overflow") of the hearts of various mammals (monkey
and dog: Nishikawa & Tsujimoto, 1975; cat: Bevan & Haeusler,
1975; rabbit: Löffelholz, 1970a; guinea-pig: Bhagat, Robinson &
West, 1967; Westfall & Hunter, 1974). A comparison of the latter
studies and the results obtained on the rat and chicken heart

(see above) suggests that the cardio-sensitivity to release
catecholamines in response to nicotine is relatively high in the
dog and non-existent in the chicken and possibly in the rat.
The concentrations of nicotinic drugs which evoked a half-maximal
overflow of noradrenaline from the rabbit heart (Löffelholz,
1970a) were $2.1 \times 10^{-5}M$ DMPP, $2.4 \times 10^{-5}M$ nicotine and $1.1 \times 10^{-4}M$
acetylcholine (in the presence of atropine). Hence, nicotine and
DMPP were approximately equally effective, whereas about a 5-fold
higher concentration of acetylcholine was required to evoke noradrenaline release. A recently introduced agonist p-aminophen-
ethyltrimethylammonium iodide (PAPETA) (Barlow & Franks, 1971)
seemed to cause a maximal overflow of catecholamines from the
isolated rabbit heart at a concentration of $3.2 \times 10^{-5}M$ (Muscholl,
1973a; Fuder, Muscholl & Wegwart, 1976).

Adrenaline was detected in mammalian hearts in concentrations very
much smaller than those of noradrenaline (reviewed by Holzbauer &
Sharman, 1972). Nicotine caused the release of both noradrenaline
and adrenaline from the hearts of the dog and the monkey
(Nishikawa & Tsujimoto, 1975). Similarly, DMPP, acetylcholine
(in the presence of atropine) and PAPETA caused the release of
noradrenaline and of false transmitters, such as alpha-methyl-
adrenaline (Muscholl, 1973a; Fuder *et al.*, 1976), dihydroxy-
pseudoephedrine (Lindmar, Muscholl & Sprenger, 1967), (-)-alpha-
methyldopamine (Kilbinger, Lindmar, Löffelholz, Muscholl & Patil,
1971) and alpha-methylnoradrenaline (Muscholl & Maitre, 1963;
Kilbinger *et al.*, 1971). These experiments on the isolated
rabbit heart unequivocally showed that the ratio of false transmitter to noradrenaline released was the same as that found in
the heart. This observation was also obtained using sympathetic
nerve stimulation, but not when release was induced by indirectly
acting amines (reviewed by Muscholl, 1972).

Other organs. Of extracardiac tissues, the spleen of the dog and
the cat has been studied most intensively in research on the
nicotinic release of the adrenergic transmitter. The *in vivo*-
effects of acetylcholine on the volume of the spleen have been a
matter of controversy for decades (reviewed by Daly & Scott,
1961). Isolation of the spleen from the circulation reduced the
possible sites of drug action. It was finally concluded on the
basis of pharmacological evidence and of denervation experiments
that the splenic contraction following intravenous application of
acetylcholine is caused by the release of noradrenaline (Farber,
1936; Daly & Scott, 1961; Brandon & Rand, 1961).

The overflow of noradrenaline from the cat spleen in response to
injections of acetylcholine or DMPP was measured in the perfusate
(reviewed by Starke, 1977). The effective doses usually ranged
between 0.05 and 0.25 mg acetylcholine, but much higher doses
were also applied (1 - 3 mg: Blakeley, Brown & Ferry, 1963;
Krauss, Carpenter & Kopin, 1970).

At present, heart and spleen are organs known to release the
endogenous transmitter in amounts that could be determined by
conventional biological or chemical assay procedures. The

overflow from isolated smooth muscle preparations, such as dog or
rabbit arteries or veins, guinea-pig intestine or vas deferens
was detected only after radioactive labelling of the vesicular
noradrenaline store.

The effects of nicotinic agonists on veins and arteries have been
reviewed recently (Shepherd & Vanhoutte, 1975). The constriction
of the isolated central ear artery of the rabbit produced by
nicotinic agonists was mediated by the release of noradrenaline
from adrenergic nerve terminals (Steinsland & Furchgott, 1975a).
Moreover, nicotine was more effective when applied extraluminally
than intraluminally presumably because the terminals within the
arterial wall are located mainly at the medio-adventitial border
and therefore are closer to the external than to the internal
surface (Bevan, Osher & Bevan, 1969; reviewed by Trendelenburg,
1972). Nicotine (1.5 x 10^{-5}M - 1.5 x 10^{-3}M) caused a concentration-dependent constriction of spiral strips of the rabbit pulmonary artery, an effect that was mediated by the release of noradrenaline (Su & Bevan, 1970). In this preparation 10^{-5}M nicotine
appeared to be a threshold concentration for the transient contraction and release of [^{3}H]noradrenaline and [^{3}H]metabolites
(Nedergaard & Schrold, 1977). Acetylcholine (10^{-4} - 10^{-3}M; 10^{-6}M
atropine present) also increased the tension and the [^{3}H]outflow
in this preparation, effects that were blocked by hexamethonium
(Endo *et al.*, 1977). The concentrations of nicotine and acetylcholine that were required to release noradrenaline from the
rabbit pulmonary artery in a concentration-dependent manner were
identical to those used in the rabbit heart (Löffelholz, 1970a).
The [^{3}H]efflux from rabbit aortic strips preincubated with [^{3}H]-
noradrenaline was increased by 10^{-3}M acetylcholine (Kiran &
Khairallah, 1969). Dog mesenteric and pulmonary arteries
(Vanhoutte, 1974), dog saphenous vein (Vanhoutte, Lorenz & Tyce,
1973), ear artery (Allan, Glover, McCulloch, Rand & Story, 1975)
and portal vein of the rabbit (Hughes & Roth, 1971) showed no or
very weak acetylcholine-induced [^{3}H]noradrenaline release, probably due to the low concentrations of acetylcholine used ($\leq$ 7 x
10^{-5}M). Direct vasodilator or vasoconstrictor effects of acetylcholine (reviewed by Vanhoutte, 1977) may obscure vasoconstriction due to liberation of noradrenaline.

The proposal by Ambache (1951) that the inhibitory action of
ganglionic stimulating drugs on the intestinal musculature is
caused by excitation of adrenergic neurons fits into the classical
view of cholinergic and adrenergic neurons as the ultimate antagonists in the peripheral autonomic nervous system. Recently,
the inhibitory effects of nicotine and of DMPP on the taenia of
the guinea-pig caecum have been attributed to stimulation of
intramural non-adrenergic neurons, which release ATP or a closely
related nucleotide (reviewed by Burnstock, 1972). However, the
finding that inhibition of the taenia of the guinea-pig intestine
in response to nicotine (10^{-4} - 10^{-3}M) was dissociated from [^{3}H]-
nucleotide release, but was proportional to [^{3}H]noradrenaline
release, supports the classical view that adrenergic neurons are
primarily responsible for the inhibitory control of the mammalian
intestinal tract (Kuchii, Miyahara & Shibata, 1973). There is

also pharmacological evidence for a catecholamine being the inhibitory neurotransmitter in the relaxation of guinea-pig taenia
coli (Weisenthal, Hug, Weisbrodt & Bass, 1971). In the latter
study, nicotine was effective in concentrations ranging from
$3 \times 10^{-5}M$ to $3 \times 10^{-4}M$.

The possibility of the existence of presynaptic cholinoceptors
on the adrenergic nerves of the vas deferens deserves a particular
mention, since this organ is innervated by "short" adrenergic
neurons. Marked differences in the secretory excitability of
short and long adrenergic neurons have been described recently
(Stjärne, 1977). In the guinea-pig, using electrophysiological
methods, the ganglionic relay has been localized between the
hypogastric and the vas deferens nerves (Ferry, 1967). The
ganglia were located in the hypogastric plexus which is situated
about 0.5 cm from the vas deferens (Wakade & Kirpekar, 1971).
Acetylcholine (up to $5 \times 10^{-6}M$) caused an atropine-sensitive
inhibition of the efflux of [^{3}H]noradrenaline induced by field
stimulation, but evidence indicating a nicotinic release of noradrenaline was not obtained in this study (Stjärne, 1975) or in a
study using the sucrose gap technique (Sjöstrand, 1973).

Intra-arterial injections of 2.5 to 10 µg nicotine to the superior
cervical ganglion of the cat evoked contractions of the nictitating membrane that were mediated via stimulation of nicotine
receptors of the ganglion (Trendelenburg, 1957). However, the
contractions observed after direct application of acetylcholine
to the nictitating membrane were abolished by atropine, but were
unaffected by nicotinic antagonists (Thompson, 1958) and by pretreatment of the animals with reserpine (Trendelenburg, 1962).

III   MECHANISM OF RELEASE

Knowledge of the events leading to the neuronal release of catecholamines by nicotinic agonists is incomplete. The following
outline is based on the recognition of classical presynaptic
nicotine receptors which when stimulated lead to an exocytotic
expulsion of the vesicle content.

Evidence for the nicotinic type of cholinoceptor responsible for
the acetylcholine-induced release of catecholamines is based upon
the observation that the release was evoked by several nicotinic
agonists, e.g., nicotine and DMPP, and was blocked by typical
nicotinic antagonists, e.g., hexamethonium, chlorisondamine and
pempidine (reviewed by Starke, 1977). In rare cases, where DMPP,
but not nicotine, caused a release of catecholamines (rat atria,
chicken heart), the release was found to be evoked by a tyramine-
like action and nicotinic effects were not detected (see section
II). The various non-nicotinic effects of DMPP were reviewed
recently (Muscholl, 1970, 1973b; Holbach, Lindmar & Löffelholz,
1977). At present, it seems justified to assume that the presynaptic nicotine receptor is essentially similar to the ganglionic and the endplate receptors. The extensive studies on the
two latter receptors do not yet allow the distinction of different

types of nicotine receptors (reviewed by Brimblecombe, 1974).
The potency of nicotinic agonists to depolarize the superior
cervical ganglion of the cat (Haefely, 1974) and to elicit the
release of noradrenaline in the rabbit heart (Löffelholz, 1970a)
was about equal for nicotine and DMPP and was found to be less
for acetylcholine in both preparations.

"Desensitization of the nicotine receptor mechanism" (see below)
cutting short nicotinic stimulation is a well known feature of
autonomic ganglia (reviewed by Trendelenburg, 1967; Haefely, 1974)
and of the end plate of skeletal muscle (reviewed by Hubbard,
1973, and Hubbard & Quastel, 1973). The phenomenon was also
found in postganglionic sympathetic nerves and appeared as a
transient release of the transmitter followed by a period of
insensitivity towards nicotinic agonists (Löffelholz, 1970a;
Ross, 1973; Steinsland & Furchgott, 1975b). Since this desensitization (synonymously called "autoinhibition") had been expected
to occur at the receptor level (Löffelholz, 1970b; critical discussion see below), it was not surprising that noradrenaline
release evoked by orthodromic action potentials was not affected
and that suppression of the nicotinic release by concomitant
stimulation of muscarine receptors did not interfere with the
development of the desensitization (Löffelholz, 1970a).

In the cat heart, desensitization caused by infusion of nicotine
(about $2 \times 10^{-4}M$) for one min disappeared with a half-time of about
5 min as indicated by the increase in ventricular pressure in
response to brief applications of acetylcholine (Bevan & Haeusler,
1975). The latter authors found, moreover, that the tachycardia
produced by nerve stimulation at 12 Hz for 30 sec was blocked at
the end of the 1-min period of infusion of nicotine and recovered
at the same rate as the response to acetylcholine (half-time
about 5 min). It is unfortunate that the overflow of noradrenaline was not measured in these experiments since the results are
in sharp contrast to the above reports obtained by measuring
release of noradrenaline (rabbit heart) or postsynaptic responses
(dog heart, rabbit ear artery).

Analysis of the time course of noradrenaline appearance in the
effluent of the isolated rabbit heart during continuous infusion
of nicotine, acetylcholine or DMPP unequivocally showed that the
release of the transmitter from the nerve into the extracellular
space was abruptly turned on and off; the overall duration of the
release was only 5 - 10 sec and was independent of the amount of
noradrenaline liberated (Löffelholz, 1970a; Lindmar & Löffelholz,
1974). The period of release from a single varicosity must be
considerably shorter than 5 - 10 sec, because the varicosities
distributed throughout the heart are affected by the drug succes-
sively over a period of several seconds. Exocytosis is a process
that requires only a fraction of one second (reviewed by
Baldessarini, 1975). The "explosive" type of release as an
immediate result of the contact of the nicotinic agonists with
the nerve is strong evidence that the nicotine receptors are a
readily accessible part of the axon membrane.

The amine uptake system or any other inward transport system does not seem to be involved in nicotinic release (reviewed by Starke, 1977). Such an involvement was suggested by Su and Bevan (1970) because of the inhibition of nicotinic release by uptake inhibitors (see section IV). Those parts of the adrenergic nerve which lack an amine uptake system, namely the preterminal axon and the cell body, are nevertheless stimulated by nicotinic agonists. It has been suggested that these drugs may "deform" receptors or may produce allosteric effects on the "receptor mechanism" (Maxwell & Eckhardt, 1973). Recent investigations on the noradrenaline release from the rabbit heart evoked by DMPP (Holbach et al., 1977) indicated that the displacement of noradrenaline from extravesicular binding sites was governed by the rate of neuronal uptake of DMPP, whereas the nicotinic release evoked by DMPP was not.

The notion that nicotine and acetylcholine cause the release of noradrenaline by increasing the Ca^{2+} influx (Burn & Gibbons, 1964; see below) is generally assumed as an essential process leading to exocytotic release of the transmitter (reviewed by Smith & Winkler, 1972; Cubeddu, Barnes, Langer & Weiner, 1974). The release of noradrenaline caused either by a nicotinic drug or by electrical nerve stimulation is dependent on $[Ca^{2+}]_o$ in contrast to the release evoked by indirectly acting amines (rabbit heart: Lindmar, Löffelholz & Muscholl, 1967; cat iris: Thoenen, Huerlimann & Haefely, 1969).

The recognition that receptor stimulation and activation of Ca^{2+} entry are not directly coupled, leads to the question whether electrical events are associated causally with nicotinic release. Under physiological conditions (reviewed by Nishi, 1976) acetylcholine released from preganglionic fibres impinges on the postsynaptic nicotine receptors, an interaction which greatly increases the ionic permeability and gives rise to a local graded depolarization of the ganglionic cell membrane (fast EPSP) (Haefely, 1974). After spreading electrotonically along the dentrites to the soma, the EPSP generates propagated impulses, if it is large enough to excite the soma membrane. The action potentials are conducted along the axon to the postganglionic nerve terminal resulting in the release of the postganglionic transmitter. The mechanism of release should be identical whether action potentials are generated in the ganglion by nicotinic agonists (e.g. Trendelenburg, 1957; Chinn & Hilton, 1976) or by direct electrical stimulation of the preterminal axons. Since the nicotinic release of catecholamines has been usually studied by application of nicotinic drugs directly to the terminals (see section I), the inward movement of Ca^{2+} (see above), as a presumptive link in the events leading to the nicotinic release of the transmitter, may be accelerated by nicotine via action potentials and also via a local graded depolarization.

Analogous to the EPSP recorded from the cell body, it is assumed that the amplitude of the local graded depolarization of the terminal axon is dependent upon the concentration of nicotine and the number of nicotine receptors activated. Thus with higher concentrations of nicotine the significance of the local depolarization will increase and even dominate the contribution made by action potentials to the release of catecholamines. Thus, with increasing concentrations of nicotine the integral of antidromic asynchronous discharges in the adrenergic neurons of the isolated cat heart decreased, whereas the transmitter overflow was gradually enhanced (Bevan & Haeusler, 1975). The inhibition of transmitter release by tetrodotoxin (indicated by postsynaptic responses) is gradually reduced with increasing concentrations of nicotine (Furchgott, Steinsland & Wakade, 1975) indicating that the presumed Ca^{2+} movement during the non-propagated depolarization is tetrodotoxin-insensitive. Indeed, the mechanism of transmitter release has many features in common with the tetrodotoxin-insensitive Ca^{2+} permeability channel which seems to be responsible for a net inward movement of Ca^{2+} necessary to initiate secretion (reviewed by Baker, 1975). Douglas, Kanno and Sampson (1967) have shown that the hormone secretion from the adrenal medulla in response to acetylcholine persisted even in a Na^+-free medium. Clearly, both propagated action potentials and local graded depolarization can trigger an exocytotic release process in the nerve terminals. Although generation of action potentials has not been observed in chromaffin cells, nicotinic release of medullary hormones is associated merely with a graded depolarization of the cell membrane (Douglas et al., 1967). Since the ionic requirements for the depolarization and the release process are different, the latter authors demonstrated that the two events were not directly related to each other and could be dissociated by manipulation of the ionic environment. In cardiac sympathetic nerves, a dissociation between the changes in membrane potential and the release of noradrenaline was also observed, although conclusions about the membrane potentials were only based on indirect measurements, namely of the antidromic firing along the preterminal axons (Cabrera, Torrance & Viveros, 1966; Haeusler, Thoenen, Haefely & Huerlimann, 1968). Firstly, omission of Ca^{2+} from the perfusion fluid of the cat heart moderately increased the amplitude of DMPP-evoked discharges and blocked the release of noradrenaline (Haeusler et al., 1968). Secondly, the nerves responded to nicotinic agonists by antidromic discharges and presumably by a graded depolarization, both of which under certain conditions seem to be maintained over one min or more (Haeusler et al., 1968; Bevan & Haeusler, 1975), whereas the release of noradrenaline (and presumably the Ca^{2+} entry) ceased after less than 5 sec due to desensitization. These results cast some doubt on the assumption that the desensitization simply is due to a transition of the receptor from an active to an inactive state (reviewed by Trendelenburg, 1967, and Rang & Ritter, 1970). The findings rather point to an action subsequent to the receptor activation as was proposed for desensitization at the muscle endplate (Magazanik & Vyskocil, 1973; Nastuk & Parsons, 1970).

Exposure of the adrenal medulla to high K^+ concentration evoked a transient secretion of hormones although repolarization of the membrane potential did not occur (Baker & Rink, 1975). In the latter study, the transient activation of the secretion was traced back to a phasic entry of Ca^{2+} which was terminated by an inactivation of a potential-dependent Ca^{2+} conductance. The authors speculate that the inactivation of the Ca^{2+} conductance may be the basis for the transient response of the adrenal medulla on prolonged exposure to acetylcholine (Douglas & Rubin, 1961), although desensitization to acetylcholine may play a determining role. In general, future studies should consider the possibility that transmitter release by nicotinic agonists may be modulated by the removal of Ca^{2+} from sites critically involved in the exocytotic process. Ca^{2+} may be inactivated by removal within the cell or by extrusion from the cell (reviewed by Rink & Baker, 1975, and by Baldessarini, 1975).

Stimulation of presynaptic muscarine receptors counteracts not only the depolarization (Haeusler *et al.*, 1968) probably by hyperpolarizing the membrane (Fozard & Muscholl, 1972), but also decreases the nicotinic release of noradrenaline (Lindmar, Löffelholz & Muscholl, 1968) presumably by lowering the inward-movement of Ca^{2+}. If this concept is true, the finding that muscarinic agonists do not change the desensitization of nicotinic release (Löffelholz, 1970a) is in favor of the view that the site of desensitization is not linked into the chain of events subsequent to the presumptive activation of the Ca^{2+} conductance, but, as was discussed above, is placed after receptor activation.

There is good evidence that the release of the adrenergic transmitter evoked by electrical nerve stimulation occurs by exocytosis (reviewed by Baldessarini, 1975), and there is good reason to believe that nicotinic release has the same mechanism. Firstly, nicotinic agonists cause an exocytotic release of hormones from the adrenal medulla (reviewed by Smith & Winkler, 1972); secondly, nicotinic agonists probably stimulate receptors in the axon plasma membrane, the release follows receptor stimulation instantaneously in an "explosive" manner and is Ca^{2+}-dependent (see section III); thirdly, nicotinic agonists and electrical nerve stimulation cause the release of false transmitters and noradrenaline in the same proportion as the two amines are stored. In contrast, indirect sympathomimetics, like tyramine, preferentially liberate the false transmitter (see section II), presumably because of a pronounced release from extravesicular compartments which are believed to contain relatively large amounts of the false transmitter (reviewed by Muscholl, 1972, and Baldessarini, 1975).

IV   EFFECTS OF DRUGS AND IONS ON NICOTINIC RELEASE

There have been so many publications on this subject that a detailed review is not possible.

The effects of drugs on nicotinic release are very varied: nicotinic antagonists, like hexamethonium (see section III), are most specific. Thus both effects mediated by receptor stimulation, i.e., the generation of propagated impulses and the release of transmitter, were blocked (Davey, Hayden & Scholfield, 1968),

whereas release by electrical nerve stimulation was not affected
(Blakeley *et al.*, 1963; Hertting & Widhalm, 1965; Davey *et al.*,
1968). The least specific are drugs that deplete the transmitter
store, such as 6-hydroxydopamine and reserpine, since the release
of noradrenaline evoked by any kind of stimulation must then be
abolished.

Three groups of drugs inhibit nicotinic release, but, under
certain conditions, do not depress the release evoked by electrical stimulation. (1) Inhibitors of amine uptake, such as cocaine
and desipramine (see section III), (2) anaesthetics, such as
halothane (chapter by Göthert), and (3) d-amphetamine (Löffelholz
& Muscholl, 1970). Ad (1) and (2): The possibility that inhibition of amine uptake is related by some unknown mechanism to the
depression of nicotinic release is very unlikely for both halothane (Göthert, 1974) and the uptake inhibitors (see section III).
Instead, a conformational change of the receptor (Göthert, 1974;
Göthert, Kennerknecht & Thielecke, 1976) or of a site linked
between receptor stimulation and the presumptive increase in Ca^{2+}
conductance (see section III), has been proposed as possible
mechanisms. Ad (3): d-amphetamine ($2 \times 10^{-5}M$) acts similarly to
the above drugs in that it also inhibits the nicotinic release of
noradrenaline (Löffelholz & Muscholl, 1970), but it behaves
differently because it strongly potentiates the release evoked by
electrical nerve stimulation (Löffelholz & Muscholl, 1970; Starke,
Wagner & Schumann, 1972).

There are a number of drugs that cause inhibition of the catecholamine release evoked by nicotinic drugs and by electrically
induced orthodromic impulses. These drugs may act, therefore, on
the presynaptic neuronal Ca^{2+} entry (see section III) or may
affect a subsequent link in the events leading to exocytosis:
(1) α-adrenoceptor agonists, (2) muscarinic agonists, (3) prostaglandins, (4) local anaesthetics, (5) adrenergic neuron blocking
drugs, and (6) agents modifying neurotubules. Ad (1): The
nicotinic release of noradrenaline was reduced by oxymetazoline
(Starke & Montel, 1974) and increased (as indicated by postsynaptic responses) in the presence of α-adrenolytic drugs (Furchgott
et al., 1975). Ad (2): The release of noradrenaline evoked by
nicotinic agonists, high K^+ concentrations or electrical nerve
stimulation is inhibited by concomitant stimulation of presynaptic
muscarine receptors. Even after maximal activation of the muscarine receptors, acetylcholine (Lindmar *et al.*, 1968) and electrical nerve stimulation (Löffelholz & Muscholl, 1969) still produced
a small release of noradrenaline. A similar persistence was
observed for the inhibition via presynaptic α-adrenoceptor stimulation (reviewed by Starke, 1977). It would be worthwhile to
find out whether the small noradrenaline release resistant to
muscarinic inhibition can be further reduced by α-adrenergic
inhibition and vice versa. Ad (3): Nicotine when infused into
the rabbit heart caused a concomitant and transient overflow of
noradrenaline and of a prostaglandine-like substance (assayed on
the stomach strip); the observation that indomethacin increased
the nicotine-induced release was interpreted as evidence for a
direct stimulation by nicotine of the synthesis of prostaglandins

(Wennmalm & Junstad, 1976; Wennmalm, 1977). The mechanism and
significance of the overflow of prostaglandins from isolated
organs upon mechanical, electrical or pharmacological manipulations is, however, obscure and needs further clarification
(reviewed by Baldessarini, 1975; chapter by Stjärne). There is,
nevertheless, unequivocal evidence that the exogenous prostaglandins E_1 and E_2 inhibit nicotine-induced release of noradrenaline
(Westfall & Brasted, 1974). Ad (4): Tetracaine blocked the
release of noradrenaline evoked by acetylcholine (cat heart:
Haeusler, Thoenen, Haefely & Huerlimann, 1969) and by nerve stimulation (rabbit heart: Hukovic & Muscholl, 1962), but not by
high K^+ concentrations (rabbit heart: Göthert, 1974). There is
strong evidence, nevertheless, that inhibition of the nicotinic
release of catecholamines is produced by stabilization of the
membrane including inhibition of both Na^+ and Ca^{2+} conductance.
Ad (5): Bretylium blocked the nicotinic release of noradrenaline
in several tissues (Davey et al., 1968; Westfall & Brasted, 1974;
Haeusler, Haefely & Huerlimann, 1969). The mechanism of the
depression produced by bretylium seems to be similar to that of
local anaesthetics. In this context, the adrenergic neuron
blockade by a nicotinic drug, DMPP, should be mentioned
(Birmingham & Wilson, 1965). The DMPP-evoked release of noradrenaline (see section II) was clearly dissociated from the
effect on neuronal amine uptake (Holbach et al., 1977) and from
adrenergic neuron blockade (Löffelholz, 1970b). Ad (6): In the
heart and vas deferens of the guinea-pig, colchicine and vinblastine inhibited the release of noradrenaline evoked by nicotine
(Sorimachi, Oesch & Thoenen, 1973) or by nerve stimulation (Thoa,
Wooten, Axelrod & Kopin, 1972), respectively. Conclusions about
the kind of inhibition produced by colchicine and vinblastine
should take into account an anticholinergic effect of these
drugs reported for the secretion of adrenal hormones (Trifaro,
Collier, Lastowecka & Stern, 1972).

Ca^{2+}-dependence is a crucial feature in stimulus-secretion
coupling (Douglas, 1968) and may be due to increased Ca^{2+}-
permeability producing an increased Ca^{2+} entry (see section III).
Changes in the ionic environment exert effects upon this Ca^{2+}-
dependent release that are similar to the various methods used
to depolarize the membrane (reviewed by Baldessarini, 1975) with
the exception of those conditions that change amplitude or even
propagation of action potentials. Thus, blockade of impulse
propagation by lowering the Na^+ concentration below 50 mM
(Kirpekar & Misu, 1967) or by tetrodotoxin (see section III) is
not compatible with transmitter release that is exclusively
caused by action potentials. The Ca^{2+}-dependent release evoked
by local graded depolarization (i.e., by nicotinic agonists in
high concentrations or by elevated K^+ concentrations) was enhanced
by low Na^+ concentrations (Löffelholz, 1967; Kirpekar & Wakade,
1968). However, low Na^+ concentrations caused only an approximately 2-fold increase of this release, an effect that was only
observed at a reduced Ca^{2+} concentration using acetylcholine as
stimulus (Löffelholz, 1967).

V   BIOLOGICAL OCCURRENCE AND DISTRIBUTION OF NICOTINE
     RECEPTORS

The ontogenetic occurrence of presynaptic nicotine receptors has
been studied in the isolated chick heart (Pappano, 1976). This
preparation, although extremely valuable for studying the ontogenesis of autonomic cardiac innervation (reviewed by Pappano,
1977), seems rather inappropriate as a tool for investigating
presynaptic nicotine receptors, because these receptors were not
detected in the heart of 1-week old chicks or of adult chickens
(Engel & Löffelholz, 1976). Nevertheless, small positive chronotropic effects evoked by nicotine were seen for the first time
after doubling the Ca^{2+} concentration of the medium on the day of
hatching (21st incubation day) (Pappano, 1976), i.e., at the
onset of adrenergic neuroeffector transmission which had been
determined using field stimulation (Pappano & Löffelholz, 1974)
and tyramine (Pappano, 1976). In the neonatal adrenal medulla
of the rat, nicotine receptors were detected before the development of a functional splanchnic innervation (Rosenthal & Slotkin,
1977). This result and work done by others (Pappano & Löffelholz,
1974; Black & Mytilineou, 1976) indicate that the onset of neuro-
effector transmission is determined by the transsynaptic regulation of the development of transmitter synthesis and release
rather than by receptor development.

The phylogenetic occurrence of nicotine receptors at peripheral
neurons has not been systematically studied. That the heart of the
chicken failed to develop presynaptic postganglionic receptors
could point to a phylogenetical acquisition of presynaptic regulatory receptors. However, the presence of presynaptic nicotine
receptors on preganglionic sympathetic nerves of amphibia is well
established (Nishi, 1976). If the presynaptic nicotine receptors
are carried from the cell body to the periphery by the out-growing
axons, their peripheral scarcity in the chicken heart should
reflect a reduced importance of nicotine receptors in ganglionic
transmission. This view is supported by the finding that hexamethonium only partially inhibited transmission through the
avian ciliary (Martin & Pilar, 1963) and avian cardiac parasympathetic ganglion (Dieterich, Kaffei, Kilbinger & Löffelholz, 1976).
Moreover, Ledbetter and Kirshner (1975) found, during exposure to
acetylcholine, an atropine-sensitive secretion of catecholamines
from chick adrenals (in culture), which did not respond to nicotine.

A comparison of the effects of nicotinic agonists on the cell
body with those on the terminals of the peripheral adrenergic
nerve (see section III) raises the important question of the
distribution of the nicotine receptors. The term "presynaptic"
receptor implicates a strategical position in synaptic impulse
transmission. The nicotine receptors of the adrenergic nerve
should then be localized only at the functional sites, namely
the cell body and the terminal axon. However, the axonal part
of the internal carotid nerve of the rabbit superior cervical
ganglion was depolarized upon exposure to acetylcholine
(Kosterlitz, Lees & Wallis, 1968). Accordingly, fibres of

mammalian vagus nerves responded to nicotinic agonists by a local hexamethonium-sensitive depolarization, which blocked impulse transmission (Armett & Ritchie, 1961; Hancock & Volle, 1969).

"Presynaptic nicotine receptors" are not exclusive to the post-ganglionic sympathetic neuron. The terminal region of the pre-ganglionic nerve is endowed also with presynaptic nicotine receptors (reviewed by Nishi, 1976). Nicotinic agonists caused a transient depolarization that lasted for several minutes and was followed by "desensitization". Nishi emphasized that desensitization of presynaptic nicotine receptors developed much more rapidly than that of the postsynaptic ganglionic receptors.

The well known observation that sensory nerve endings (see section VII) are equipped with nicotine receptors (e.g. Brown & Gray, 1948; Haeusler *et al.*, 1969) represents an example of an extrasynaptic occurrence of nicotine receptors.

VI   SPECULATIONS ON A PHYSIOLOGICAL SIGNIFICANCE

The widespread distribution of the nicotine receptor on afferent and efferent nerves, at pre-, post- and extrasynaptic sites suggests that these receptors may represent an integral part of the axon membrane with either no physiological meaning or a very general one. In the sympathetic nervous system, a physiological role for presynaptic nicotine receptors has not yet been shown inspite of an enormous effort to elucidate their role.

Koelle (1962) suggested that the ganglionic presynaptic receptors are stimulated by the released acetylcholine which, in turn, releases further acetylcholine. Another theory (Nishi, 1976) is based on the observation that the presynaptic depolarization elicited by the released acetylcholine counteracts the post-tetanic hyperpolarization of the presynaptic membrane and thereby maintains the constancy of transmitter output during and after preganglionic firing.

The postganglionic presynaptic nicotine receptors of the adrenergic neuron are an essential part of the "cholinergic link" theory (reviewed by Burn & Rand, 1965, and Burn, 1977), which is similar to Koelle's theory in that in both theories acetylcholine is regarded as the primary stimulus (cholinergic link) for the release of the transmitter that leads finally to the suprathreshold postsynaptic stimulation. This "second" transmitter is acetylcholine in Koelle's view of ganglionic release and noradrenaline in Burn's theory of postganglionic release. Hardly compatible with a "cholinergic link" are observations reviewed in sections II and III: Blockade of the nicotine receptors by nicotinic antagonists or by desensitization (critical replication by Burn, 1971) or even absence of the receptors (chicken heart) has no depressant effect on postganglionic transmission. The various arguments for or against the theory have not changed in recent years and the reader is referred to previous critical reviews (Ferry, 1966; Kosterlitz & Lees, 1972; Baldessarini, 1975).

VII   TOXICOLOGICAL ASPECTS

Stimulation of nicotine receptors on peripheral adrenergic
neurons resulting in sympathomimetic effects (see section II)
certainly will contribute to the picture of severe nicotine
poisoning. Nicotine may be accidentally ingested with insecti-
cides or with tobacco products. A marked rise in the plasma
level of acetylcholine, as was observed after severe poisoning
with cholinesterase inhibitors in animals (Stewart, 1952) and in
man (Okonek & Kilbinger, 1974) can be expected to stimulate all
peripheral nicotine receptors. In fact, the urinary excretion
of catecholamines was markedly increased in patients poisoned
with an organophosphate (Okonek, 1975). Since these patients
were treated with high doses of atropine, the sympathomimetic
effect of acetylcholine would be mediated not only via postsynaptic receptors of the ganglion but also via presynaptic
receptors of the terminal axon of the adrenergic neuron. Atropine markedly increases acetylcholine-evoked release of noradrenaline by blocking presynaptic muscarinic inhibition.

Injection of nicotine (0.4 - 1.0 mg) into the brachial artery
caused dilatation followed by constriction of the blood vessels
of hand and forearm in man (Fewings, Rand, Scroop & Whelan,
1966). The vasoconstriction was, at least partially, caused by
stimulation of the sympathetic terminal axons. Systemic application of nicotine evoked a rise in the blood pressure and an
increase in the urinary excretion of catecholamines (see section
I). However, acute cardiovascular effects of tobacco smoking are
an exception (reviewed by Löffelholz, 1971), because the maximal
nicotine concentration of the arterial blood in regular cigarette
smokers who inhaled was only about $2 \times 10^{-7}M$ (Armitage, Dollery,
George, Houseman, Lewis & Turner, 1975). Acute cardiovascular
effects may consist of bradycardia or tachycardia and vasoconstriction and are exclusively mediated by stimulation of sensory
nerves, mainly those of the carotid and aortic bodies (Comroe,
1960; Silvette, Hoff, Larson & Haag, 1962; Zapata, Zuazo &
Llados, 1976).

VIII   REFERENCES

Allen, G.S., Glover, A.B., McCulloch, M.W., Rand, M.J. & Story,
    D.F. (1975). Modulation by acetylcholine of adrenergic trans-
    mission in the rabbit ear artery. *Br. J. Pharmacol.* 54, 49-
    53.

Ambache, N. (1951). Unmasking after cholinergic paralysis of
    botulinum toxin, of a reversed action of nicotine on the
    mammalian intestine, revealing the probable local inhibitory
    ganglion cells in the enteric plexuses. *Br. J. Pharmacol.* 6,
    51-67.

Armett, C.J. & Ritchie, J.M. (1961). The action of acetylcholine
    and some related substances on conduction in mammalian non-
    myelinated nerve fibres. *J. Physiol. (Lond.)* 155, 372-384.

Armitage, A.K., Dollery, C.T., George, C.F., Houseman, T.H., Lewis, P.J. & Turner, D.M. (1975). Absorption and metabolism of nicotine from cigarettes. *Br. Med. J.* 4, 313-316.

Baker, P.F. (1975). Transport and metabolism of calcium ions in nerve. In: *Calcium Movement in Excitable Cells* (eds.) P.F. Baker & H. Reuter, pp. 9-53, Pergamon Press, Oxford.

Baker, P.F. & Rink, T.J. (1975). Catecholamine release from bovine adrenal medulla in response to maintained depolarization. *J. Physiol. (Lond.)* 253, 593-594.

Baldessarini, R.J. (1975). Release of catecholamines. In: *Handbook of Psychopharmacology* (eds.) L.L. Iversen, S.D. Iversen & S.H. Snyder, Vol. 3, pp. 37-137, Plenum Press, New ·York - London.

Barlow, R.B. & Franks, F. (1971). Specificity of some ganglion stimulants. *Br. J. Pharmacol.* 42, 137-142.

Bassett, A.L., Wiggins, J.R., Danilo, Jr., P., Nilsson, K. & Gelbard, H. (1974). Direct and indirect inotropic effects of nicotine on cat ventricular muscle. *J. Pharmacol. Exp. Pathol.* 188, 148-156.

Bevan, J.A. & Haeusler, G. (1975). Electrical events associated with the action of nicotine at the adrenergic nerve terminals. *Arch. Int. Pharmacodyn. Ther.* 218, 84-95.

Bevan, J.A., Osher, I.V. & Bevan, R.D. (1969). Distribution of bound norepinephrine in the arterial wall. *Eur. J. Pharmacol.* 5, 299-301.

Bhagat, B. (1966). Responses of isolated guinea-pig atria to various ganglion-stimulating agents. *J. Pharmacol. Exp. Pathol.* 154, 264-270.

Bhagat, B., Robinson, J.M. & West, W.L. (1967). Mechanism of sympathomimetic responses of isolated guinea-pig atria to nicotine and dimethylphenylpiperazinium iodide. *Br. J. Pharmacol.* 30, 470-477.

Birmingham, A.T. & Wilson, A.B. (1965). An analysis of the blocking action of dimethylphenylpiperazinium iodide on the inhibition of isolated small intestine produced by stimulation of the sympathetic nerves. *Br. J. Pharmacol.* 24, 375-386.

Black, I.B. & Mytilineou, C. (1976). Trans-synaptic regulation of the development of endorgan innervation by sympathetic neurons. *Brain Res.* 101, 503-521.

Blakeley, A.G.H., Brown, G.L. & Ferry, C.B. (1963). Pharmacological experiments on the release of the sympathetic transmitter. *J. Physiol. (Lond.)* 167, 505-514.

Brandon, K.W. & Rand, M.J. (1961). Acetylcholine and the sympathetic innervation of the spleen. *J. Physiol. (Lond.)* 157, 18-32.

Brimblecombe, R.W. (1974). Drug actions at peripheral sites. In: *Drug Actions on Cholinergic Systems* (ed.) R.W. Brimblecombe, pp. 43-62, The MacMillan Press, London.

Brown, G.L. & Gray, J.A.B. (1948). Some effects of nicotine-like substances and their relation to sensory nerve endings. *J. Physiol. (Lond.)* 107, 306-317.

Buccino, R.A., Sonnenblick, E.H., Cooper, T. & Braunwald, E. (1966). Direct positive inotropic effect of acetylcholine on myocardium. *Circ. Res.* 19, 1097-1108.

Burn, J.H. (1971). Acetylcholine and "auto-inhibition". *J. Pharm. Pharmacol.* 23, 470-471.

Burn, J.H. (1977). Evidence that acetylcholine releases noradrenaline in the sympathetic fibre. *J. Pharm. Pharmacol.* 29, 325-329.

Burn, J.H. & Gibbons, W.R. (1964). The part played by calcium in determining the response to stimulation of sympathetic postganglionic fibres. *Br. J. Pharmacol.* 22, 540-548.

Burn, J.H. & Rand, M.J. (1965). Acetylcholine in adrenergic transmission. *Ann. Rev. Pharmacol.* 5, 163-182.

Burnstock, G. (1972). Purinergic nerves. *Pharmacol. Rev.* 24, 509-581.

Cabrera, R., Torrance, R.W. & Viveros, H. (1966). The action of acetylcholine and other drugs upon the terminal parts of the postganglionic sympathetic fibre. *Br. J. Pharmacol.* 27, 51-63.

Chiang, T.S. & Leaders, F.E. (1968). Mechanism of the secondary positive effect of nicotine in rat atria. *Arch. Int. Pharmacodyn. Ther.* 172, 333-346.

Chiba, S., Tamura, K., Kubota, K. & Hashimoto, K. (1972). Pharmacologic analysis of nicotine and dimethylphenylpiperazinium on pacemaker activity of the SA node in the dog. *Jap. J. Pharmacol.* 22, 645-651.

Chinn, C. & Hilton, J.G. (1976). Selective activation of nicotinic and muscarinic transmission in cardiac sympathetic ganglia of the dog. *Eur. J. Pharmacol.* 40, 77-82.

Comroe, J.H. (1960). The pharmacological actions of nicotine. *Ann. NY Acad. Sci.* 90, 48-51.

Cubeddu, X., Barnes, E.M., Langer, S.Z. & Weiner, N. (1974). Release of norepinephrine and dopamine-β-hydroxylase by nerve stimulation. I. Role of neuronal and extraneuronal uptake and of alpha presynaptic receptors. *J. Pharmacol. Exp. Ther.* 190, 431-450.

Daly, M. DeB. & Scott, M.J. (1961). The effects of acetylcholine on the volume and vascular resistance of the dog's spleen. *J. Physiol. (Lond.)* 156, 246-259.

Davey, M.J., Hayden, M.L. & Scholfield, P.C. (1968). The effects of bretylium on C fibre excitation and noradrenaline release by acetylcholine and electrical stimulation. *Br. J. Pharmacol.* 34, 377-387.

Dieterich, H.A., Kaffei, H., Kilbinger, H. & Löffelholz, K. (1976). The effects of physostigmine on cholinesterase activity, storage and release of acetylcholine in the isolated chicken heart. *J. Pharmacol. Exp. Ther.* 199, 236-246.

Douglas, W.W. (1968). Stimulus-secretion coupling: The concept and clues from chromaffin and other cells. *Br. J. Pharmacol.* 34, 451-474.

Douglas, W.W. & Rubin, R.P. (1961). The role of calcium in the secretory response of the adrenal medulla to acetylcholine. *J. Physiol. (Lond.)* 159, 40-57.

Douglas, W.W., Kanno, T. & Sampson, S.R. (1967). Effects of acetylcholine and other medullary secretagogues and antagonists on the membrane potential of adrenal chromaffin cells: An analysis employing techniques of tissue culture. *J. Physiol. (Lond.)* 188, 107-120.

Endo, T., Starke, K., Bangerter, A. & Taube, H.D. (1977). Presynaptic receptor systems on the noradrenergic neurones of the rabbit pulmonary artery. *Naunyn Schmiedebergs Arch. Pharmacol.* 296, 229-247.

Engel, U. & Löffelholz, K. (1976). Presence of muscarinic inhibitory and absence of nicotinic excitatory receptors at the terminal sympathetic nerves of chicken heart. *Naunyn Schmiedebergs Arch. Pharmacol.* 295, 225-230.

Farber, S. (1936). The action of acetylcholine on the volume of the spleen of the dog. *Arch. Int. Pharmacodyn. Ther.* 53, 367-376

Ferry, C.B. (1966). Cholinergic link hypothesis in adrenergic neuroeffector transmission. *Physiol. Rev.* 46, 420-456.

Ferry, C.B. (1967). The innervation of the vas deferens of the guinea-pig. *J. Physiol. (Lond.)* 192, 463-478.

Fewings, J.D., Rand, M.J., Scroop, G.C. & Whelan, R.F. (1966). The action of nicotine on the blood vessels of the hand and forearm in man. *Br. J. Pharmacol.* 26, 567-579.

Fozard, J.R. & Muscholl, E. (1972). Effects of several muscarinic agonists on cardiac performance and the release of noradrenaline from sympathetic nerves of the perfused rabbit heart. *Br. J. Pharmacol.* 45, 616-629.

Franko, B.Y., Ward, J.W. & Alphin, R.C. (1963). Pharmacologic studies of N-benzyl-3-pyrrolidyl acetate methobromide (AHR-602), a ganglion stimulating agent. *J. Pharmacol. Exp. Ther.* 39, 25-30.

Fuder, H., Muscholl, E. & Wegwart, R. (1976). The effects of methacholine and calcium deprivation on the release of the false transmitter, α-methyladrenaline, from the isolated rabbit heart. *Naunyn Schmiedebergs Arch. Pharmacol.* 293, 225-234.

Furchgott, R.F., Steinsland, O.S. & Wakade, T.D. (1975). Studies on prejunctional muscarinic and nicotinic receptors. In: *Chemical Tools in Catecholamine Research* (eds.) O. Almgren, A. Carlsson & J. Engel, Vol. 2, pp. 167-174, North Holland, Amsterdam - Oxford.

Ginzel, K.H. & Kottegoda, S.R. (1953). Nicotine-like actions in auricles and blood vessels after denervation. *Br. J. Pharmacol.* 8, 348-351.

Ginzel, K.H. & Kottegoda, S.R. (1954). Die Wirkung von Nicotin und Hexamethonium am normalen und chronisch denervierten Herzvorhofpräparat und am Kaninchenohr. *Naunyn Schmiedebergs Arch. Exp. Pathol. Pharmacol.* 222, 178-180.

Göthert, M. (1974). Effects of halothane on the sympathetic nerve terminals of the rabbit heart. Differences in membrane actions of halothane and tetracaine. *Naunyn Schmiedebergs Arch. Pharmacol.* 286, 125-143.

Göthert, M., Kennerknecht, E. & Thielecke, G. (1976). Inhibition of receptor-mediated noradrenaline release from the sympathetic nerves of the isolated rabbit heart by anaesthetics and alcohols in proportion to their hydrophobic property. *Naunyn Schmiedebergs Arch. Pharmacol.* 292, 145-152.

Haefely, W. (1974). The effects of various "nicotine-like" agents in the cat superior cervical ganglion *in situ*. *Naunyn Schmiedebergs Arch. Pharmacol.* 281, 93-117.

Haeusler, G., Haefely, W. & Huerlimann, A. (1969). On the mechanism of the adrenergic nerve blocking action of bretylium. *Naunyn Schmiedebergs Arch. Pharmacol.* 265, 260-277.

Haeusler, G., Thoenen, H., Haefely, W. & Huerlimann, A. (1968). Electrical events in cardiac adrenergic nerves and noradrenaline release from the heart induced by acetylcholine and potassium chloride. *Naunyn Schmiedebergs Arch. Pharmacol. Exp. Pathol.* 261, 389-411.

Haeusler, G., Thoenen, H., Haefely, W. & Huerlimann, A. (1969).
  Electrosecretory coupling at the release of noradrenaline from
  adrenergic nerve fibers by nicotine-like acting substances.
  Naunyn Schmiedebergs Arch. Pharmacol. Exp. Pathol. 263, 217-
  218.

Hancock, J.C. & Volle, R.L. (1969). Blockade of conduction in
  vagal fibers by nicotinic drugs. *Arch. Int. Pharmacodyn.
  Ther.* 178, 85-98.

Hertting, G. & Widhalm, S. (1965). Über den Mechanismus der
  Noradrenalin-Freisetzung aus sympathischen Nervenendigungen.
  Naunyn Schmiedebergs Arch. Exp. Pathol. Pharmacol. 250, 257-
  258.

Hoffmann, F., Hoffmann, E.F., Middleton, S. & Talesnik, J.
  (1945). The stimulating effect of acetylcholine on the
  mammalian heart and the liberation of an epinephrine-like
  substance by the isolated heart. *Am. J. Physiol.* 144, 189-
  198.

Holbach, H.J., Lindmar, R. & Löffelholz, K. (1977). DMPP and the
  adrenergic nerve terminal: Mechanisms of noradrenaline
  release from vesicular and extravesicular compartments.
  Naunyn Schmiedebergs Arch. Pharmacol. 300, 131-138.

Holzbauer, M. & Sharman, D.F. (1972). The distribution of cate-
  cholamines in vertebrates. In: *Catecholamines, Handbook of
  Experimental Pharmacology* (eds) H. Blaschko & E. Muscholl,
  Vol. 33, pp. 110-185, Springer, Berlin-Heidelberg-New York.

Hubbard, J.I. (1973). Microphysiology of vertebrate neuromuscular
  transmission. *Physiol. Rev.* 53, 674-723.

Hubbard, J.I. & Quastel, D.M.J. (1973). Micropharmacology of
  vertebrate neuromuscular transmission. *Ann. Rev. Pharmacol.*
  13, 199-216.

Hughes, J. & Roth, R.H. (1971). Evidence that angiotensin
  enhances transmitter release during sympathetic nerve stimulation. *Br. J. Pharmacol.* 41, 239-255.

Huković, S. & Muscholl, E. (1962). Die Noradrenalin-Abgabe aus
  dem isolierten Kaninchenherzen bei sympathischer Nervenreizung
  und ihre pharmakologische Beeinflussung. *Naunyn Schmiedebergs
  Arch. Exp. Pathol. Pharmacol.* 244, 81-96.

Iversen, L.L. (1967). The discovery of the sympathetic neuro-
  transmitter. In: *The Uptake and Storage of Noradrenaline in
  Sympathetic Nerves* (ed.) L.L. Iversen, pp. 23-29, University
  Press, Cambridge.

Jones, A., Gomez Alonso De La Sierra, B. & Trendelenburg, U.
  (1963). The pressor response of the spinal cat to different
  groups of ganglion-stimulating agents. *J. Pharmacol. Exp.
  Ther.* 139, 312-320.

Kilbinger, H., Lindmar, R., Löffelholz, K., Muscholl, E. & Patil, P.N. (1971). Storage and release of false transmitters after infusion of (+)- and (-)-α-methyldopamine. *Naunyn Schmiedebergs Arch. Pharmacol*. 271, 234-248.

Kiran, B.K. & Khairallah, P.A. (1969). Angiotensin and nor-epinephrine efflux. *Eur. J. Pharmacol*. 6, 102-108.

Kirpekar, S.M. & Misu, Y. (1967). Release of noradrenaline by splenic nerve stimulation and its dependence on calcium. *J. Physiol. (Lond.)* 188, 219-234.

Kirpekar, S.M. & Wakade, A.R. (1968). Release of noradrenaline from the cat spleen by potassium. *J. Physiol. (Lond.)* 194, 595-608.

Koelle, G.B. (1962). A new general concept of the neurohumoral functions of acetylcholine and acetylcholinesterase. *J. Pharm. Pharmacol*. 14, 65-90.

Kosterlitz, H.W., Lees, G.M. & Wallis, D.I. (1968). Resting and active potentials recorded by the sucrose-gap method in the superior cervical ganglion of the rabbit. *J. Physiol. (Lond.)* 195, 39-53.

Kosterlitz, H.W. & Lees, G.M. (1972). Interrelationships between adrenergic and cholinergic mechanisms. In: *Catecholamines, Handbook of Experimental Pharmacology* (eds.) H. Blaschko & E. Muscholl, Vol. 33, pp. 762-812, Springer, Berlin-Heidelberg-New York.

Krauss, K.R., Carpenter, D.O. & Kopin, I.J. (1970). Acetyl-choline-induced release of norepinephrine in the presence of tetrodotoxin. *J. Pharmacol. Exp. Ther*. 173, 416-421.

Kuchii, M., Miyahara, J.T. & Shibata, S. (1973). (^{3}H)-adenine nucleotide and (^{3}H)-noradrenaline release evoked by electri-cal field stimulation, perivascular nerve stimulation and nicotine from the taenia of the guinea-pig caecum. *Br. J. Pharmacol*. 49, 258-267.

Ledbetter, F.H. & Kirshner, N. (1975). Studies of chick adrenal medulla in organ culture. *Biochem. Pharmacol*. 24, 967-974.

Lindmar, R. (1962). Die Wirkung von 1,1-Dimethyl-4-phenyl-piperazinium-jodid am isolierten Vorhof im Vergleich zur Tyramin- und Nicotinwirkung. *Naunyn Schmiedebergs Arch. Exp. Pathol. Pharmacol*. 242, 458-466.

Lindmar, R. & Löffelholz, K. (1974). Neuronal and extraneuronal uptake and efflux of catecholamines in the isolated rabbit heart. *Naunyn Schmiedebergs Arch. Pharmacol*. 284, 63-92.

Lindmar, R., Löffelholz, K. & Muscholl, E. (1967). Unterschiede zwischen Tyramin und Dimethylphenylpiperazin in der Ca^{2+}-Abhängigkeit und im zeitlichen Verlauf der Noradrenalin-Freisetzung am isolierten Kaninchenherzen. *Experientia* 23, 933-934.

Lindmar, R., Löffelholz, K. & Muscholl, E. (1968). A muscarinic mechanism inhibiting the release of noradrenaline from peripheral adrenergic nerve fibres by nicotinic agents. *Br. J. Pharmacol*. 32, 280-294.

Lindmar, R., Muscholl, E. & Sprenger, E. (1967). Funktionelle Bedeutung der Freisetzung von Dihydroxyephedrin und Dihydroxypseudoephedrin als "falschen" sympathischen Überträgerstoffen am Herzen. *Naunyn Schmiedebergs Arch. Pharmacol. Exp. Pathol*. 256, 1-25,

Löffelholz, K. (1967). Untersuchungen über die Noradrenalin-Freisetzung durch Acetylcholin am perfundierten Kaninchenherzen. *Naunyn Schmiedebergs Arch. Pharmacol. Exp. Pathol*. 258, 108-122.

Löffelholz, K. (1970a). Auto-inhibition of nicotinic release of noradrenaline from postganglionic sympathetic nerves. *Naunyn Schmiedebergs Arch. Pharmacol*. 267, 49-63.

Löffelholz, K. (1970b). Nicotinic drugs and postganglionic sympathetic transmission. *Naunyn Schmiedebergs Arch. Pharmacol*. 267, 64-73.

Löffelholz, K. (1971). Die akuten Kreislaufwirkungen des Tabakrauchens. *Hippokrates* 42, 461-470.

Löffelholz, K. & Muscholl, E. (1969). A muscarinic inhibition of the noradrenaline release evoked by postganglionic sympathetic nerve stimulation. *Naunyn Schmiedebergs Arch. Pharmacol*. 265, 1-15.

Löffelholz, K. & Muscholl, E. (1970). Der Einfluß von d-Amphetamin auf die Noradrenalin-Abgabe aus dem isolierten Kaninchenherzen. *Naunyn Schmiedebergs Arch. Pharmacol*. 266, 393.

Magazanik, L.G. & Vyskocil, F. (1973). Desensitization of the motor end-plate. In: *Drug Receptors* (ed.) H.P. Rang, pp. 105-119, University Park Press, Baltimore.

Martin, R.A. & Pilar, G. (1963). Transmission through the ciliary ganglion of the chick. *J. Physiol. (Lond.)* 168, 464-475.

Maxwell, R.A. & Eckhardt, S.B. (1973). The case for a postjunctional action of several inhibitors of norepinephrine uptake. *Proc. 5th Int. Cong. Pharmacol*. 4, 418-432. Karger, Basel.

Muscholl, E. (1970). Cholinomimetic drugs and release of the adrenergic transmitter. In: *New Aspects of Storage and Release Mechanisms of Catecholamines* (eds.) H.J. Schumann & G. Kroneberg, pp. 168-186, Springer, Berlin-Heidelberg-New York.

Muscholl, E. (1972). Adrenergic false transmitters. In: *Catecholamines, Handbook of Experimental Pharmacology* (eds.) H. Blaschko & E. Muscholl, Vol. 33, pp. 618-660, Springer, Berlin-Heidelberg-New York.

Muscholl, E. (1973a). Regulation of catecholamine release. The muscarinic inhibitory mechanism. In: *Frontiers in Catecholamine Research*, pp. 537-542, Pergamon Press, Oxford.

Muscholl, E. (1973b). Muscarinic inhibition of the norepinephrine release from peripheral sympathetic fibres. *Proc. 5th Int. Cong. Pharmacol.* 4, 440-457, Karger, Basel.

Muscholl, E. & Maitre, L. (1963). Release by sympathetic stimulation of α-methylnoradrenaline stored in the heart after administration of α-methyldopa. *Experientia* 19, 658-659.

Nastuk, W. & Parsons, R.L. (1970). Factors in the inactivation of postjunctional membrane receptors of frog skeletal muscle. *J. Gen. Physiol.* 56, 218-249.

Nedergaard, O.A. & Schrold, J. (1977). The mechanism of action of nicotine on vascular adrenergic neuroeffector transmission. *Eur. J. Pharmacol.* 42, 315-329.

Nishi, S. (1976). Cellular pharmacology of ganglionic transmission. In: *Advances in General and Cellular Pharmacology* (eds.) T. Narahashi & C.P. Bianchi, Vol. 1, pp. 179-245, Plenum Press, New York-London.

Nishikawa, T. & Tsujimoto, A. (1975). Comparison of the cardiostimulatory effects of nicotine in dogs and monkeys. *J. Pharm. Pharmacol.* 27, 716-717.

Okonek, S. (1975). Aktuelle Gesichtspunkte zur Intoxikation durch Alkylphosphate. Biochemische Befunde, Symptomatik und Therapie. *Internist* 16, 123-130.

Okonek, S. & Kilbinger, H. (1974). Determination of acetylcholine, nitrostigmine and acetylcholinesterase activity in four patients with severe nitrostigmine (E 605 forte[R]) intoxication. *Arch. Toxicol.* 32, 97-108.

Otten, U. & Thoenen, H. (1976). Mechanisms of tyrosine hydroxylase and dopamine β-hydroxylase induction in organ cultures of rat sympathetic ganglia by potassium depolarization and cholinomimetics. *Naunyn Schmiedebergs Arch. Pharmacol.* 292, 153-159.

Pappano, A.J. (1976). Onset of chronotropic effects of nicotinic drugs and tyramine on the sino-atrial pacemaker in chick embryo heart: Relationship to the development of autonomic neuroeffector transmission. *J. Pharmacol. Exp. Ther.* 196, 676-684.

Pappano, A.J. (1977). Ontogenetic development of autonomic neuroeffector transmission and transmitter reactivity in embryonic and fetal hearts. *Pharmacol. Rev.* 29, 1-65.

Pappano, A.J. & Löffelholz, K. (1974). Ontogenesis of adrenergic and cholinergic neuroeffector transmission in chick embryo heart. *J. Pharmacol. Exp. Ther.* 191, 468-478.

Patrick, R.L. & Kirshner, N. (1971). Effect of stimulation on the levels of tyrosine hydroxylase, dopamine-β-hydroxylase and catecholamines in intact and denervated rat adrenal glands. *Mol. Pharmacol.* 7, 87-96.

Priola, D.V., Spurgeon, H.A. & Geis, W.P. (1977). The intrinsic innervation of the canine heart. A functional study. *Circ. Res.* 40, 50-56.

Rang, H.P. & Ritter, J.M. (1970). On the mechanism of desensitization at cholinergic receptors. *Mol. Pharmacol.* 6, 357-382.

Richardson, J.A. & Woods, E.F. (1959). Release of norepinephrine from the isolated heart. *Proc. Soc. Exp. Biol.* 100, 149-151.

Rink, T.J. & Baker, P.F. (1975). The role of the plasma membrane in the regulation of intracellular calcium. In: *Calcium Transport in Contraction and Secretion* (eds.) E. Caratoli, F. Clementi, W. Drabikowski & A. Margreth, pp. 235-242, North-Holland, Amsterdam-Oxford.

Rosenthal, R.N. & Slotkin, T.A. (1977). Development of nicotinic responses in the rat adrenal medulla and long-term effects of neonatal nicotine administration. *Br. J. Pharmacol.* 60, 59-64.

Ross, G. (1973). Effects of intracoronary infusions of acetylcholine and nicotine on the dog heart *in vivo*. *Br. J. Pharmacol.* 48, 612-619.

Rubin, R.P. & Warner, W. (1975). Nicotine-induced stimulation of steroidogenesis in adrenocortical cells of the cat. *Br. J. Pharmacol.* 53, 357-362.

Seidler, F.J. & Slotkin, T.A. (1976). Effects of chronic nicotine administration on the denervated rat adrenal medulla. *Br. J. Pharmacol.* 56, 201-208.

Shepherd, J.T. & Vanhoutte, P.M. (1975). Pharmacology of the adrenergic nerve ending. In: *Veins and Their Control* (eds.) J.T. Shepherd & P.M. Vanhoutte, pp. 86-98, W.B. Saunders, London-Philadelphia-Toronto.

Silvette, H., Hoff, E.C., Larson, P.S. & Haag, H.B. (1962). The actions of nicotine on central nervous system functions. *Pharmacol. Rev.* 14, 137-173.

Sjöstrand, N.O. (1973). Effect of acetylcholine and some other smooth muscle stimulants on the electrical and mechanical responses of the guinea-pig vas deferens to nerve stimulation. *Acta Physiol. Scand.* 89, 1-9.

Smith, A.D. & Winkler, H. (1972). Fundamental mechanisms in the release of catecholamines. In: *Catecholamines, Handbook of Experimental Pharmacology* (eds.) H. Blaschko & E. Muscholl, Vol. 33, pp. 538-617, Springer, Berlin-Heidelberg-New York.

Sorimachi, M., Oesch, F. & Thoenen, H. (1973). Effects of colchicine and cytochalasin B on the release of ^{3}H-norepinephrine from guinea-pig atria evoked by high potassium, nicotine and tyramine. *Naunyn Schmiedebergs Arch. Pharmacol.* 276, 1-12.

Starke, K. (1977). Regulation of noradrenaline release by presynaptic receptor systems. *Rev. Physiol. Biochem. Pharmacol.* 77, 1-124.

Starke, K. & Montel, H. (1974). Influence of drugs with affinity for α-adrenoceptors on noradrenaline release by potassium, tyramine and dimethylphenylpiperazinium. *Eur. J. Pharmacol.* 27, 273-280.

Starke, K., Wagner, J. & Schümann, H.J. (1972). Adrenergic neuron blockade by clonidine: Comparison with guanethidine and local anaesthetics. *Arch. Int. Pharmacodyn. Ther.* 195, 291-308.

Steinsland, O.S. & Furchgott, R.F. (1975a). Vasoconstriction of the isolated rabbit ear artery caused by nicotinic agonists acting on adrenergic neurons. *J. Pharmacol. Exp. Ther.* 193, 128-137.

Steinsland, O.S. & Furchgott, R.F. (1975b). Desensitization of the adrenergic neurons of the isolated rabbit ear artery to nicotinic agonists. *J. Pharmacol. Exp. Ther.* 193, 138-148.

Stewart, W.C. (1952). Accumulation of acetylcholine in brain and blood of animals poisoned with cholinesterase inhibitors. *Br. J. Pharmacol.* 7, 270-276.

Stjärne, L. (1975). Pre- and post-junctional receptor-mediated cholinergic interactions with adrenergic transmission in guinea-pig vas deferens. *Naunyn Schmiedebergs Arch. Pharmacol.* 288, 305-310.

Stjärne, L. (1977). Differences in secretory excitability between short and long adrenergic neurons: Comparison of ³H-noradrenaline secretion evoked by field stimulation of guinea-pig vas deferens and human blood vessels. *Acta Physiol. Scand.* 100, 264-266.

Su, C. & Bevan, J.A. (1970). Blockade of the nicotine-induced norepinephrine release by cocaine, phenoxybenzamine and desipramine. *J. Pharmacol. Exp. Ther.* 175, 533-540.

Thoa, N., Wooten, G., Axelrod, J. & Kopin, I. (1972). Inhibition of release of dopamine-β-hydroxylase and norepinephrine from sympathetic nerves by colchicine, vinblastine or cytochalasin-B. *Proc. Natl. Acad. Sci. USA* 69, 520-522.

Thoenen, H., Huerlimann, A. & Haefely, W. (1969). Cation dependence of the noradrenaline-releasing action of tyramine. *Eur. J. Pharmacol.* 6, 29-37.

Thompson, J.W. (1958). Studies on the responses of the isolated nictitating membrane of the cat. *J. Physiol. (Lond.)* 141, 46-72.

Trendelenburg, U. (1957). The action of morphine on the superior cervical ganglion and on the nictitating membrane of the cat. *Br. J. Pharmacol.* 12, 79-85.

Trendelenburg, U. (1962). The action of acetylcholine on the nictitating membrane of the spinal cat. *J. Pharmacol. Exp. Ther.* 135, 39-44.

Trendelenburg, U. (1967). Some aspects of the pharmacology of autonomic ganglion cells. *Ergebn. der Physiol.* 59, 1-85.

Trendelenburg, U. (1972). Factors influencing the concentration of catecholamines at the receptors. In: *Catecholamines, Handbook of Experimental Pharmacology* (eds.) H. Blaschko & E. Muscholl, Vol. 33, pp. 726-761, Springer, Berlin-Heidelberg-New York.

Trifaró, J.M., Collier, B., Lastowecka, A. & Stern, D. (1972). Inhibition by colchicine and vinblastine of acetylcholine-induced catecholamine release from the adrenal gland: An anticholinergic action, not an effect upon microtubules. *Mol. Pharmacol.* 8, 264-267.

Vanhoutte, P.M. (1974). Inhibition by acetylcholine of adrenergic neurotransmission in vascular smooth muscle. *Circ. Res.* 34, 317-326.

Vanhoutte, P.M. (1977). Cholinergic inhibition of adrenergic transmission. *Fed. Proc.* 36, 2444-2449.

Vanhoutte, P.M., Lorenz, R.R. & Tyce, G.M. (1973). Inhibition of norepinephrine-^{3}H release from sympathetic nerve endings in veins by acetylcholine. *J. Pharmacol. Exp. Ther*. 185, 386-394.

Wakade, A.R. & Kirpekar, S.M. (1971). Chemical and histochemical studies on the sympathetic innervation of the vas deferens and seminal vesicle of the guinea-pig. *J. Pharmacol. Exp. Ther*. 178, 432-441.

Weisenthal, L.M., Hug, Jr., C.C., Weisbrodt, N.W. & Bass, P. (1971). Adrenergic mechanisms in the relaxation of guinea-pig taenia coli *in vitro*. *J. Pharmacol. Exp. Ther*. 178, 497-508.

Wennmalm, Å. (1977). Nicotine stimulates prostaglandin formation in the rabbit heart. *Br. J. Pharmacol*. 59, 95-100.

Wennmalm, Å. & Junstad, M. (1976). Nicotine mediated release of prostaglandin E from the rabbit heart. *Acta Physiol. Scand*. 96, 281-282.

Westfall, T.C. (1965). Effect of nicotine and nicotine analogues on tissue and urinary catecholamines in the rat. *Acta Physiol. Scand*. 63, 77-83.

Westfall, T.C. & Brasted, M. (1974). Specificity of blockade of the nicotine-induced release of ^{3}H-norepinephrine from adrenergic neurons of the guinea-pig heart by various pharmacological agents. *J. Pharmacol. Exp. Ther*. 189, 659-664.

Westfall, T.C. & Hunter, P.E. (1974). Effect of muscarinic agonists on the release of (^{3}H)noradrenaline from the guinea-pig perfused heart. *J. Pharm. Pharmacol*. 26, 458-460.

Wilson, S.P. & Kirshner, N. (1977). The acetylcholine receptor of the adrenal medulla. *J. Neurochem*. 28, 687-695.

Zapata, P., Zuazo, A. & Llados, F. (1976). Acute changes in ventilation and blood pressure induced by inhalation of tobacco smoke. *Arch. Int. Pharmacodyn. Ther*. 219, 116-127.

RELEASE INDUCED BY CALCIUM IONOPHORES

D. J. Triggle

I   INTRODUCTION

The ionophores (ion-bearers; Pressman *et al.*, 1967) represent an
increasingly large group of agents, both natural and synthetic,
that possess the ability to complex ions and transport them across
cell and artificial membranes.   Several reviews of the chemical
and biological properties of these agents are available (Pressman,
1973, 1976; Pressman & de Guzman, 1974; Gomez-Puyou & Gomez-
Lojero, 1977).   Many of these ionophores exhibit considerable
discriminatory ability in ion transport.   Thus, the antibiotic
agent valinomycin (a cyclic depsipeptide) exhibits a 10,000-fold
preference for K^+ (ionic radius, 1.33 $\overset{o}{A}$) over Na^+ (ionic radius,
0.95 $\overset{o}{A}$).

A detailed analysis of the physicochemical basis of ionophore
function lies outside the scope of this chapter, but detailed
reviews are available (Lehn, 1973; Simon *et al.*, 1973; Pressman,
1976).   Nonetheless, some brief general discussion of their ligand
complexing activities will be helpful to provide a basis for the
analysis of catecholamine releasing activities of ionophores.   In
very general terms, ionophores possess both hydrophobic and hydro-
philic groups (dominantly oxygen functions) which, in the complex,
are directed externally and internally respectively.   The hydro-
philic groups serve to replace the solvation shell of the cation
and the hydrophobic exterior permits passage across lipid phases.
The ion selectivity of a given ionophore is determined by the
energy of desolvation of the cation, the energy of complexation
of the cation with the ionophore and by the conformational flexibility of the ionophore.   The greater the flexibility, the less
rigidly determined is the cation coordination geometry and the
less selective is the ionophore (Lehn, 1973; Simon *et al.*, 1973;
Pfeiffer & Lardy, 1976).

Ionophores can be classified into neutral and carboxylic species,
the former representing a group of diverse cyclic structures,
from antibiotic cyclic peptides to synthetic polyethers whilst
the latter are variants on a common linear structure of hetero-
cyclic rings with a terminal carboxylic group which are, however,
also cyclic in the complexed state.   Included in this latter
group are the important "calcium ionophores", X-537A (I) and
A 23187 (II).   Neutral species form charged complexes and hence
may generate transmembrane current whilst the carboxylic ionophores form, in their negatively charged state, neutral 1:1 or

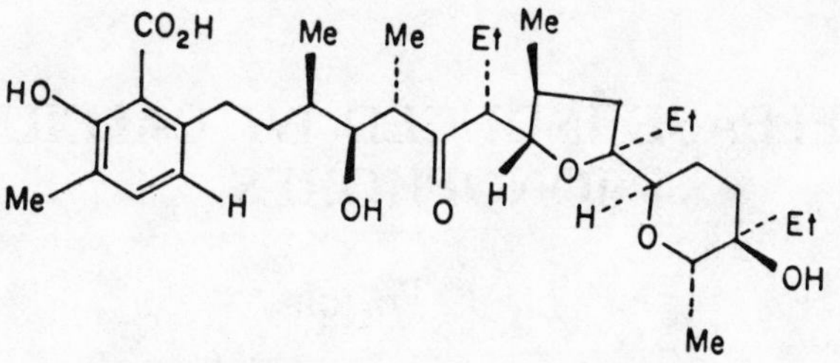

I

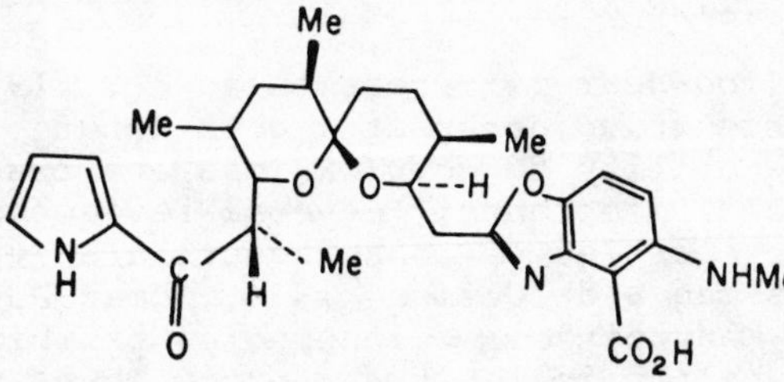

II

2:1 complexes and generally mediate electrically neutral processes (Fig. 1).

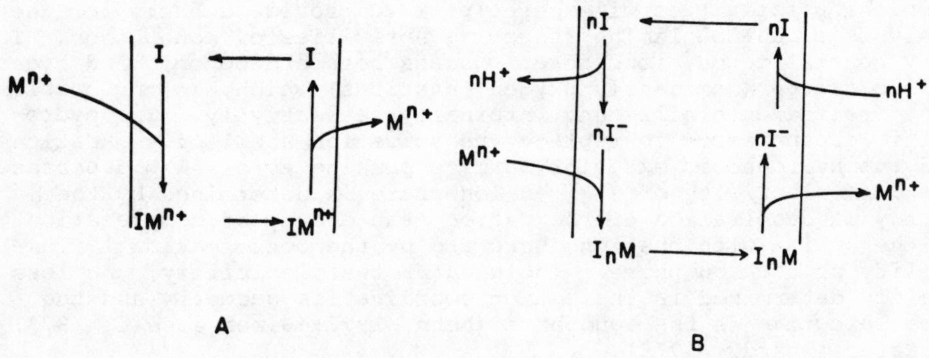

A   B

Fig. 1.   Models for ionophore-mediated cation transport.
          I = ionophore, M^{n+} – monovalent cation (n = 1)
          or divalent cation (n = 2).   A, transport by a
          neutral ionophore showing the deposition of a
          positive charge on one side of the membrane.   B,
          transport by a carboxylic ionophore, showing the
          exchange mediation of positive charges.

II   CALCIUM IONOPHORES

Both X-537A and A 23187 serve as carriers of Ca^{2+} and are able to
initiate a wide variety of Ca^{2+}-dependent events in a fashion
independent of specific receptor activation. Such events include
stimulus-secretion and excitation-contraction coupling in a
variety of systems, lymphocyte activation, increased K^+ permeability, inhibition of cell agglutination, neutrophil chemotaxis,
inhibition of microtubule assembly, egg cell activation, etc.,
(Pressman, 1976; Rosenberger & Triggle, 1977). There is often a
very close similarity between the events initiated by the ionophores and those initiated by specific receptor activation indicating that a major function of these ionophores is to permit
Ca^{2+} entry into the cell by a process (or processes) that bypasses
the physiological entry.

However, neither ionophore shows absolute selectivity for Ca^{2+}
and both can complex and transport other divalent and monovalent
cations, the latter property being best demonstrated with X-537A
(Pressman, 1973, 1976; Celis *et al.*, 1974; Degani & Friedman,
1974). Figure 2 shows the dependence of formation constant for
ionophore - M^{2+} complexation upon cation ionic radius revealing
the stability sequences, X-537A, $Ba^{2+} > Sr^{2+} > Ca^{2+} > Mn^{2+} >$
Mg^{2+} and A 23187, $Mn^{2+} > Ca^{2+} > Mg^{2+} > Sr^{2+} > Ba^{2+}$. Table 1 lists

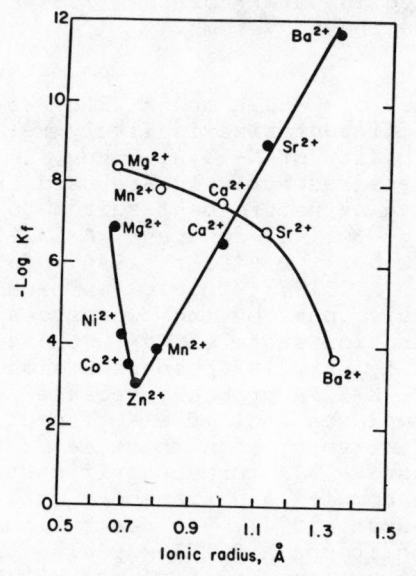

Fig. 2.   The negative logarithms of the overall binding
          constants for divalent cations with ionophores
          X-537A and A 23187.   Decreasing values for -
          LOG K_f indicate increasing stability. The data
          for A 23187 are from Pfeiffer and Lardy (1976)
          and refer to toluene-butanol-water and the data
          for X-537A are from Degani and Freedman (1974)
          and refer to methanol. (Reproduced with per-
          mission from Pfeiffer and Lardy, 1976).

the corresponding data for univalent cations showing again that
these two ionophores give quite different orders of ion selectivity.

TABLE 1   Formation Constants for Complexation of Monova-
           lent Cations with X-537A and A 23187 (Degani &
           Friedman, 1974; Pfeiffer & Lardy, 1976).

	$-$ Log K_f			
	Li^+	Na^+	K^+	Complex
X-537A[1]	6.2	5.7	5.6	MX
A-23187[2]	6.11	$-$	$-$	MX
A-23187[2]	1.31	3.22	4.14	MHX_2

[1] Hexane at 25°.

[2] Determined in water/toluene (70%) - butanol
    (30%) two phase systems.

The relative abilities of X-537A and A 23187 to discriminate
between cations of different size is likely related to the greater
conformational flexibility of X-537A. Thus, in the Ba^{2+}-$(X-537A)_2$
complex 6 and 3 oxygens respectively are used from each ionophore
molecule to generate a structure best suited to the complexation
of large cations (Fig. 3).   In contrast, A 23187 is conformation-
ally less flexible (Deber & Pfeiffer, 1976; Pfeiffer & Lardy,
1976) and the Ca^{2+} - $(A\ 23187)_2$ complex is highly symmetrical,
each ionophore molecule contributing two oxygen and one nitrogen
to the 6-fold coordination state of Ca^{2+} (Chaney *et al.*, 1976;
(Fig. 4).   Additionally, A 23187 possesses higher divalent cation
selectivity than does X-537A probably because of its greater ten-
dency to form 2:1 complexes and, if electroneutral complexes are
transported more effectively, then the ease of transport will be
$M^{2+} > M^+$.   In contrast X-537A forms significant 1:1 complexes and
a greater ability to complex and transport monovalent cations is
found (Degani & Freedman, 1974).   It seems likely, however, that
under appropriate conditions A 23187 may also transport significantly the monovalent cations Li^+, Na^+ and K^+ (Pfeiffer & Lardy,
1976).

In addition to their ability to complex and transport inorganic
cations, both X-537A and A 23187 can complex a number of organic
cations. This property is most marked with X-537A as might be
expected from its lower cation selectivity. Thus X-537A has
marked ability to complex and transport biogenic amines including dopamine and 5-hydroxytryptamine. Primary amines complex

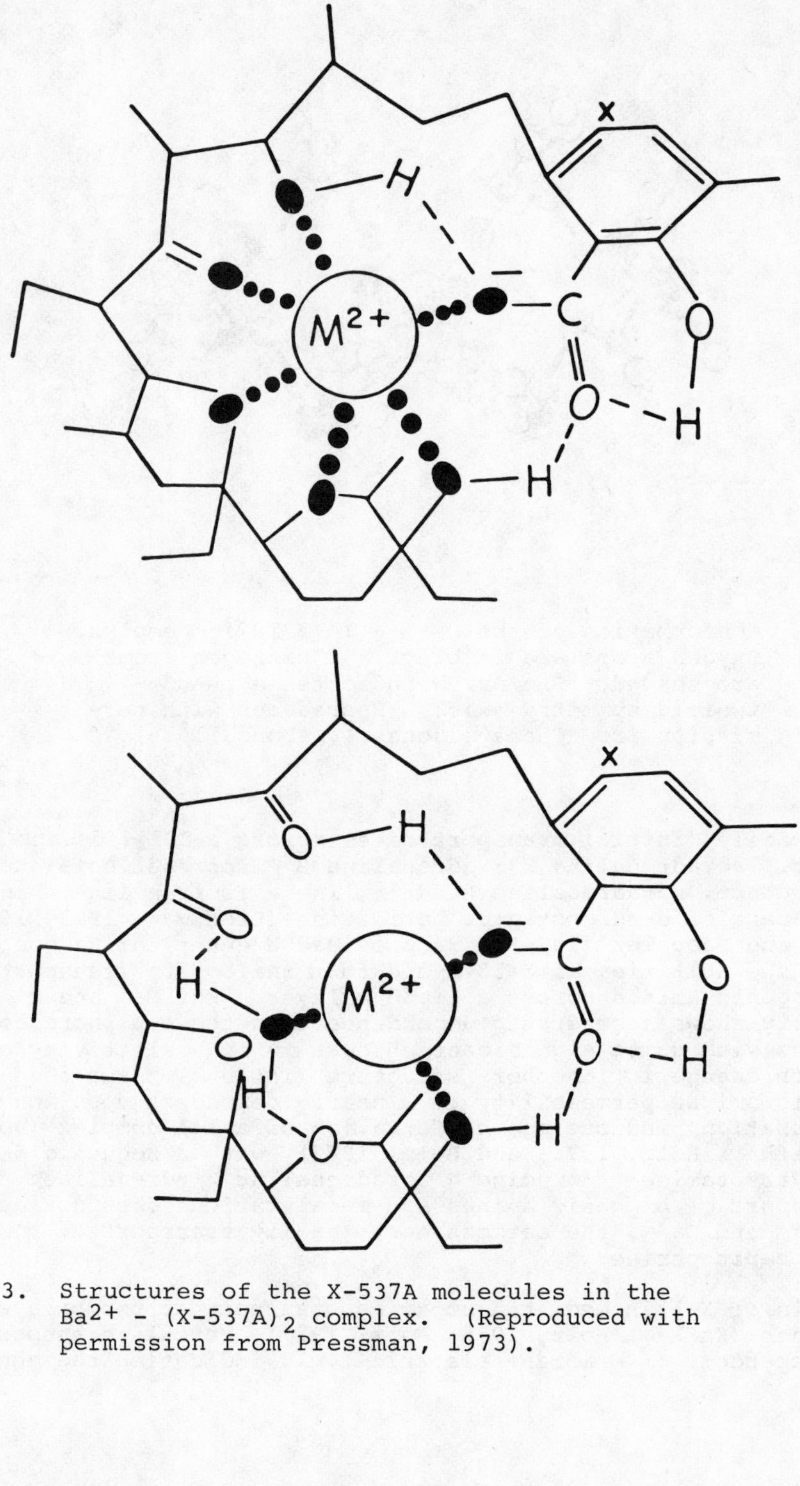

Fig. 3.   Structures of the X-537A molecules in the
          Ba^{2+} - $(X-537A)_2$ complex. (Reproduced with
          permission from Pressman, 1973).

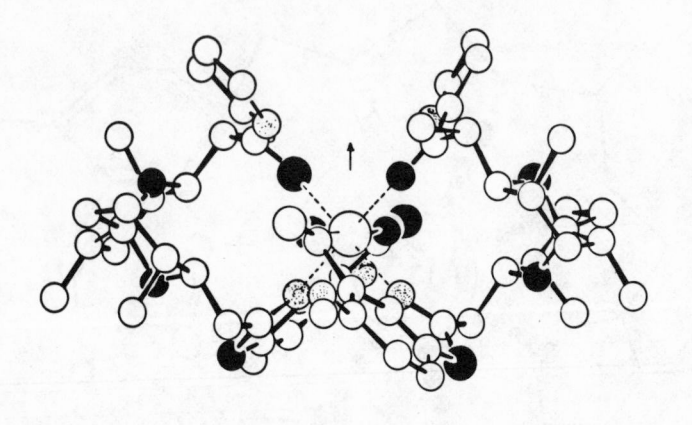

Fig. 4.   Conformation of the Ca^{2+} - (A 23187)$_2$ complex.
         Oxygen atoms are in black and nitrogen atoms
         are shaded. The arrow indicates a pseudo-
         twofold symmetry axis. (Reproduced with per-
         mission from Chaney, Jonas & Debono, 1976).

most readily (initial transport rates across a CCl_4: decane layer,
nmol/hr., noradrenaline 29; adrenaline 9; isoprenaline 6) to give
the sequence, noradrenaline > adrenaline > isoprenaline, highly
reminiscent of α-adrenoceptor activation (Pressman, 1973, 1976).
Schadt and Haeusler (1974) have provided a quantitative comparison of the abilities of X-537A and four analogs to transport ions
and biogenic amines across a lipid bilayer. For M^{2+} and M^+ con-
ductivity shows a quadratic dependence upon the ionophore concentrations with quite significant changes in ion selectivity occur-
ing with change in ionophore structure (Table 2). For the
biogenic amines permeability is linearly dependent upon ionophore
concentration, indicating the formation of a 1:1 complex (see
also Kafka & Holz, 1976; and Holz, 1977), with a sequence 5-
hydroxytryptamine > dopamine > noradrenaline > adrenaline.
Cotransport of biogenic amines and metal cations does not occur
since K^+ and Ca^{2+}, the cations most readily transported, compete
with norepinephrine.

Analysis of X-537A mediated dopamine transport across bilayer
membranes (Kafka & Holz, 1976; Holz, 1977), reveals transport to
be independent of membrane electric field indicating the absence

TABLE 2 Ionic Conductivities (M^{2+}, M^+) and Permeability Coefficients (Biogenic Amines) Measured in Lipid Bilayer Membranes for X-537A and Related Compounds (Schadt & Haeusler, 1974)

Ionophore	Ca[a], (M)	Ionic Conductivities ($\times 10^{11}$), ohm^{-1};					Permeability coefficients (p) $\times 10^3$, μ sec^{-1}			
		LiCl	NaCl	KCl	MgCl$_2$	CaCl$_2$	5-HT	DA	NA	A
X-537A	1×10^{-7}	45	45	200	45	200	1300	750	190	18
Br-X537A	1.1×10^{-7}	420	420	3800	420	420	1300	750	190	18
X-537A-oxime	$> 10^{-5}$	360	360	360	360	360	3.8	< 0.5	< 0.5	< 0.5
Nitro-X-537A	3.9×10^{-6}	5.9	5.9	5.9	5.9	5.9	14	4.8	2.2	< 0.5
Acetyl-X-537A	2.4×10^{-6}	15	15	77	15	15	210	160	100	< 0.5
Lipid bilayer	–	5.9	5.9	5.9	5.9	5.9	1.4	< 0.5	< 0.5	< 0.5

a   Concentration required to increase contractile force of cat heart by 50%.

of significant net charge transport. That this transport is an
exchange diffusion process (Fig. 1B) is suggested not only by the
absence of any electric field effect but also by the dopamine
conductance which is orders of magnitude higher than the $[^{14}C]$
dopamine flux. Furthermore, dopamine transport is enhanced by
trans-addition of dopamine and other ions including tyramine, H^+
and K^+, to the membrane system and when unequal dopamine concentrations are present cis and trans equal unidirectional fluxes
are measured.

As will be noted later many of the catecholamine-releasing
actions in tissues of X-537A are Ca^{2+}-independent and it is likely
therefore that this ionophore mediates an exchange diffusion process of catecholamine release probably by inducing a cytoplasmic
H^+ and K^+ exchange for vesicular catecholamine following which
the cytoplasmic catecholamine may leave the nerve terminal by
membrane leakage, by the membrane catecholamine transport system,
via a second ionophore-mediated exchange diffusion across the
nerve terminal membrane or by leakage after intracellular metabolism. Evidence for exchange diffusion by Br-X537-A has been
obtained for adrenal medullary chromaffin granules (Papadopoulou-
Daifotis et al., 1977) where noradrenaline and adrenaline release
are promoted by the cations, H^+, Na^+, K^+ and Ca^{2+} and where at
low extravesicular cation concentrations ($< 2 \times 10^{-3}M$) a selective release of norepinephrine can be seen.

A 23187 is reported to form lipid soluble complexes with amino
acids and to facilitate their uptake into human lymphocytes
(Hovi et al., 1975). The amino acids show increasing relative
affinity for the ionophore in the following order, Glu << Asp <
Lys < Gly < Leu. Additionally, A 23187 complexes with the ammonium ion with a stability sequence, $Ca^{2+} > NH_4^+ > K^+$ (Wong, 1976).

These several properties of X-537A and A 23187 clearly make
incorrect any automatic assumption that their actions are due
only to the equilibration of Ca^{2+} gradients across cell membranes.
Analysis of the actions of these two agents must take into
account that they can transport a variety of monovalent and divalent cations, both inorganic and organic, although it is clear
that of the two ionophores A 23187 is substantially more selective towards Ca^{2+}.

A further complexity in the actions of both X-537A and A-23187
arises from their ability to enter the cell and to mobilize Ca^{2+}
from intracellular sources. Thus, in a number of systems these
agents have been shown to activate (partially or totally) Ca^{2+}-
dependent events in the absence of extracellular Ca^{2+} (Rosenberger,
& Triggle, 1977). Included in such events are egg cell activation
(Chambers et al., 1974), histamine release from mast cells
(Foreman et al., 1973), platelet secretion and aggregation
(Feinstein & Fraser, 1975), frog egg contractility (Schroeder &
Strickland, 1974) and skeletal and smooth muscle contraction
(Desmedt & Hainaut, 1976; Murray et al., 1975). Such findings
accord with the several demonstrations that both X-537A and
A 23187 can release Ca^{2+} from mitochondria (Babcock et al., 1976)

and sarcoplasmic reticulum (Scarpa *et al.*, 1972). Additionally, the abilities of these agents to enter the cell and to promote Ca^{2+} utilization to a possibly non-physiological extent is perhaps responsible for the extensive cellular damage seen in some but not all systems (Chandler & Williams, 1977; Goldstein *et al.*, 1974; Lichtenstein, 1975).

Finally, there are some extremely interesting qualitative differences between X-537A and A 23187 action in a number of tissues. In rat glioma cell A 23187 is a potent protein synthesis inhibitor whilst X-537A is very much more effective in promoting acetylcholine release at neuromuscular junctions (Kita & Van der Kloot, 1974; Kita *et al.*, 1976), in causing vasopressin release (Nakazato & Douglas, 1974), in promoting cardiac contractility (Schaffer *et al.*, 1974) and whilst X-537A causes contractions of rat vas deferens but not of guinea-pig ileum, A 23187 has the opposite selectivity (Swamy *et al.*, 1975). Other similar differences of action between X-537A and A 23187 have been reported but no single satisfactory explanation of such differences yet appears available.

III   CATECHOLAMINE RELEASE BY THE CALCIUM IONOPHORES

Several studies have demonstrated the abilities of X-537A and A 23187 to release catecholamines from a variety of preparations, ranging from adrenal glands to cardiac muscle. A summary of the findings is presented in Table 3. The evidence for catecholamine release ranges from direct measurements of output, including in a few instances both free amines and deaminated metabolites, to indirect demonstrations that the actions of the ionophore are sensitive to catecholamine depletion or to α- or β-receptor antagonists.

From the available data on catecholamine release it is immediately apparent that X-537A is generally more effective than A 23187 and that in a number of instances the latter ionophore is without effect despite its higher divalent cation selectivity. Furthermore, the actions of X-537A are generally much less dependent upon Ca^{2+}_{EXT} suggesting that the ability to transport Ca^{2+} across the plasma membrane is not the dominant factor in catecholamine release promoted by this ionophore.

Studies on the adrenal gland serve as fairly representative of the contrasting actions of X-537A and A 23187. In the cat adrenal gland X-537A ($7 \times 10^{-7} - 2 \times 10^{-5}M$) releases catecholamines at a rate which, at the higher ionophore concentrations, is comparable to that produced by acetylcholine or K^+ depolarization, namely a 100-200 fold increase above basal level (to - 5 µg/ml). The actions of X-537A are not greatly reduced by atropine or hexamethonium and are thus due to direct stimulation of the chromaffin cell (Cochrane *et al.*, 1975). Although the activity of X-537A is reduced by 90% after 45 min of Ca^{2+} - free perfusion this effect of Ca^{2+} removal is far less dramatic than that seen when ACh or K^+ are used as stimulants. In contrast, Cochrane *et al.*,

(1975) reported A 23187 to be an erratic and weak catecholamine releaser, a concentration of 10^{-4}M producing only a ~ 5 fold increase in catecholamine output by a Ca^{2+}_{EXT} -dependent process. However, in the same preparation Garcia *et al.* (1975) noted that A 23187 produces a concentration-dependent catecholamine release reaching ~ 0.75 µg/min in response to 10^{-5}M A 23187. In frog adrenal gland A 23187 (5 x 10^{-5}M) was found to be without effect whilst X-537A (2 x 10^{-5}M) released catecholamines by a Ca^{2+}_{EXT} - independent process (Ricci *et al.*, 1975). In this preparation the ratio of noradrenaline:adrenaline liberated by X-537A was the same as that (NA:A 1:4) during spontaneous release, and the cate- cholamines were accompanied by dopamine-β-hydroxylase suggesting that X-537A is promoting, at least partially, an exocytotic release process. Since X-537A, but not A 23187, has been shown to release catecholamines from adrenal chromaffin granules (Johnson & Scarpa, 1974; Holz, 1975) it is likely that the effec- tiveness of X-537A in perfused adrenal preparations resides in its ability to affect the granule membrane.

The actions of both X-537A and A 23187 have been examined in a number of brain synaptosome preparations derived from both whole brain and discrete brain areas. In rat striatium synaptosomes both agents are approximately equipotent in releasing dopamine (Holz, 1975), but are clearly acting by different mechanisms since the actions of X-537A are Ca^{2+}_{EXT}-independent, whilst those of A-23187 show an absolute Ca^{2+}-dependence at 10^{-7}M, but some Ca^{2+}-independence at higher concentrations. Additionally, deter- mination of the release of deaminated dopamine shows that A 23187 behaves like veratridine whilst X-537A releases more deaminated material and behaves intermediately between veratridine and reserpine. Since veratridine causes exocytotic release it is likely that a major function of X-537A is to promote dopamine transport across the granule membrane into the cytoplasm from whence it is released in both free and deaminated form. Essen- tially similar conclusions have been drawn by Colburn *et al.* (1974) using synaptosomes from whole rat brain. Additionally, A 23187 action was found to be greatly reduced at 0° whilst that of X-537A was not affected.

A similar difference in action of X-537A and A 23187 has been reported for the rat vas deferens (Thoa *et al.*, 1974) where X-537A, although significantly more potent than A 23187, releases proportionately less dopamine-β-hydroxylase.

In rat atrial segments X-537A is again more potent than A 23187 and X-537A behaves like reserpine in releasing approximately 50% deaminated products whereas A 23187 releases less (35%) deaminated product (Thoa *et al.*, 1974). The remaining studies of ionophore action on cardiac tissue have been largely concerned with their effects on cardiac performance and it is of interest that, with the exception of one report (Holland *et al.*, 1975), A 23187 is ineffective in enhancing cardiac contractility. As judged by the sensitivity of X-537A responses to propranolol (Levy *et al.*, 1973; DeGuzman & Pressman, 1974; Schaffer *et al.*, 1974; Osborne *et al.*, 1977), or reserpine (Levy *et al.*, 1973; Schaffer *et al.*,

1974; Schwartz *et al.*, 1974; Schadt & Haeusler, 1974) at least some component of the action of X-537A in enhancing cardiac contractility is due to catecholamine release. However, the imperfect correlation between the noradrenaline-transporting ability of X-537A analogs and their positive inotropic effects (Schadt & Haeusler, 1974; Table 2) indicates that noradrenaline transport is not the sole mode of action of these agents (Pressman, 1976).

It is clear that X-537A and A 23187 release catecholamines by at least two distinct processes. The actions of A 23187 are probably largely exerted by a Ca^{2+}-dependent stimulation of exocytosis whilst X-537A acts, in addition, through its ability to complex and transport catecholamines directly by a Ca^{2+}-independent process. Furthermore, the importance of these two actions of X-537A will be dependent upon ionophore concentration since X-537A forms 1:1 complexes with catecholamines but 2:1 complexes with calcium (and other divalent cations). Additionally, both ionophores can cause Ca^{2+} mobilization from internal stores. It is interesting that the relative effectiveness of X-537A and A 23187 appears to vary significantly between preparations. Thus, in adrenal gland and adrenal chromaffin granules, X-537A >> A 23187 whereas in brain synaptosome preparations this large difference in activity is not observed. Several factors may contribute to these differences in activity. There may exist significant differences in partitioning behaviour of these two ionophores with different membranes. Of probable larger importance, however, is the greater ability of X-537A to transport monovalent cations and thus produce membrane depolarization (Cochrane *et al.*, 1975; Rosenberger & Triggle, 1977). Consistent with this is the observation that X-537A promptly depolarizes frog skeletal muscle whereas A 23187 has only a weak depolarizing action (Cochrane & Douglas, 1975). Hence, in some tissues a combination of Ca^{2+} entry/mobilization plus depolarization may be a necessary prerequisite for catecho-amine secretion. It is possible that in the absence of such enhanced Ca^{2+} entry the normal cellular Ca^{2+} sequestering/pumping processes are able to maintain a low intracellular Ca^{2+} concentration despite the ionophore-induced entry of Ca^{2+}.

TABLE 3 Catecholamine Release by Ionophores X-537A and A 23187

System	Ionophore	Conc. (M)a	Effectb	Ca2+ dependence	Nature of released amine	Ref.
Bovine adrenal chromaffin granules	X-537A	$5.5-27.5 \times 10^{-6}$	NA/A release	No	-	Johnson & Scarpa, 1974
	A 23187	2.4×10^{-5}	Ineffective	-		
Bovine adrenal chromaffin granules	Br-X-537A	$10-6-10^{-4}$	NA/A release	No	-	Papadopoulou-Daifatis et al., 1977
Rat adrenal chromaffin granules	X-537A	$10^{-7}-10^{-6}$	DA release	-	-	Holz, 1975
Cat adrenal	A 23187	$10^{-7}-10^{-5}$	Ineffective	-	-	1975
Cat adrenal	X-537A	$10-6-2 \times 10^{-5}$	Release	Partial	-	Cochrane et al., 1975
	A 23187	$4 \times 10^{-6}-10^{-4}$	Release (X-537A > A 23187)	Yes		
Cat adrenal	A 23187	$10-6-10^{-5}$	Release	Yes	-	Garcia et al., 1975
Frog Adrenal	X-537A	2.5×10^{-5}	Release	No	-	Ricci et al., 1975
	A 23187	5×10^{-5}	Ineffective			

Table 3 (Continued)

System	Ionophore	Conc. (M)[a]	Effect[b]	Ca^{2+} dependence	Nature of released amine	Ref.
Rat striatium Synaptosomes	X-537A A 23187	5x10^{-8}-5x10^{-7} 3x10^{-8}-10^{-6}	DA release DA release (X-537A ~ A 23187)	No Partial	Deaminated Free amine	Holz, 1975
Rat brain Synaptosomes	X-537A A 23187	10^{-7}-10^{-5} 10^{-7}-10^{-5}	NA release NA release (X-537A > A 23187)	No Yes	Deaminated Free Amine	Colburn et al., 1976
Mouse forebrain Synaptosomes	A 23187	2x10^{-6}-10^{-5}	NA release	Yes	-	Cotman et al., 1976; Levy et al., 1976
Rat cerebrum Synaptosomes	A 23187	2x10^{-5}	NA release	-	-	Levi et al. 1976
Rabbit brain synaptosomes	X-537A A 23187	10^{-6} 10^{-5}	NA release NA release (X-537A > A 23187)	- -	- -	Fairhurst, et al., 1976
Rat neocortex slices	A 23187	5x10^{-4}	Ineffective	-	-	Vargas et al., 1976

Release induced by calcium ionophores

Table 3 (Continued)

System	Ionophore	Conc. (M)a	Effectb	Ca2+ dependence	Nature of released amine	Ref.
Mouse brain (*in vivo*)	X-537A	15mg/kg	NA release	-	-	Fairhurst *et al.*, 1976
	A 23187	2.5mg/kg	No DA release	-	-	
Guinea-pig vas deferens	X-537A	10^{-5}	NA release	No	Deaminated	Thoa *et al.* 1974; Swamy *et al.*, 1975
	A 23187	10^{-4}	NA release (X-537A > A 23187)	Yes	Partially-deaminated	
Rat vas deferens	X-537A	5×10^{-6}-3×10^{-5}	NA release	-	-	Swamy *et al.* 1975
	A 23187	10^{-6}-10^{-4}	Ineffective	-	-	
Rat atria	X-537A	3×10^{-7}-3×10^{-5}	NA release	No	Deaminated	Thoa *et al.* 1974
	A 23187	3×10^{-5}-3×10^{-4}	NA release	Yes	Partially-deaminated	
Rabbit atrium	X-537A	5×10^{-6}	CA release	-	-	Levy *et al.* 1973
Dog heart	X-537A	0.75-1.0 mg/kg	CA release	-	-	DeGuzman & Pressman, 1974; Schwartz *et al.*, 1974.
Rat heart	X-537A	10-150 μg/heart	CA release	-	-	Schaffer *et al.*, 1974
	A 23187	50 μg/heart	Ineffective	-	-	

Table 3 (Continued)

System	Ionophore	Conc. (M)a	Effectb	Ca2+ dependence	Nature of released amine	Ref.
Rabbit heart	X-537A	9x10-6	CA release	-	-	Schwartz, et al., 1974
	A 23187	varied	Ineffective	-	-	
Rabbit, cat atria	X-537A	1-3x10-6	CA release	-	-	Schwartz et al., 1974
	A 23187	varied	Ineffective	-	-	
Beagle heart	X-537A	1mg/kg	CA release	-	-	Osborne et al., 1975

a Solvent vehicle (usually ethanol or dimethylsulfoxide) apparently without effect in all cases.

b Release refers to nature of catecholamine, noradrenaline (NA), noradrenaline plus adrenaline (CA) or dopamine (DA). In the last seven entries of the table (smooth muscle and heart preparations) evidence for the release of CA is inferential and is based upon blockade of ionophore action by reserpine, propranolol, phenoxybenzamine, etc.

IV   REFERENCES

Babcock, D.F., First, N.L. & Lardy, H.A. (1976). Action of iono-
    phore A 23187 at the cellular level. Separation of effects at
    the plasma and mitochondrial membranes. *J. Biol. Chem.* 251,
    3381-3386.

Bottenstein, J.E. & de Vellis, J. (1976). Divalent cation iono-
    phore A 23187: A potent protein synthesis inhibitor. *Biochem.
    Biophys. Res. Commun.* 73, 486-493.

Celis, H., Estrado-O, S. & Montal, M. (1974). Model translocators
    for divalent and monovalent ion transport in phospholipid
    membranes. I. The ion permeability induced in lipid bilayers
    by the antibiotic X-537A. *J. Membr. Biol.* 18, 187-199.

Chandler, E.D. & Williams, J.A. (1977). Intracellular uptake and
    α-amylase and lactate dehydrogenase releasing actions of the
    divalent cation ionophore A 23187 in dissociated pancreatic
    acinar cells. *J. Membr. Biol.* 32, 201-230.

Chambers, E.L., Pressman, B.C. & Rose, B. (1974). The activation
    of sea-urchin eggs by the divalent cation ionophores A 23187
    and X-537A. *Biochem. Biophys. Res. Commun.* 60, 126-132.

Chaney, M.O., Jones, N.D. & Debono, M. (1976). The structure of
    the calcium complex of A 23187, a divalent cation ionophore
    antibiotic. *J. Antibiot.* 29, 424-427.

Cochrane, D.E. & Douglas, W.W. (1975). Depolarizing effects of
    the ionophores X-537A and A 23187 and their relevance to secre-
    tion. *Br. J. Pharmacol.* 54, 400-402.

Cochrane, D.E., Douglas, W.W., Mouri, T. & Nakazato, Y. (1975).
    Calcium and stimulus-secretion coupling in the adrenal medulla:
    Contrasting stimulating effects of the ionophores X-537A and
    A 23187 on catecholamine output. *J. Physiol. (Lond.)* 252,
    363-378.

Colburn, R.W., Thoa, N.B. & Kopin, J.J. (1976). Influence of
    ionophores which bind calcium on the release of norepinephrine
    from synaptosomes. *Life Sciences* 17, 1395-1400.

Cotman, C.W., Haycock, J.W. & White, W.F. (1976). Stimulus-
    secretion coupling processes in brain: Analyses of noradrena-
    line and gamma-aminobutyric acid release. *J. Physiol.* 254,
    475-505.

Deber, C.M. & Pfeiffer, D.R. (1976). Ionophore A 23187. Solu-
    tion conformations of the calcium complex and free acid
    deduced from proton and carbon-13 nuclear magnetic resonance
    studies. *Biochemistry* 15, 132-141.

Degani, H. & Friedman, H.L. (1974). Ion binding by X-537A. Formulas, formation constants and spectra of complexes. *Biochemistry* 13, 5022-5032.

Desmedt, J.E. & Hainaut, K. (1976). The effect of A 23187 iono-phore on calcium movements and contraction processes in single barnacle muscle fibres. *J. Physiol. (Lond.)* 257, 87-107.

Fairhurst, A.S., Julien, R.M. & Whittaker, M.L. (1976). Effects of ionophores A 23187 and X-537A on brain calcium, catechol-amines and excitability. *Life Sciences* 17, 1433-1444.

Feinstein, M.B. & Fraser, C. (1975). Human platelet secretion and aggregation induced by calcium ionophores. *J. Gen. Physiol.* 66, 561-581.

Foreman, J.C., Mongar, J.L. & Gomperts, B.D. (1973). Calcium ionophores and movement of calcium ions following the physio-logical stimulus to a secretory process. *Nature* 245, 249-251.

Garcia, A.G., Kirkepar, S.M. & Prat, J.C. (1975). A calcium ionophore stimulating the secretion of catecholamines from the cat adrenal. *J. Physiol. (Lond.)* 244, 253-262.

Goldstein, J.M., Horn, J.K., Kaplan, H.B. & Weissman, G. (1974). Calcium-induced lyoszyme secretion from human polymorphonuclear leucocytes. *Biochem. Biophys. Res. Commun.* 60, 807-812.

Gomez-Puyou, A. & Gomez-Lojero, C. (1977). The use of ionophores and channel formers in the study of biological membranes. Curr. Top. Cell. Regul. 8, 221-257.

DeGuzman, N.T. & Pressman, B.C. (1974). The inotropic effects of the calcium ionophore X-537A in the anesthetized dog. *Circula-tion* 69, 1072-1077.

Holland, D.R., Steinberg, M.I. & Armstrong, W.McD. (1975). A 23187: A calcium ionophore that directly increases cardiac contractility. *Proc. Soc. Exp. Biol. Med.* 148, 1141-1145.

Holz, R.W. (1975). The release of dopamine from synaptosomes from rat striatum by the ionophores X-537A and A 23187. *Biochim. Biophys. Acta* 375, 138-152.

Holz, R.W. (1977). Exchange diffusion of dopamine induced in planar lipid bilayer membranes by the ionophore X-537A. *J. Gen. Physiol.* 69, 633-653.

Hovi, T., Williams, S.C. & Allison, A.C. (1975). Divalent cation ionophore A 23187 forms lipid soluble complexes with leucine and other amino acids. *Nature* 256, 70-72.

Johnson, R.G. & Scarpa, A. (1974). Catecholamine equilibration gradients of isolated chromaffin vesicles induced by the iono-phore X-537A. *FEBS Lett.* 47, 117-121.

320   D. J. Triggle

Kafka, M.S. & Holz, R.W. (1976). Ionophores X-537A and A 23187.
    Effects on the permeability of lipid bimolecular membranes to
    dopamine and calcium. *Biochim. Biophys. Acta* 426, 31-37.

Kita, H. & Van der Klott, W. (1974). Calcium ionophore X-537A
    increases spontaneous and phasic quantal release of acetylcho-
    line at frog neuromuscular junction. *Nature* 250, 658-660.

Kita, H., Madden, K. & Van der Kloot, W. (1976). Effects of the
    "calcium ionophore" A 23187 on transmitter release at the frog
    neuromuscular junction. *Life Sciences* 17, 1837-1842.

Lehn, J.M. (1973). Design of organic complexing agents. Strate-
    gies towards properties. *Structure and Bonding* 16, 1-70.

Levi, G., Roberts, P.J. & Raiteri, M. (1976). Release and
    exchange of neurotransmitters in synaptosomes: Effects of the
    ionophore A 23187 and of ouabain. *Neurochem. Res.* 1, 409-416.

Levy, J.V., Cohen, J.A. & Inesi, G. (1973). Contractile effects
    of a calcium ionophore. *Nature* 242, 461-463.

Levy, W.B., Haycock, J.W. & Cotman, C.W. (1976). Stimulation-
    dependent depression of readily releasable neurotransmitter
    pools in brain. *Brain Res.* 115, 243-256.

Lichtenstein, L.M. (1975). The mechanism of basophil histamine
    release induced by antigen and by the calcium ionophore
    A 23187. *J. Immunol.* 114, 1692-1699.

Murray, J.W., Reed, P.W. & Fay, F.S. (1975). Contraction of
    isolated smooth muscle cells by ionophore A 23187. *Proc. Natl.
    Acad. Sci. USA* 72, 4459-4463.

Nakazato, Y. & Douglas, W.W. (1974). Vasopressin release from
    the isolated neurohypophysis induced by a calcium ionophore
    X-537A. *Nature (Lond.)* 249, 479-481.

Osborne, M.W., Wenger, J.W. & Zanko, M.T. (1977). The cardio-
    vascular pharmacology of the antibiotic ionophore Ro 2-2985
    (X-537A). *J. Pharmacol. Exp. Ther.* 200, 195-206.

Papadopoulou-Daifotis, Z.P., Morris, S.J. & Schober, R. (1977).
    Differential lysis of adrenaline- and noradrenaline-containing
    chromaffin granules promoted by the ionophore Br-X-537 A.
    Neuroscience 2, 609-619.

Pfeiffer, D.R. & Lardy, H.A. (1976). Ionophore A 23187: The
    effect of H^+ concentration on complex formation with divalent
    and monovalent cations and the demonstration of K^+ transport
    in mitochondria mediated by A 23187. *Biochemistry* 15, 935-
    943.

Pressman, B.C. (1973). Properties of ionophores with broad range
    cation selectivity. *Fed. Proc.* 32, 1698-1703.

Pressman, B.C. (1976). Biological applications of ionophores. *Ann. Rev. Biochem.* 45, 501-530.

Pressman, B.C. & de Guzman, N.T. (1974). New ionophores for old organelles. *Ann. N.Y. Acad. Sci.* 227, 380-397.

Pressman, B.C., Harris, E.J., Jagger, W.S. & Johnson, J.H. (1967). Antibiotic-mediated transport of alkali ions across lipid barriers. *Proc. Natl. Acad. Sci. USA* 58, 1949-1956.

Ricci, A., Sanders, K.M., Portmore, J. & Van der Kloot, W.G. (1975). Effects of the ionophores X-537A and A 23187 on catecholamine release from the *in vitro* frog adrenal. *Life Sciences* 16, 177-184.

Rosenberger, L. & Triggle, D.J. (1977). Calcium, calcium translocation and specific calcium antagonists. In: *Calcium and Drug Action* (ed.) G.B. Weiss, Plenum Press, New York.

Scarpa, A., Baldassare, J. & Inesi, G. (1972). The effect of calcium ionophores in fragmented sarcoplasmic reticulum. *J. Gen. Physiol.* 60, 735-749.

Schadt, M. & Haeusler, G. (1974). Permeability of lipid bilayer membranes to biogenic amines and cations: Changes induced by ionophores and correlation with biological activities. *J. Membr. Biol.* 18, 277-294.

Schaffer, S.W., Safer, B., Scarpa, A. & Williamson, J.R. (1974). Mode of action of the calcium ionophores X-537A and A 23187 on cardiac contractility. *Biochem. Pharmacol.* 23, 1609-1617.

Schroeder, T.E. & Strickland, D.L. (1974). Ionophore A 23187, calcium and contractility in frog eggs. *Exp. Cell Res.* 83, 139-142.

Schwartz, A., Lewis, R.M., Hanley, H.G., Munson, R.G., Dial, F.D. & Ray, M.V. (1974). Hemodynamic and biochemical effects of a new positive inotropic agent. Antibiotic ionophore Ro 2-2985. *Circ. Res.* 34, 102-111.

Simon, W., Morf, W.E. & Meier, P.Ch. (1973). Specificity for alkali and alkaline earth cations of synthetic and natural organic complexing agents in membranes. *Structure and Bonding* 16, 113-160.

Swamy, V.C., Ticku, M., Triggle, C.R. and Triggle, D.J. (1975). The actions of the ionophores X-537A and A 23187 on smooth muscle. *Can. J. Physiol. Pharmacol.* 53, 1108-1114.

Thoa, N.B., Costa, J.L., Moss, J. & Kopin, I.J. (1974). Mechanism of release of norepinephrine from peripheral adrenergic neurones by the calcium ionophores X-537A and A 23187. *Life Sciences* 14, 1705-1719.

Vargas, O., Miranda, R. & Orrego, F. (1976). Effects of sodium-
    deficient media and of a calcium ionophore (A 23187) on the
    release of [^{3}H]noradrenaline, [^{14}C]-α-aminoisobutyrate and
    [^{3}H]-γ-aminobutyrate from superfused slices of rat neocortex.
    Neuroscience 1, 137-145.

Wong, D.T. (1976). Complexation of ammonium ions by the poly-
    ethermonocarboxylic acid ionophore A 23187. *FEBS Lett.* 71,
    175-177.

RELEASE INDUCED BY ALTERATIONS IN EXTRACELLULAR POTASSIUM AND SODIUM AND BY VERATRIDINE AND SCORPION VENOM

D. M. Paton

I   INTRODUCTION

A number of procedures and drugs cause the release of noradrenaline from adrenergic neurons, possibly as a result of membrane depolarization. These include: increasing the extracellular concentration of potassium $[K]_0$; veratridine; scorpion venom; inhibition of the sodium pump by ouabain or omission of extracellular potassium; and reducing the extracellular concentration of sodium $[Na]_0$. In this chapter, the characteristics of release produced by these procedures will be reviewed. A brief summary is provided at the end of each section.

Only release from tissues with intact vesicular function will be considered. The reason for this is that when vesicular function is impaired by reserpine and monoamine oxidase is inhibited, subsequent exposure to noradrenaline results in accumulation of the amine in the cytoplasm of adrenergic neurons. Under these conditions, the procedures listed above all accelerate the loss of noradrenaline from adrenergic neurons (i.e., cause release from the cytoplasm or extravesicular compartment) by a process that is not dependent on extracellular calcium and is inhibited by drugs that block the neuronal transport of noradrenaline, e.g., cocaine, desipramine. These findings have indicated that, under these conditions, release occurs by means of carrier-mediated transport out of the neuron. This mechanism clearly differs from that operating in tissues with intact vesicular function and will not be considered further here. The topic has been recently reviewed elsewhere (Paton, 1976).

II   RELEASE INDUCED BY POTASSIUM

Numerous studies have demonstrated that increasing the extracellular concentration of potassium, $[K]_0$, causes the release of noradrenaline from both peripheral and central adrenergic neurons. This effect has a threshold concentration for $[K]_0$ of about 15-25 mM and above this threshold release increases linearly with $[K]_0$ (Blaustein, Johnson & Needleman, 1972; Carpenter & Nash, 1976).

Evidence that elevated $[K]_0$ causes membrane depolarization
Increasing $[K]_0$ to 50-160 mM caused a brisk but very short period of firing in sympathetic nerves to the isolated cat heart; the release of noradrenaline was not, however, restricted to this short period of firing (Haeusler, Thoenen, Haefely & Huerlimann,

1968). It was concluded that the release produced by increasing
$[K]_0$ was dependent on sustained depolarization rather than the
production of action potentials.

The voltage-sensitive fluorescent probe, 3,3'-dipentyl 2,2'-oxa-
carbocyanine, has been used to estimate the changes in membrane
potential in rat brain synaptosomes resulting from changes in
$[K]_0$ (Blaustein & Goldring, 1975). When the fluorescence of
synaptosomes was plotted as a function of log $[K]_0$, an approximately linear relationship was observed at concentrations greater
than 10 mM. This effect was not due to changes in $[Cl]_0$ because
similar changes were observed when chloride was replaced by the
impermeant anion, methylsulphate. Rubidium was about as effective as potassium in increasing fluorescence while caesium was
only about one-fourth as effective. These studies provided evidence that there is normally a large potassium gradient across
the plasma membranes of synaptosomes and that synaptosomes are
depolarized when $[K]_0$ is increased.

Evidence for activation of a calcium channel
Potassium-evoked release of noradrenaline from both peripheral
(Kirpekar & Wakade, 1968) and central noradrenergic neurons
(Blaustein et al., 1972) is dependent upon the presence of extracellular calcium. Omission of calcium did not, however, alter
the membrane depolarization produced by increasing $[K]_0$ (Blaustein
& Goldring, 1975). When $[K]_0$ was increased above 15-20 mM, the
rate of calcium uptake in rat brain synaptosomes increased with
maximal stimulation occurring when $[K]_0$ was about 60 mM
(Blaustein, 1975). This effect of potassium on calcium uptake
was quantitatively mimicked by rubidium, but caesium was only
about one-fourth as effective. The Q_{10} for potassium-stimulated
calcium uptake was about 1.4, which the author (Blaustein, 1975)
concluded was compatible with a physical process such as diffusion
through a water-filled pore. In rat brain synaptosomes, exposure
to 50 mM KCl increased the uptake of calcium and sodium; tetrodotoxin reduced the increased uptake of sodium but not that of calcium (Goddard & Robinson, 1976). These results may be interpreted
in terms of a voltage-dependent increase in calcium permeability;
depolarization due to an increase in $[K]_0$ would tend to open membrane channels which are selectively permeable to calcium ions
(Blaustein, 1975).

Additional evidence for a calcium channel has been obtained from
studies of the effects on potassium-evoked release of agents that
block the sodium and potassium channels. Most studies have found
that such release is not inhibited by tetrodotoxin (Blaustein et
al., 1972; Torack & LaValle, 1973). However, tetrodotoxin did
reduce but not abolish, potassium-induced release in rat brain
slices (Taube, Starke & Borowski, 1977). Similarly, tetraethylammonium (Kirpekar, Wakade & Prat, 1976) and 4-aminopyridine
(Paton, Golko & Johns, 1977), agents that block the potassium
channel, failed to abolish potassium-evoked release of noradrenaline.

When $[K]_0$ is increased, release of noradrenaline occurs immediately and the rate of release was maximal initially, progressively declining thereafter (Carpenter & Nash, 1976; Garcia, Kirpekar & Sanchez-Garcia, 1976). It appears unlikely that this results from depletion of the transmitter stores available for release (Garcia *et al*., 1976). These investigators suggested rather that there was an initial activation of calcium channels on exposure to an elevated $[K]_0$ followed by inactivation of these channels. In keeping with this proposal was their observation that when spleens were continuously depolarized by potassium in the absence of extracellular calcium, the subsequent introduction of calcium caused a reduced release of noradrenaline. By contrast, the ability of tyramine to cause release was not reduced.

Potassium-induced release of noradrenaline from adrenergic neurons was inhibited by manganese, cobalt, lanthanum, thulium and by high concentrations of magnesium, and by the calcium antagonist, verapamil (Wakade & Kirpekar, 1974; Paton *et al*.,1977), and these inhibitory effects were observed in the presence of tetrodotoxin and 4-aminopyridine (Paton *et al*., 1977). These findings suggest that these cations and verapamil may inhibit release by preventing the increased calcium uptake resulting from depolarization by potassium, possibly by an action at the level of the calcium channel.

Mechanism of release
Exposure of guinea-pig vasa deferentia to elevated $[K]_0$ caused release of both noradrenaline and dopamine-β-hydroxylase, their ratio being similar to that obtained by nerve stimulation and that found in tissue homogenates (Thoa, Wooten, Axelrod & Kopin, 1975)'. Omission of extracellular calcium abolished the release not only of noradrenaline but also of dopamine-β-hydroxylase by potassium. These findings provided evidence th at the potassium-evoked release of noradrenaline occurs by exocytosis.

The potassium-induced release of noradrenaline was reduced in isolated guinea-pig atria by $10^{-4}M$ cytochalasin B and $10^{-3}M$ colchicine (Sorimachi, Oesch & Thoenen, 1973) and in guinea-pig vasa deferentia by $10^{-3}M$ colchicine (Thoa *et al*., 1975). It is possible, therefore, that neurofilaments and/or neurotubules may be involved in potassium-evoked release of transmitter.

The potassium-induced release of noradrenaline and dopamine in rat hypothalamic synaptosomes was not inhibited by inhibitors of the neuronal uptake of these amines (Mulder, Van Den Berg & Stoof, 1975; Raiteri, del Carmine, Bertollini & Levi, 1977). Since these agents inhibit both the inward and outward carrier-mediated transport of noradrenaline in adrenergic neurons (Paton, 1976), this finding indicates that such release does not involve the neuronal carrier system.

Studies of the metabolic fate of noradrenaline have also provided support for the view that release occurs by exocytosis in rat brain synaptosomes; elevated $[K]_0$ caused the release of noradrenaline with no change in the rate of loss of deaminated metabolites

(Raiteri, Levi & Federico, 1975). Any increase in the level of
free amine in the cytoplasm would result in an increase in deaminated metabolites.

Evidence for presynaptic regulation of potassium-induced release
There has been considerable interest in the possible role of presynaptic receptors in the regulation of release of noradrenaline
by potassium. Since potassium produces a sustained depolarization of nerves, such studies also provide information on how activation of presynaptic receptors may alter the release of noradrenaline or dopamine. The concentration of potassium used in such
studies is important. It has been found, for example, that α-ad-
renoceptor agonists and antagonists modify potassium-induced release in brain cortical slices when $[K]_0$ is 13-26 mM (Dismukes,
de Baer & Mulder, 1977) and 50 mM in perfused rabbit hearts
(Starke & Montel, 1974) but not at higher concentrations.

Evidence has been obtained for inhibitory presynaptic α-adreno-
ceptor, opiate and prostaglandin receptors that modulate the release of noradrenaline from central and peripheral neurons.
α-Adrenoceptor agonists (e.g., oxymetazoline, tramazoline and noradrenaline) reduced and α-adrenoceptor antagonists (e.g., phentolamine, yohimbine) increased potassium-evoked release from perfused
rabbit hearts (Starke & Montel, 1974) and from rat brain slices
(Dismukes & Mulder, 1976; Dismukes et al., 1977; Taube et al.,
1977). Opiate agonists (e.g., morphine, methionine-enkephalin,
fentanyl) reduced the potassium-induced release of noradrenaline
and dopamine in rat brain slices (Taube et al., 1977; Subramanian,
Mitznegg, Sprugel, Domschke, Domschke, Wunsch & Demling, 1977).
The inhibitory effects of opiate antagonists were antagonized by
the opiate antagonist naloxone, but not by the α-adrenoceptor
antagonist, phentolamine (Taube et al., 1977).

There is evidence for muscarinic presynaptic receptors that inhibit potassium-evoked release of noradrenaline in peripheral
neurons, but the evidence for central neurons is conflicting.
Muscarinic agonists (e.g., methacholine, acetylcholine) reduced
release in perfused rabbit hearts (Dubey, Muscholl & Pfeiffer,
1975) and canine saphenous veins (Vanhoutte & Verbeuren, 1976).
Acetylcholine reduced such release in rat cerebellar slices
(Westfall, 1974) but did not alter release in the rat hypothalamus (Taube et al., 1977).

An interesting aspect of such studies has been the demonstration
that presynaptic modulation (i.e., muscarinic, α-adrenoceptor) of
potassium-evoked release of noradrenaline was more marked at lower extracellular concentrations of calcium (Dubey et al., 1975;
Dismukes et al., 1977) suggesting that such modulation of release
may result from reducing calcium uptake.

There is also evidence that the potassium-evoked release of dopamine from rat striatal slices is modulated by presynaptic dopaminergic receptors (Westfall, Besson, Giorguieff & Glowinski,
1976), since the dopaminergic receptor antagonist, fluphenazine,
potentiated the release of dopamine.

Conclusions
Increases in $[K]_0$ above about 20 mM cause release of noradrenaline and dopamine from noradrenergic and dopaminergic neurons.
This apparently results from membrane depolarization and a result-
ant activation of a calcium channel. The entry of calcium then
initiates release of amine by exocytosis. Potassium-evoked release can be modulated by activation of certain presynaptic receptors.

   III   RELEASE INDUCED BY VERATRIDINE AND BY SCORPION VENOM

The alkaloid, veratridine and the venoms of certain scorpions
depolarize cells with a sodium action potential by blocking inactivation of the sodium conductance mechanism; this effect is
prevented by tetrodotoxin (for references see Blaustein, 1975;
Blaustein & Goldring, 1975).

Both veratridine and scorpion venom cause the release of noradrenaline and dopamine from neurons (Blaustein *et al.*, 1972;
Blaustein, 1975; Mulder *et al.*, 1975). This effect was dependent
on extracellular calcium and was inhibited by tetrodotoxin. Both
agents markedly stimulated calcium uptake in synaptosomes, this
effect being prevented by tetrodotoxin (Blaustein, 1975). In
order for veratridine to stimulate calcium uptake, $[Na]_0$ had to
be high and $[Na]_i$ low. Studies using the fluorescent probe,
3,3'-dipentyl 2,2'-oxocarbocyanine have provided evidence that
veratridine depolarizes rat brain synaptosomes (Blaustein &
Goldring, 1975).

In guinea-pig vasa deferentia, veratridine caused the proportional
release of noradrenaline and dopamine-β-hydroxylase, their ratios
being similar to that obtained following nerve stimulation and
exposure to increased $[K]_0$ and that present in tissue homogenates
(Thoa *et al.*, 1975). The veratridine-induced release of both noradrenaline and dopamine-β-hydroxylase was abolished by removal of
extracellular calcium, and greatly reduced by tetrodotoxin or
colchicine.

These studies suggest that both veratridine and scorpion venom
depolarize adrenergic neurons by preventing inactivation of sodium
conductance. Depolarization results in an activation of a calcium
channel. Entry of calcium initiates release of amine by exocytosis.

   IV   RELEASE PRODUCED BY PROCEDURES
         THAT INHIBIT SODIUM PUMPING

Procedures that inhibit sodium pumping (e.g., ouabain, omission
of extracellular potassium) caused the release of noradrenaline
from adrenergic neurons (Gillis & Paton, 1967; Bogdanski & Brodie,
1969), increased the uptake of calcium and sodium in synaptosomes
(Goddard & Robinson, 1976) and appeared to depolarize synaptosomes
(Blaustein, 1975). Inhibition of sodium pumping also causes the

release of acetylcholine from cholinergic neurons (Vizi, 1972; Baker & Crawford, 1975). It is interesting to note that noradrenaline and dopamine increase the activity of the NaK-ATPase in brain, apparently by reversal of divalent cation inhibition of the enzyme (Hexum, 1977).

V   RELEASE PRODUCED BY LOWERING THE
     EXTERNAL SODIUM CONCENTRATION

Numerous studies have demonstrated that a reduction in the external concentration of Na, $[Na]_0$, causes the release of noradrenaline from adrenergic nerves (Bogdanski & Brodie, 1969; Keen & Bogdanski, 1970). The effect on release is dependent on $[Na]_0$; release does not occur when $[Na]_0$ is 75 mM or greater (Bogdanski & Brodie, 1969). Release is observed whether sucrose, choline chloride or lithium chloride are used to substitute for sodium chloride in the medium.

When $[Na]_0$ was severely reduced and replaced by sucrose, lithium or choline, the uptake of calcium in synaptosomes was increased (Blaustein, 1975; Goddard & Robinson, 1976). However, complete replacement of $[Na]_0$ with lithium did not depolarize synaptosomes as judged by fluorescence (Blaustein & Goldring, 1975).

The time course of release induced by a reduction in $[Na]_0$ is quite different from that produced by an increase in $[K]_0$, being more gradual in onset (Nakazato, Onoda & Ohga, 1977). In rat brain slices, substitution of $[Na]_0$ by choline or lithium produced an initial small release of $[^3H]$noradrenaline lasting about 8 min followed by an extremely large release that gradually subsided (Vargas, Miranda & Orrego, 1976). These workers concluded that the initial release represented reduced re-uptake of amine rather than true release while the second major release period was considered to result from a large increase in calcium influx.

Most studies have found that the release produced by a reduction in $[Na]_0$ is calcium-dependent (Bogdanski & Brodie, 1969; Keen & Bogdanski, 1970; Vargas et al., 1976). For example, in rat brain slices, the secondary large release component was abolished when calcium was omitted (Vargas et al., 1976). However, in cat spleen slices, low sodium-induced release was reported to be calcium-independent and was not abolished by the addition of EGTA (Garcia & Kirpekar, 1973). In guinea-pig vasa deferentia, the calcium-dependence of release was influenced by the substitute used for sodium (Nakazato et al., 1977); choline substitution was more calcium dependent than sucrose-substitution. It is interesting to note that, in rat brain slices, prolonged exposure to a solution containing 26 mM $[Na]_0$ with choline-substitution and no extracellular calcium caused a delayed release of noradrenaline, this effect being potentiated by the addition of EGTA (Vargas et al., 1976). The authors concluded that this represented a non-specific increase in membrane permeability.

In those systems which were calcium-dependent, calcium could be replaced by strontium and barium (Keen & Bogdanski, 1970; Vargas *et al.*, 1976). Magnesium has been reported to inhibit release produced by a reduction in $[Na]_0$ (Keen & Bogdanski, 1970) or to have no effect (Garcia & Kirpekar, 1973; Nakazato *et al.*, 1977).

Exposure of cat splenic slices to a sodium-free medium caused release of noradrenaline without a concomitant release of dopamine-β-hydroxylase (Garcia & Kirpekar, 1975). The authors concluded that release did not occur by exocytosis. In synaptosomes, a sodium-free medium caused release of noradrenaline that was partially antagonized by desipramine suggesting that the establishment of an outward downhill sodium gradient facilitated the outward carrier-mediated transport of noradrenaline (Raiteri *et al.*, 1977).

It seems clear from the published studies that a reduction in $[Na]_0$ increases the outward carrier-mediated transport of any noradrenaline present in the cytoplasm and also causes the release of noradrenaline from vesicles. How this latter process occurs is still unknown. It is possible that some of the variable results that have been reported may reflect differences in the methods used (Vargas *et al.*, 1976).

VI   REFERENCES

Baker, P.F. & Crawford, A.C. (1975). A note on the mechanism by which inhibitors of the sodium pump accelerate spontaneous release of transmitter from motor nerve terminals. *J. Physiol.* 247, 209-226.

Blaustein, M.P. (1975). Effects of potassium, veratridine and scorpion venom on calcium accumulation and transmitter release by nerve terminals *in vitro*. *J. Physiol.* 247, 617-655.

Blaustein, M.P. & Goldring, J.M. (1975). Membrane potentials in pinched-off presynaptic nerve terminals monitored with a fluorescent probe: evidence that synaptosomes have potassium diffusion potentials. *J. Physiol.* 247, 589-615.

Blaustein, M.P., Johnson, E.M. Jr. & Needleman, P. (1972). Calcium-dependent norepinephrine release from presynaptic nerve endings *in vitro*. *Proc. Nat. Acad Sci.* [*USA*] 69, 2237-2240.

Bogdanski, D.F. & Brodie, B.B. (1969). The effects of inorganic ions on the storage and uptake of H^3-norepinephrine by rat heart slices. *J. Pharmacol. Exp. Ther.* 165, 181-189.

Carpenter, J.R. & Nash, C.W. (1976). Release of [^3H]noradrenaline from perfused rat hearts by potassium and its modifications by 6-hydroxydopamine and reserpine. *Can. J. Physiol. Pharmacol.* 54, 907-915.

Dismukes, K., De Boer, A.A. & Mulder, A.H. (1977). On the mechanism of alpha-receptor mediated modulation of ^3H-noradrenaline release from slices of rat brain neocortex. *Naunyn-Schmiedeberg's Arch. Pharmacol.* 299, 115-122.

Dismukes, R.K. & Mulder, A.H. (1976). Cyclic AMP and α-receptor-mediated modulation of noradrenaline release from rat brain slices. *Eur. J. Pharmacol*. 39, 383-388.

Dubey, M.P., Muscholl, E. & Pfeiffer, A. (1975). Muscarinic inhibition of potassium-induced noradrenaline release and its dependence on the calcium concentration. *Naunyn-Schmiedeberg's Arch. Pharmacol*. 291, 1-15.

Garcia, A.G. & Kirpekar, S.M. (1973). Release of noradrenaline from the cat spleen by sodium deprivation. *Br. J. Pharmacol*. 47, 729-747.

Garcia, A.G. & Kirpekar, S.M. (1975). On the mechanism of release of norepinephrine from cat spleen slices by sodium deprivation and calcium pretreatment. *J. Pharmacol. Exp. Ther*. 192, 343-350.

Garcia, A.G., Kirpekar, S.M. & Sanchez-Garcia, P. (1976). Release of noradrenaline from the cat spleen by nerve stimulation and potassium. *J. Physiol*. 261, 301-317.

Gillis, C.N. & Paton, D.M. (1967). Cation dependence of sympathetic transmitter retention by slices of rat ventricle. *Br. J. Pharmacol. Chemother*. 29, 309-318.

Goddard, G.A. & Robinson, J.D. (1976). Uptake and release of calcium by rat brain synaptosomes. *Brain Res*. 110, 331-350.

Haeusler, G., Thoenen, H., Haefely, W. & Huerlimann, A. (1968). Electrical events in cardiac adrenergic nerves and noradrenaline release from the heart induced by acetylcholine and KCl. *Naunyn-Schmiedeberg's Arch. Pharmacol. Exp. Path*. 261, 389-411.

Hexum, T.D. (1977). The effect of catecholamines on transport (Na,K) adenosine triphosphatase. *Biochem. Pharmacol*. 26, 1221-1222.

Keen, P.M. & Bogdanski, D.F. (1970). Sodium and calcium ions in uptake and release of norepinephrine by nerve endings. *Am. J. Physiol*. 219, 677-682.

Kirpekar, S.M. & Wakade, A.R. (1968). Release of noradrenaline from the cat spleen by potassium. *J. Physiol*. 194, 595-608.

Kirpekar, S.M., Wakade, A.R. & Prat, J.C. (1976). Effect of tetraethylammonium and barium on the release of noradrenaline from the perfused cat spleen by nerve stimulation and potassium. *Naunyn-Schmiedeberg's Arch. Pharmacol*. 294, 23-29.

Mulder, A.H., Van den Berg & Stoof, J.C. (1975). Calcium-dependent release of radiolabeled catecholamines and serotonin from rat brain synaptosomes in a superfusion system. *Brain Res*. 99, 419-424.

Nakazato, Y., Onoda, Y. & Ohga, A. (1977). Role of calcium in the release of noradrenaline induced by sodium deprivation from the guinea-pig vas deferens. *Pfluger's Arch.* 372, 63-67.

Paton, D.M. (1976). Characteristics of efflux of noradrenaline from adrenergic neurons. In: *The Mechanism of Neuronal and Extraneuronal Transport of Catecholamines* (ed.) D.M. Paton, Raven Press, New York, pp. 155-174.

Paton, D.M., Golko, D.S. & Johns, A. (1977). Characteristics of the calcium channel in peripheral adrenergic neurons. *Proc. Can. Fedn. Biol. Soc.* 20, 166.

Raiteri, M., del Carmine, R., Bertollini, A. & Levi, G. (1977). Effect of desmethylimipramine on the release of [^{3}H]norepinephrine induced by various agents in hypothalamic synaptosomes. *Mol. Pharmacol.* 13, 746-758.

Raiteri, M., Levi, G. & Federico, R. (1975). Stimulus-coupled release of unmetabolized ^{3}H-norepinephrine from rat brain synaptosomes. *Pharmacol. Res. Commun.* 7, 181-187.

Sorimachi, M., Oesch, F. & Thoenen, H. (1973). Effects of colchicine and cytochalasin B on the release of ^{3}H-norepinephrine from guinea-pig atria evoked by high potassium, nicotine and tyramine. *Naunyn-Schmiedeberg's Arch. Pharmacol.* 276, 1-12.

Starke, K. & Montel, H. (1974). Influence of drugs with affinity for α-adrenoceptors on noradrenaline release by potassium, tyramine and dimethylphenylpiperazinium. *Eur. J. Pharmacol.* 27, 273-280.

Subramanian, N., Mitznegg, P., Sprugel, W., Domschke, W., Domschke, S., Wunsch, E. & Demling, L. (1977). Influence of enkephalin on K$^+$-evoked efflux of putative neurotransmitters in rat brain. *Naunyn-Schmiedeberg's Arch. Pharmacol.* 299, 163-165.

Taube, H.D., Starke, K. & Borowski, E. (1977). Presynaptic receptor systems on the noradrenergic neurones of rat brain. *Naunyn-Schmiedeberg's Arch. Pharmacol.* 299, 123-141.

Thoa, N.B., Wooten, G.F., Axelrod, J. & Kopin, I.J. (1975). On the mechanism of release of norepinephrine from sympathetic nerves induced by depolarizing agents and sympathomimetic drugs. *Mol. Pharmacol.* 11, 10-18.

Torack, R.M. & LaValle, M. (1973). The role of norepinephrine in the function of the area postrema. II. *In vitro* incubation and stimulated release of tritiated norepinephrine. *Brain Res.* 61, 253-265.

Vanhoutte, P.M. & Verbeuren, T.J. (1976). Inhibition by acetylcholine of the norepinephrine release evoked by potassium in canine saphenous veins. *Circ. Res.* 39, 263-269.

Vargas, O., Miranda, R. & Orrego, F. (1976). Effects of sodium-
    deficient media and of a calcium ionophore (A-23187) on the
    release of (^{3}H)-noradrenaline, (^{14}C)-α-aminoisobutyrate, and
    (^{3}H)-γ-aminobutyrate from superfused slices of rat neocortex.
    Neuroscience 1, 137-145.

Vizi, E.S. (1972). Stimulation by inhibition of (Na$^+$ - K$^+$ - Mg^{2+})
    -activated ATPase of acetylcholine release in cortical slices
    from rat brain. *J. Physiol.* 226, 95-117.

Wakade, A.R. & Kirpekar, S.M. (1974). Calcium-independent re-
    lease of ^{3}H-norepinephrine from reserpine-pretreated guinea-
    pig vas deferens and seminal vesicle. *J. Pharmacol. Exp. Ther.*
    190, 451-458.

Westfall, T.C. (1974). Effect of muscarinic agonists on the re-
    lease of ^{3}H-norepinephrine and ^{3}H-dopamine by potassium and
    electrical stimulation from rat brain slices. *Life Sci.* 14,
    1641-1652.

Westfall, T.C., Besson, M.-J., Giorguieff, M.-F. & Glowinski, J.
    (1976). The role of presynaptic receptors in the release and
    synthesis of ^{3}H-dopamine by slices of rat striatum. *Naunyn-
    Schmiedeberg's Arch. Pharmacol.* 292, 279-287.

RELEASE INDUCED BY
PHENETHYLAMINES

U. Trendelenburg

I   INTRODUCTION

Six years ago a review dealing with the noradrenaline-releasing
action of certain phenetylamines was titled "Classification of
Sympathomimetic Amines" (Trendelenburg, 1972) and dealt with all
the factors which determine whether a sympathomimetic amine acts
directly on the alpha- and beta-adrenoceptors or rather releases
noradrenaline from adrenergic nerve endings, an effect that is
often or always subject to tachyphylaxis. No doubt, a very careful
sifting of the experimental evidence published since then would
enable one to complement the old review and to present a long list
of predominantly minor corrections. However, the major points
that are being discussed presently have barely been touched upon
in that review. It is the aim of the present review to discuss
these points. There are two questions of major importance: a)
Is the efflux of noradrenaline from the adrenergic nerve ending
carrier-mediated? b) Is noradrenaline bound to extravesicular
binding sites? The reader will notice that both questions deal
with the physiology of the adrenergic nerve ending rather than
primarily with the mode of action of phenethylamines. However, it
is necessary to critically discuss these points here, since phenethylamines presently are very important tools used in experiments
dealing with these two questions.

The reader will find this review rather critical. The main reason
for presenting a predominantly critical review lies in the fact
that we have reached a stage in this field of research, where we
are able to refine our questions to a considerable degree, although
the state of the art is such that there is very little evidence
available that can be interpreted in one way only. While there is
good justification for such a critical approach, it should be
emphasized that the aim of this review is not negative in the sense
that its author takes pleasure in demonstrating "errors" or "faults"
in the work of others. The reader would misunderstand the aim of
the review, if such an impression were to arise. On the contrary,
the discerning reader should detect that the author is not only
fascinated by the complexities of the adrenergic nerve ending, but
actually convinced that the next few years will bring the answers
that this review cannot yet provide. Such optimism is justified,
since the kinetic methods introduced into this field by a number
of different people will in all probability eventually yield the
desired results. Moreover, correct answers will be obtained the
earlier, the sooner the complexities of the adrenergic nerve
endings are fully understood (and taken into consideration when

experiments are designed).

It is not surprising that kinetic experiments performed some 5 or
10 years ago often failed to take into consideration certain complexities of adrenergic nerve endings that were then not known
(or the importance of which had not yet been fully realized). In
spite of some critical analysis of such earlier experiments, it
should be emphasized that we owe a great debt to those who introduced kinetic analysis into this field.

There has not been any reason to revise the established view that,
in normal preparations, phenythylamines with an indirect sympathomimetic action are able to enter not only the adrenergic nerve
ending but also the storage vesicles, that they are able to
increase the efflux of noradrenaline from the vesicles into the
axoplasma, and that the axoplasmatic noradrenaline then leaves
the nerve ending to exert its effect at the adrenoceptors. Since
noradrenaline is a rather polar compound which does not easily
penetrate cell membranes, it is of considerable interest to find
out how free axoplasmatic noradrenaline is able to leave the nerve
ending so quickly that there is a nearly instantaneous response
of the effector organ to such indirectly acting amines. In
experiments designed to study this question, it is desirable to
simplify the system as much as possible. Hence, most studies
dealing with the mechanism responsible for neuronal efflux of noradrenaline are carried out after pretreatment of the animal with
reserpine (to exclude vesicularly stored noradrenaline) and often
also after inhibition of intraneuronal monoamine oxidase (MAO) or
(for safety's sake) of MAO and catechol-O-methyl transferase
(COMT). However, it should be realized that such studies deal
with artificial systems which bear little resemblance to the nerve
endings of a "normal" preparation, such as for instance the nictitating membrane of an untreated cat which is injected with tyramine. In such a normal system most of the endogenous noradrenaline is stored in the vesicles; since MAO is intact, the chance
for free axoplasmatic noradrenaline to survive for any length of
time is very low. Moreover, even if there existed extravesicular
binding sites (see below for discussion), it is unlikely that any
substantial extravesicular binding of endogenous noradrenaline can
take place when vesicular uptake and MAO are intact. Therefore,
it is likely that indirect sympathomimetic effects exerted on such
"normal" tissues are mainly due to the release of the transmitter
from storage vesicles.

When, on the other hand, experiments are performed with the simplified systems mentioned above, and when adrenergic nerve endings
are loaded with labelled noradrenaline (after pretreatment with
reserpine and after inhibition of MAO), very high concentrations
of free axoplasmic noradrenaline can be reached; if extravesicular
binding sites exist, binding of noradrenaline might then be quite
pronounced. However, even if we were able to demonstrate the
existence of such extravesicular binding sites as well as an
ability of tyramine to accelerate the net dissociation of noradrenaline from the binding sites, it would be false to conclude that
this represents the mode of action of tyramine in the "normal"

nictitating membrane alluded to above.

II   IS AMINE EFFLUX CARRIER-MEDIATED?

When we disregard exocytosis as a mechanism of release of noradrenaline, two mechanisms may be responsible for any efflux of noradrenaline (or related amines) from the adrenergic nerve ending
into the extracellular space: an outward transport of the amine
by a carrier mechanism (either by the same carrier that is responsible for the inward transport or by a different carrier) and
passive diffusion (in the following to be called a "leak"). The
evidence for or against these two possibilities will be discussed.
For this discussion it is important to stress that the efflux of
noradrenaline elicited by indirectly acting sympathomimetic amines
involves the existence of a normal sodium gradient. As discussed
by Paton (this volume), any reduction or reversal of the sodium
gradient (by lowering of the external sodium concentration, by
ouabain, by prolonged depolarization, or by certain metabolic
inhibitors) elicits an efflux of noradrenaline from the nerve ending. In this context it is important to realize that the neuronal
carrier is sodium-sensitive insofar as sodium either decreases the
Km of the carrier for noradrenaline or increases the Vmax of the
carrier (for discussion, see White, 1976). According to the model
proposed by Bogdanski (Bogdanski, Tissari & Brodie, 1968, 1970;
Bogdanski & Brodie, 1969) the carrier has a very low Km when
exposed to the extracellular fluid (which contains a high concentration of sodium), while the Km is high on the inside of the
cell membrane (where the sodium concentration is very low).
According to this model, any increase in the internal sodium concentration (such as brought about by the experimental procedures
enumerated above) would greatly reduce the normally high Km of the
carrier for the <u>outward</u> transport of noradrenaline.

Such considerations lead to the conclusion that any evidence indicating that amine efflux is carrier-mediated when the internal
sodium concentration is increased, does not necessarily prove that
amine efflux is also carrier-mediated when the sodium gradient is
normal.

Evidence for a carrier-mediated efflux of a solute can be obtained
by the observation of any of the following phenomena:

A.   Saturability of Efflux

Whenever the efflux of phenethylamines from adrenergic nerve endings has been studied, saturability of efflux was not observed.
For instance, efflux curves (obtained with isolated organs first
loaded with labelled amine and then washed out with amine-free
solution) have always been found to be multiphasic exponential;
they never have exhibited a convex shape. This absence of any
convexity in efflux is worth emphasizing, since convex curves
(indicating the involvement of a saturable process) have indeed
been observed for the efflux of O-methylated catecholamines from
the rat heart (Uhlig, Bönisch and Trendelenburg, 1974, for

isoprenaline; Mekanontchai & Trendelenburg, unpublished observations, for noradrenaline); however, in this case the metabolizing enzyme, COMT, was found to be saturable, not the mechanism responsible for efflux. Moreover, no saturability of the efflux of [^{3}H]noradrenaline was observed when the degree of initial filling of the neurone with the amine was varied over a wide range (Henseling, Eckert & Trendelenburg, 1976a).

These negative results cannot be taken as evidence that efflux is not carrier-mediated (i.e., that it occurs through passive diffusion out of the nerve ending, i.e., through a "leak"). Since it is quite possible that the Km for carrier-mediated efflux is much higher than the Km for carrier-mediated inflow (uptake), our failure to observe saturability of the efflux of noradrenaline would be compatible with the view that efflux is mediated by a carrier characterized by a very high Km.

If it is correct that any increase in the internal sodium concentration greatly decreases the Km for carrier-mediated efflux, it can be predicted that the demonstration of saturability of carrier-mediated efflux should be much easier when the internal sodium concentration is increased than when it is normal. However, even such positive evidence would not prove conclusively that efflux is carrier-mediated when the internal sodium concentration is normal. This may be so, because efflux of noradrenaline from nerve endings may well be both carrier-mediated and due to a "leak"; in that case, efflux might be predominantly carrier-mediated when the internal sodium concentration is increased, but mainly due to a "leak" when it is normal.

B.   The Preloading Effect

In systems in which a carrier transports the solute in both directions and in which there is no accumulation of the solute above a tissue/medium ratio of 1, the phenomenon of "countertransport" has been observed: an uphill transport of the "driven" substrate takes place when there is a downhill transport of the "driving" substrate (Rosenberg & Wilbrandt, 1957; Wilbrandt & Rosenberg, 1961; Heinz & Walsh, 1958). Such considerations may be applicable to the adrenergic nerve ending, though it is able to concentrate the amine. For instance, the initial rate of uptake of any amine that is transported by the neuronal carrier in both directions might be accelerated after "preloading" of the adrenergic nerve endings with the same or another amine.

In experiments with perfused hearts of reserpine-pretreated rabbits, Bönisch (unpublished observations) tried to obtain evidence for countertransport. The hearts were first loaded with amine by perfusion of the hearts with a high concentration of unlabelled metaraminol (3 μM). Soon after this initial loading (which aimed at achieving a high concentration of free amine in the axoplasm) the initial rate of neuronal uptake of [^{3}H]metaraminol was determined for a low concentration (0.03 μM) of the amine (by measuring arterio-venous differences for [^{3}H]metaraminol from the 2nd to the 10th min of perfusion, and by extrapolation to zero time). If countertransport were to exist, the initial rate of neuronal uptake of the labelled amine should have been higher after the preloading than in control hearts which were not pre-loaded. No indication for any acceleration of initial uptake was obtained. It is very unlikely that extraneuronal uptake interfered in these experiments, since the extraneuronal uptake system is very poorly developed in the rabbit heart (Graefe, Bönisch, Fiebig & Trendelenburg, 1975; Graefe, Bönisch & Keller, 1978).

Although such negative findings do not prove the absence of carrier-mediated efflux of metaraminol, the experiments clearly failed to provide any evidence for the existence of carrier-mediated efflux from adrenergic nerve endings.

C. Accelerated Exchange Diffusion

Whenever a carrier is responsible for inward and outward movement of a solute, the phenomenon of "accelerated (or facilitated) exchange diffusion" may be observed (Stein, 1967). For this phenomenon to occur, a one-compartmental system is needed which is filled with an amine. As soon as the same (or another) amine is offered to the outside, the carrier-mediated inward (i.e., uphill) movement of the driving amine increases the unidirectional outward movement of the driven amine (i.e., the downhill movement is accelerated). Any conclusion that an experimental observation represents accelerated exchange diffusion is justified only if two conditions are met: a) the "driving" (or releasing) amine must be transported by the carrier responsible for the transport of the driven amine; and b) the system must be a one-compartmental one. If condition a) is not met, the phenomenon cannot represent accelerated exchange diffusion, and if condition b) is not met, there are alternative explanations.

While there is general agreement that phenethylamines of low lipid solubility require a carrier for uptake into the adrenergic nerve ending, there is justifiable doubt whether this applies to phen-ethylamines with high lipid solubility (i.e., to amphetamine and related amines). This problem will be further discussed in section II D.

In order to obtain the required "one-compartmental system", Paton (1973, 1976) used isolated atria obtained from reserpine-pretreated rabbits (so as to avoid any vesicular distribution of [3H]nor-adrenaline). Moreover, both noradrenaline-metabolizing enzymes were inhibited. The atria were loaded with [3H]noradrenaline and subsequently washed with amine-free solution until the efflux of total radioactivity became monophasic exponential (i.e., until the fractional rate of loss or the rate coefficient for efflux became constant).   The addition of any of a large number of phenethylamines to the wash out solution (including those of either low or high lipid solubility) then elicited an efflux of radioactivity.

The validity of the conclusion that this elicited efflux of total radioactivity represents accelerated exchange diffusion stands

and falls with the assumption that the neurone represents a one-
compartmental system. While it is very likely that the pretreatment with reserpine prevented any substantial vesicular distribution of [^{3}H]noradrenaline, we cannot - at the present time - be
certain that there are no extravesicular binding sites for [^{3}H]
noradrenaline for which the various phenethylamines might compete.
In fact, some evidence in favour of the existence of such extravesicular binding sites will be presented below (see section III).

It might well be argued that the existence of a second compartment
was already excluded by the fact that the observations were made
when the fractional rate of loss of radioactivity was constant.
However, although this is indicative of the fact that there is
only one factor limiting the rate of efflux, it does not necessarily prove the system to be one-compartmental. There are at
least two two-compartmental systems which can generate an efflux
characterized by a constant fractional rate of loss of radioactivity: a) the two compartments ("free" amine and amine "bound
to extravesicular binding sites") are arranged in series, and the
rate limiting step for the efflux from the neurone is located in
the cell membrane (i.e., is associated with the carrier); or b)
the two compartments are arranged in the same way, but the rate
constant for net efflux from the neurone is so much higher than
that for the net dissociation of the amine from extravesicular
binding sites, that the rapid efflux of "free" amine coincides
with the rapid efflux from extraneuronal compartments. In this
case, the so-called "late" or "neuronal" efflux of radioactivity
(Paton, 1973; Henseling *et al.*, 1976a) does not represent the
total neuronal efflux (since most of the "free" amine has left
the neurone much earlier). Moreover, the apparent half time for
this late efflux would then reflect the net dissociation of the
amine from extravesicular binding sites. Both hypothetical models
represent two-compartmental systems which generate a late efflux
that is characterized by a constant fractional rate of loss of
radioactivity.

Moreover, it should be realized that in the experiments of Paton
(1973, 1976) the efflux of total radioactivity was measured, not
the efflux of [^{3}H]noradrenaline. At this time it was justified
to assume that inhibition of MAO should suffice to exclude the
intraneuronal deamination of noradrenaline as a major source of
error. However, in the meantime new evidence has been obtained
that suggests that incomplete inhibition of neuronal MAO may
result in a considerable error.

When the MAO of rabbit aortic strips was inhibited by an exposure
of the strips to 0.5 mM pargyline for 30 min, the formation of
deaminated metabolites (during 30 min of exposure to 1.2 μM
[^{3}H]noradrenaline) was reduced by about 90% (Henseling &
Trendelenburg, 1978). In spite of this apparent 90% inhibition
of MAO, nearly half the neuronal efflux of radioactivity (determined in aortic strips first loaded with [^{3}H]noradrenaline as
described above, and then washed with amine-free solution for
240 min) consisted of deaminated metabolites (Eckert, Henseling,
Gescher & Trendelenburg, 1976a).   This striking

discrepancy between "apparent inhibition of MAO" and the high rate of neuronal efflux of deaminated metabolites is probably explained by the following consideration. The efflux of noradrenaline from the nerve ending has a long half time, partly because a substantial proportion of the efflux of amine is subject to re-uptake. The metabolites, on the other hand, are not subject to re-uptake; hence they represent a high percentage of the late neuronal net efflux of total radioactivity.

Under these conditions the fractional rate of loss of total radio-activity is determined more by the slow metabolic degradation of the amine by the intracellular enzyme than by the rate constant for the efflux of noradrenaline. Or in other words, under such conditions the fractional rate of loss of total activity must be substantially higher than the rate constant (k) for the efflux of the amine.

Although there is no evidence to indicate that the late neuronal efflux determined by Paton (1973) contained or did not contain deaminated metabolites, it is worth emphasizing that an unexpect-edly high contribution by deaminated metabolites to the late neuronal efflux does not seem to be restricted to rabbit aortic strips. When Graefe, Stefano and Langer (1977) determined the late neuronal efflux of total radioactivity from rat vasa deferentia previously loaded with [^{3}H]noradrenaline (MAO inhibited by pargyline as described above, but no pretreatment with reser-pine), deaminated metabolites accounted for 25% of total radio-activity. Recent experiments (Fuchs & Graefe, unpublished obser-vations) indicated that this percentage increases to 80% after pretreatment of the animals with reserpine. Eckert *et al.*, (1976a) also found pretreatment with reserpine to increase the percentage contribution by deaminated metabolites to the late efflux of total radioactivity (rabbit aortic strips).

These recent observations make it obvious that the neuronal efflux of total radioactivity should be analysed for the presence of deaminated metabolites even when inhibitors of MAO had been employed. Indeed, such measurements might help to solve the pro-blem, since evidence against accelerated exchange diffusion is obtained as soon as the addition of phenethylamines to the wash out solution is found to increase not only the efflux of total radioactivity but also that of labelled deaminated metabolites. Such evidence would be indicative of an increase of the concen-tration of free axoplasmic noradrenaline (in response to the administration of phenethylamines). Unfortunately, the absence of such an increase in the efflux of labelled deaminated metabo-lites cannot be taken as conclusive evidence for the existence of accelerated exchange diffusion, since agents which inhibit the neuronal uptake of noradrenaline (such as cocaine, desipramine or the phenethylamines) are known to reduce the efflux of deaminated metabolites of labelled noradrenaline; this is so, because a con-siderable proportion of intraneuronal deamination (observed in reserpine-pretreated preparations) takes place after the re-uptake of noradrenaline that had already left the nerve ending. Or stated in kinetic terms: re-uptake of noradrenaline results in a rate

constant for the net efflux of this amine that is much lower than
the rate constant for the unidirectional efflux of noradrenaline.
Thus, re-uptake keeps the concentration of free axoplasmic noradrenaline high (Graefe *et al.*, 1977).

It should be added that phenethylamines are not only able to accelerate the neuronal efflux of other phenethylamines, but also that
of other agents that are a) substrates of the cocaine-sensitive
neuronal uptake mechanism, and b) accumulated in the axoplasm.
This has been studied in some detail for bretylium. There is good
evidence to indicate that bretylium is transported into the adrenergic nerve ending by the cocaine-sensitive uptake mechanism
(Ross & Gosztonyi, 1975) and that the efflux of bretylium from the
neurone is accelerated by amphetamine (Ross & Kelder, 1976).
However, as far as the interpretation of these results is concerned,
we face the same problems (as discussed above) in deciding whether
this represents accelerated exchange diffusion or is due to competition for extravesicular binding sites.

D.   Inhibition of Efflux by Inhibitors of Uptake

Provided an inhibitor of carrier-mediated uptake is not transported itself, such an agent should inhibit carrier-mediated
efflux as well (Stein, 1967) by arresting the carrier at the outside of the cell membrane. It is important to realize that only
non-transported inhibitors can exert this effect since inhibitors
which are transported themselves should accelerate efflux (see
preceding section). Unfortunately, it remains unknown whether or
not agents like cocaine or desipramine are transported by the
carrier into the adrenergic nerve ending. However, this is
unlikely, if we accept the theory of Häusler, Haefely and
Hürlimann (1969), according to which adrenergic neurone blocking
agents must have two properties: They must be transported into
the adrenergic neurone by the same mechanism that also transports
noradrenaline (so that they are accumulated in the nerve ending),
and they must have a local anesthetic effect (which becomes manifest only where they are accumulated, i.e., in adrenergic nerve
endings). If cocaine were actively transported into the adrenergic nerve endings, it should be a highly potent adrenergic neurone blocker, since it is a potent local anesthetic agent.
However, an adrenergic neurone blocking effect of cocaine has not
been reported.

There is a second reason why it would be interesting to determine
whether inhibitors of neuronal uptake are also inhibitors of
neuronal efflux: For the extraneuronal system it is well known
that inhibitors of uptake (corticosteroids and phenoxybenzamine;
Iversen & Salt, 1970; Iversen, Salt & Wilson, 1972) inhibit also
the efflux of catecholamines (Bönisch, Uhlig & Trendelenburg,
1974; Uhlig *et al.*, 1974; Eckert, Henseling & Trendelenburg,
1976b).

When the effect of cocaine (or desipramine) on the neuronal efflux
is considered, two facts tend to greatly complicate the analysis.
Firstly, as already mentioned above, there is a great likelihood
that a considerable proportion of the neuronal noradrenaline that

leaves the nerve ending is available for re-uptake. Hence, if
efflux is carrier-mediated, cocaine can be expected to have two
opposite effects: If it is not transported by the carrier, it
should decrease the efflux of noradrenaline by immobilizing the
carrier at the outside of the cell membrane, while it should
increase efflux by inhibiting re-uptake. The experimental observations are contradictory. While Lindmar and Löffelholz (1974,
perfused rabbit heart), Henseling, Eckert and Trendelenburg
(1976b; rabbit aortic strips) and Graefe *et al*. (1977, rat vas
deferens) found desipramine and cocaine to accelerate the late
neuronal efflux of noradrenaline (i.e., to reduce the half time
for efflux), Raiteri, Levi and Federico (1974) observed a significant slowing of the efflux of total radioactivity in the presence of cocaine. In these latter experiments a "superfused
synaptosomal preparation" (obtained from the brain of rats) was
used to minimize re-uptake of the [^{3}H]noradrenaline with which
the synaptosomes were preloaded. This conflict of evidence might
be explained by the assumption that neuronal efflux of noradrenaline is both carrier-mediated <u>and</u> due to a leak. In that case,
the experimental conditions <u>might</u> determine whether the inhibition
of re-uptake or that of carrier-mediated efflux predominates
(cocaine resulting in either an acceleration or a slowing of
efflux), especially if one entertains the possibility that the
contribution by each of the two mechanisms of efflux varies with
the height of the concentration of "free" noradrenaline in the
axoplasm. For instance, it is quite conceivable that carrier-
mediated efflux predominates at low, and efflux by "leakage" at
high internal concentrations of free noradrenaline (if, for
instance, carrier-mediated efflux were saturable).

A second complication arises whenever intraneuronal MAO is either
intact or incompletely inhibited. As pointed out in the preceding
section, an incomplete inhibition of MAO appears to go hand in
hand with the appearance of considerable amounts of deaminated
metabolites in the efflux. This surprisingly large degree of
intraneuronal deamination (observed when MAO is largely but not
completely inhibited) is at least partly due to re-uptake, since
the addition of cocaine to the wash out solution reduces the
efflux of deaminated metabolites (Eckert *et al*., 1976a). This
effect is also seen when MAO is intact. For instance, Graefe
et al. (1977) found the neuronal efflux of radioactivity from
normal rat vasa deferentia (no pretreatment with reserpine, no
enzyme inhibition; late neuronal efflux after initial loading with
[^{3}H]noradrenaline) to consist of 10% of noradrenaline and of 90%
of predominantly deaminated metabolites. On the addition of
cocaine to the wash out solution, the fractional rate of efflux
of total radioactivity neither increased nor decreased; however,
the percentage contribution by noradrenaline was greatly increased,
while that by the deaminated metabolites was correspondingly
decreased. Thus, an apparent lack of effect of cocaine on the
neuronal efflux of total radioactivity does not necessarily prove
that cocaine fails to affect the efflux of noradrenaline. It is
of interest to note that when the MAO of the rat vas deferens is
inhibited (Graefe *et al*., 1977; experiments with [^{3}H]noradrena-
line) or not able to metabolize the amine (Graefe, Stefano &

Langer, 1973; experiments with [^{3}H]metaraminol), cocaine clearly
increases the efflux of both, total radioactivity and noradrenaline.

In the experiments of Paton (1973; rabbit atria, reserpine pretreatment, COMT and MAO inhibited; neuronal efflux after initial
loading with [^{3}H]noradrenaline) cocaine failed to cause any pronounced change in the fractional rate of loss of radioactivity
from nerve endings. Since the degree of deamination of noradrenaline by the possibly not completely inhibited MAO was not determined in these experiments, the lack of effect of cocaine on the
efflux of total radioactivity does not exclude the possibility
that it increased the rate of efflux of unchanged amine (while
decreasing that of the deaminated metabolites). Consequently,
the absence of any apparent effect of cocaine on the efflux of
total radioactivity cannot be interpreted as evidence against re-
uptake of the amine (in the absence of cocaine).

Quite apart from the question whether cocaine accelerates or slows
the "spontaneous" efflux of noradrenaline from adrenergic nerve
endings, cocaine has a separate effect on the efflux of noradrenaline induced by phenethylamines. As demonstrated by Paton (1973;
rabbit atria preloaded with [^{3}H]noradrenaline), by Raiteri, del
Carmine and Bartolini (1977; superfused synaptosomal preparation
preloaded with [^{3}H]noradrenaline) and by Ross and Kelder (1976;
rat vas deferens preloaded with [^{3}H]bretylium), cocaine (or
desipramine) is able to prevent the increase in efflux of radioactivity induced by phenethylamines.

First, one should consider the efflux-increasing effect of those
indirectly acting amines which have a very low lipid solubility
and which are dependent on carrier-mediated uptake (e.g., tyramine). If the system under study is a one-compartmental one, the
results of such studies would be consistent with accelerated
exchange diffusion. However, if the system is a two-compartmental
one (i.e., if there are extravesicular binding sites for noradrenaline), the chain of events might be the following: After carrier-
mediated uptake into the nerve ending, the indirectly acting amine
might compete with the labelled noradrenaline for extravesicular
binding sites; the consequent increase in free axoplasmic noradrenaline then promotes an efflux from the nerve ending (either via the
carrier or via a leak). The inhibitory effect of cocaine (or
desipramine) can be elicited at either one of two possible sites
of action: It can prevent the neuronal uptake of the indirectly
acting amine or it can prevent the efflux of noradrenaline by
immobilization of the carrier (if efflux is carrier-mediated).

However, if the indirectly acting amine possesses high lipid
solubility (e.g., amphetamine and related amines), the amine may
well enter the neurone without the help of the carrier-mechanism.
Since cocaine is able to abolish the increase in the efflux of
noradrenaline induced by amphetamine or beta-phenethylamine
(Paton, 1973; Raiteri et al., 1977) as well as the increase in
efflux of [^{3}H]bretylium elicited by amphetamine (Ross & Kelder,
1976), it might be argued that a) only one site of action is
available for the effect of cocaine, and b) hence, that efflux

of [^{3}H]noradrenaline or [^{3}H]bretylium was carrier-mediated.

Unfortunately, this argument stands and falls with the evidence
that the highly lipid soluble phenethylamines are not subject to
carrier-mediated uptake into nerve endings. There is no doubt
that all attempts to detect a cocaine- or desipramine-sensitive
uptake of highly lipid soluble phenethylamines (e.g., amphetamine,
ephedrine, phenylpropanolamine etc.) have failed (Ross & Renyi,
1966a and b; Ross, Renyi & Brunfelter, 1968; Thoenen, Hürlimann &
Haefely, 1968; Brodie, Costa, Groppetti & Matsumoto, 1968; Jacquot,
Bralet, Cohen & Valette, 1969; Golko & Paton, 1976). Nevertheless,
this does not constitute conclusive evidence against carrier-
mediated neuronal uptake of such amines. For ephedrine, for
instance, Golko and Paton (1976) showed that its accumulation in
rabbit atria was not saturable and largely unaffected by either
cocaine or desipramine or lack of external sodium. The authors
suggested that the uptake of ephedrine occurred largely as a
result of passive diffusion into all cells, followed by extraneuronal binding (since steady-state tissue/medium ratios clearly
exceeded unity). It should be realized that the large distribution volume (i.e., the ability of highly lipid soluble phenethylamines to penetrate into all cells of the tissue) as well as the
postulated intracellular binding of such amines must make it very
difficult to determine whether or not there is carrier-mediated
neuronal uptake of the amines. If, for the sake of the argument,
the volume of the adrenergic nerve endings is assumed to amount
to 0.1% of the total tissue, and if we further simplify the
system by neglecting extraneuronal binding, then a considerable
accumulation of such an amine in nerve endings (as a result of
carrier-mediated uptake) would increase the tissue/medium ratio
from 1.00 (postulated for passive diffusion only) to 1.01 (for
passive diffusion plus 10-fold accumulation in adrenergic nerve
endings) or to 1.10 (for passive diffusion plus 100-fold accumulation in adrenergic nerve endings). If extraneuronal binding
takes place to result in a tissue/medium ratio of 3.00 (for
passive diffusion only), the corresponding "expected" tissue
medium ratios are 3.01 and 3.10. Or in other words, it would be
exceedingly difficult to prove the existence of a very considerable
accumulation of these amines in nerve endings, especially when
rather long exposures to highly lipid soluble amines are considered. Chances for the detection of carrier-mediated uptake of
such amines might be increased if initial rates of uptake were
measured with very short exposures to the amines. Unfortunately,
most of the studies quoted above were carried out many years ago,
i.e., at a time when the importance of determinations of initial
rates of uptake had not been fully realized. Thus, although the
problem might be experimentally accessible (since we now have
methods for exact determinations of initial rates of uptake during
exposures lasting for not more than 1 min; Graefe et al., 1978),
we remain in doubt whether or not the highly lipid soluble phenethylamines are subject to carrier-mediated neuronal uptake. It
should perhaps be emphasized that experiments involving very short
exposures to such amines are highly relevant to the problems discussed here, since the onset of the indirect sympathomimetic
effect of amphetamine-like amines is very quick indeed.

A second aspect of this problem should be mentioned. If it is true that amphetamine-like amines are not transported by the nor-adrenaline uptake mechanism, they should behave like "non-transport inhibitors", since their ability to inhibit the neuronal uptake of noradrenaline is well established (Iversen, 1967). Thus, amphetamine should be cocaine-like in its effect on efflux (acceleration by inhibition of re-uptake plus slowing by inhibition of efflux of noradrenaline), and it should be quite unable to elicit the phenomenon of "accelerated exchange diffusion". In Paton's experiments (1973), for instance, cocaine failed to affect the neuronal efflux of total radioactivity (rabbit atria, pretreatment with reserpine, both enzymes inhibited), while amphetamine greatly increased it. Such results are clearly not consistent with the view that the effects of amphetamine are "cocaine-like". Hence, it appears justified to continue to consider the possibliity that amphetamine-like amines are subject to carrier-mediated uptake into adrenergic nerve endings.

    E.   The Half Time for the Approach to Steady-State Filling

According to Stein (1967), the following predictions can be made for one-compartmental systems into which the amine is transported by a carrier.

(a) If the carrier is responsible for inward and outward transport (i.e., when we have a "pump and pump system"), one should see the following when this system is exposed to various concentrations of the amine: With increasing concentrations of the amine the tissue/medium ratio attained at steady state should remain constant, while the half time required for the approach to steady state should increase.

(b) If the inward movement is carrier-mediated, while the outward movement is due to passive diffusion (i.e., when we have a "pump and leak system"), the half time for the approach to steady state should be independent of the concentration of the amine, while the tissue/medium ratio should decline with increasing concentrations.

After pretreatment of the animals with reserpine and after inhibition of both noradrenaline-metabolizing enzymes, Bönisch and Graefe (1976; unpublished results) determined tissue/medium ratios and half times for the approach to steady state in rabbit hearts perfused with various concentrations of [^{3}H]noradrenaline or [^{3}H]-metaraminol. The experimental results agreed with neither of the predictions: With increasing concentrations of the amines both the tissue/medium ratio and the half time for the approach to steady state declined. Thus, the results failed to support the view that the adrenergic nerve endings of reserpine-pretreated preparations (whose MAO and COMT had been inhibited) represented a one-compartmental system. Indeed, the results indicate that there are at least two compartments (for further discussion, see section III).

F.   The Temperature-dependence of Neuronal Efflux

The Q_{10} for neuronal efflux should be greater for carrier-mediated efflux than for efflux through passive diffusion. Lindmar and Löffelholz (1972) obtained a Q_{10} of about 5 for the neuronal efflux of noradrenaline from perfused rabbit hearts (after pre-treatment with reserpine, after inhibition of MAO, after initial loading with noradrenaline), i.e., neuronal efflux was highly temperature-dependent. Paton (1973) obtained a somewhat lower Q_{10} for neuronal efflux (2.5-3.0; rabbit atria, after pretreatment with reserpine, both enzymes inhibited; initial loading with [^{3}H] noradrenaline).

Both Q_{10}-values may well be interpreted as not being in favour of passive diffusion. However, since we cannot be certain that the systems under study represent one-compartmental systems (see section IIC and III), either carrier-mediated efflux or dissocia-tion from extravesicular binding sites may represent the highly temperature-sensitive mechanism. Thus, until we know whether the system under study is one- or two-compartmental, the observed high degree of temperature-dependence remains uninterpretable.

III   ARE THERE EXTRAVESICULAR BINDING SITES FOR NORADRENALINE?

In an attempt to explain the adrenergic neurone blocking effect of agents like guanethidine as well as the fact that indirectly acting sympathomimetic amines are able to reverse an established adrenergic neurone block, extravesicular binding sites for nor-adrenaline have been postulated (Giachetti & Hollenbeck, 1976). However, since these postulated extravesicular binding sites are functionally defined (their occupation by noradrenaline ensures normal function; their occupation by agents like guanethidine results in adrenergic neurone block), their role as a possible "second axoplasmic compartment" (i.e., in addition to the free axoplasmic noradrenaline) cannot be assessed. Hence, the present discussion will not consider this type of postulated extravesicu-lar binding sites.

Evidence for the existence of extravesicular (i.e., reserpine-resistant) binding sites for phenethylamines was obtained by Bönisch and Graefe (1976, 1977). As pointed out above, in their first series of experiments they perfused rabbit hearts (after pretreatment of the animals with reserpine, and after inhibition of MAO and COMT) with various concentrations of labelled nor-adrenaline or metaraminol, so as to determine the steady-state tissue/medium ratio as well as the half time for the approach to steady-state distribution. As discussed in section IIE, the results were incompatible with the existence of a simple one-compartmental system (irrespective of whether the compartment was conceived as a "pump and pump" or as a "pump and leak" system). Moreover, when hearts were perfused with 0.3 µM labelled nor-adrenaline or metaraminol, and when the removal of the amine from the perfusion fluid was followed throughout the experiment, the

amines were clearly found to distribute into two neuronal (i.e.,
cocaine-sensitive) compartments, one of which equilibrated
quickly (half times of 6 to 8 minutes), while the other equilibrated slowly (half time of 38 minutes for noradrenaline and of
25 minutes for metaraminol). Kinetic analysis indicated that the
two compartments were in series (the quickly equilibrating compartment being in contact with the extracellular space). A
mathematical model was developed for this two-compartmental
system, and it was found that calculations of steady-state
tissue/medium ratios and of half times for the approach to steady
state were in full agreement with the experimental results: Both
parameters declined when the system was exposed to increasing
concentrations of the amines.

It is very unlikely that the slowly equilibrating compartment is
due to an insufficient pretreatment with reserpine (i.e., that
it is vesicular), since reserpine was administered both 20 h
(1 mg/kg) and 3 h (0.5 mg/kg) before the experiment. Moreover,
the slowly equilibrating compartment had a considerable space,
as it was six times greater than the quickly equilibrating compartment, when hearts were perfused with 0.3 μM [^{3}H]noradrenaline.

Since basically identical results were obtained with noradrenaline
and metaraminol, a further possible objection to results obtained
with metaraminol can be excluded. Studies of the subcellular
distribution of [^{3}H]metaraminol (rat heart; Lundborg & Waldeck,
1966) as well as of the release of [^{3}H]metaraminol by field stimulation (rat iris initially loaded with [^{3}H]metaraminol; Farnebo,
1971) clearly indicated that [^{3}H]metaraminol is able to enter the
storage vesicles of adrenergic nerves by means of a reserpine-
resistant mechanism, while this was not so for [^{3}H]noradrenaline.
While there were pronounced differences between the two amines in
the studies of the Swedish workers, the new results presented
here have revealed only minor, quantitative differences between
the two amines.

Independent evidence for extravesicular binding sites was obtained
in a second series of experiments (Bönisch & Graefe, 1977). For
rabbit hearts (experimental conditions as described above) initial
rates of the neuronal uptake of [^{3}H]noradrenaline were determined
with the recently developed method of Graefe *et al.* (1978).
This method permits an accurate determination of initial rates of
uptake during the first 1 to 2 minutes of a perfusion with [^{3}H]
noradrenaline and [^{14}C]sorbitol (the latter to correct for the
extracellular distribution of the amine). Neuronal (i.e.,
cocaine-sensitive and corticosterone-resistant) uptake was found
to be saturable and to obey Michaelis-Menten kinetics (Km of
about 5 μM). When, on the other hand, the steady-state accumulation of noradrenaline was determined for a wide range of concentrations of the amine in the perfusion fluid, kinetic analysis
revealed that two saturable components were involved. While the
low-affinity component had a Km very similar to that of neuronal
uptake, the Km of the high-affinity component was lower by about
one order of magnitude.

Such results indicate that, even after pretreatment with reserpine, the adrenergic nerve ending seems to represent a two-
compartmental system which can not only accumulate free axoplasmic noradrenaline but which can also bind noradrenaline (or
metaraminol) to extravesicular binding sites. Apparently, these
binding sites have a high affinity to noradrenaline and a
limited (saturable) capacity. As a result of the difference
between the Km-values for neuronal uptake and extravesicular
binding, most of the axoplasmic noradrenaline is bound to extravesicular sites, when the neurone is in equilibrium with low
extracellular concentrations of noradrenaline. However, the
relation between "free" and "bound" noradrenaline is reversed,
when the nerve ending equilibrates with high extracellular concentrations of noradrenaline.

It is too early to know how such results fit into the various
schemes that one can construct to explain the fact that phenethylamines accelerate the efflux of noradrenaline from adrenergic
nerve endings. However, such results illustrate two important
points: It is quite possible that noradrenaline (and other phenethylamines) distribute into two axoplasmic compartments, and it
is also possible that phenethylamines elicit an efflux of noradrenaline from the neurone by interacting with extravesicular
binding sites normally occupied by noradrenaline.

IV   UPTAKE AND RETENTION OF TYRAMINE BY AND IN ISOLATED
      STORAGE VESICLES

The view that tyramine is taken up not only into the adrenergic
nerve ending but also into the storage vesicles (so as to elicit
the release of vesicularly stored noradrenaline), was in conflict
with the fact that experiments with isolated medullary vesicles
failed to provide any evidence for an ATP-Mg^{2+}-dependent uptake
(Carlsson, Hillarp & Waldeck, 1963). Similarly negative results
were obtained by Matthaei, Lentzen and Philippu (1976) who worked
with synaptic vesicles isolated from the caudate nucleus of the
pig. This was the more surprising, as tyramine was a competitive
inhibitor of the ATP-Mg^{2+}-dependent uptake of noradrenaline,
dopamine and 5-hydroxytryptamine (Matthaei *et al.*, 1976).

This minor discrepancy between expectations and facts is explained
by the long time required for the separation of the isolated
vesicles from the incubation medium, when this is done by centrifugation. As this requires at least 60 minutes, tyramine appears
to escape from the vesicles before being analysed. When Lentzen
and Philippu (1977) separated isolated vesicles (from the same
source) from the incubation medium by means of millipore filters,
separation was achieved within 20 seconds. An ATP-Mg^{2+}-dependent
uptake of tyramine was then clearly demonstrable.

V   METABOLISM OF THE NORADRENALINE RELEASED BY INDIRECTLY
     ACTING SYMPATHOMIMETIC AMINES

When tissues are first loaded with [^{3}H]noradrenaline and then
exposed to a quickly acting reserpine-like compound (Ro 4-1284),
large amounts of DOPEG (dihydroxyphenylglycol) appear in the
incubation medium or perfusion fluid (Leitz & Stefano, 1971;
Adler-Graschinsky, Langer & Rubio, 1972). Apparently, any release
of noradrenaline from the storage vesicles leads to an extensive
intraneuronal deamination of noradrenaline. This is so as long
as the intraneuronal MAO is not inhibited.

When the releasing effects of indirectly acting sympathomimetic
amines are considered, one has to remember that most of them have
a considerable affinity for MAO, irrespective of whether or not
they are substrates of the enzyme. Hence, it was not surprising
that Leitz and Stefano (1971) found no increased efflux of [^{3}H]-
DOPEG when they exposed guinea-pig atria preloaded with [^{3}H]nor-
adrenaline to rather high concentrations of tyramine or amphetamine. On the contrary, the efflux of [^{3}H]DOPEG fell below that
seen prior to the exposure to the indirectly acting amines.
However, when Langer (personal communication) carried out similar
experiments with considerably lower concentrations of tyramine
(i.e., with concentrations which may be assumed not to inhibit
MAO), he observed not only an increase in the efflux of [^{3}H]nor-
adrenaline but also in that of [^{3}H]DOPEG. Further evidence for
intraneuronal deamination subsequent to the release of noradrenaline from vesicles was obtained by Luchelli-Fortis and Langer
(1974) who obtained for guinea-pig atria and cat nictitating
membrane an increased efflux of [^{3}H]noradrenaline and [^{3}H]DOPEG
on exposure of such preloaded tissue to phenylephrine.

Such observations (all made with adrenergic nerve endings containing intact storage vesicles) indicate that various indirectly
acting amines are able to release noradrenaline (presumably from
storage vesicles) which is then subject to deamination by intraneuronal MAO, provided the concentrations of the releasing amines
are below those which inhibit MAO. Unfortunately, no such observations have been made in preparations obtained from reserpine-
pretreated animals. In such preparations one would have to
partially inhibit MAO (so as to achieve a "loading" of the
neurone). If indirectly acting amines would then increase the
efflux of [^{3}H]DOPEG, this would be very good evidence for the
existence of a two-compartmental system.

VI   CONCLUSIONS

It is the aim of this review to emphasize that there are certain
key problems that have to be solved before we can understand the
mode of action of the indirectly acting sympathomimetic amines
(and the mechanism by which noradrenaline leaves the nerve
endings). At the present time much of the argumentation of
different groups of researchers is circulatory in the sense that
they start from different assumptions. For instance, when Paton

(1973) discussed his results in terms of accelerated exchange diffusion, he assumed that a) amphetamine was subject to carrier-mediated neuronal uptake, b) he dealt with a one-compartmental system, c) MAO was completely inhibited, and d) re-uptake of noradrenaline was not important. Ross and Kelder (1976), on the other hand, based their interpretation of basically similar results on the premises that a) the system is two-compartmental, b) amphetamine is not subject to carrier-mediated uptake (though disregarding the fact that amphetamine should then be cocaine-like), and c) re-uptake does take place.

Much of our uncertainty can be attributed to our lack of knowledge concerning the following questions of central importance:

1. Does the adrenergic nerve ending of preparations obtained from reserpine-pretreated animals constitute a one-compartmental system or are there extravesicular binding sites for phenethylamines (and bretylium)?

2. To what degree are the results of efflux experiments affected by lack of inhibition or by incomplete inhibition of neuronal MAO?

3. To what extent are results of efflux experiments affected by re-uptake of the released amine?

4. Is the neuronal efflux of phenethylamines saturable when the internal sodium concentration is normal?

5. Are phenethylamines of high lipid solubility subject to carrier-mediated uptake and, if not, should they act like "non-transported inhibitors of uptake"?

6. Are cocaine-like agents indeed not transported by the neuronal carrier?

7. Is it possible to obtain experimental evidence for the phenomena of "counter-transport"?

At least some of these questions will have to be answered before we can be certain that the efflux of noradrenaline from adrenergic nerve endings is either carrier-mediated or due to passive leakage (or due to both mechanisms). Unless they are answered, our argumentation runs the risk of remaining circular.

However, it should also be stressed that convincing evidence relevant to just one of the points enumerated above should greatly simplify our future task. It can be safely predicted, that it will be most difficult to obtain the first answers, but that further progress will then be quick, since the design of future experiments should be much easier as soon as one or two question marks have disappeared. By focussing attention onto a few important points, perhaps this review can contribute to a solution of the problem under study.

VII   REFERENCES

Adler-Graschinsky, E., Langer, S.Z. & Rubio, M.C. (1972). Metabolism of norepinephrine released by phenoxybenzamine in
   isolated guinea-pig atria. *J. Pharmacol. Exp. Ther.* 180,
   286-301.

Boenisch, H. & Graefe, K.-H. (1976). Distribution kinetics of
   ^{3}H-(-)-noradrenaline (NA) and ^{3}H-(±)-metaraminol (MA) in the
   perfused rabbit heart. *Naunyn-Schmiedeberg's Arch. Pharmacol.*
   293, R4.

Boenisch, H. & Graefe, K.-H. (1977). Saturation kinetics of
   uptake and of the neuronal steady-state accumulation of ^{3}H-
   (-)-noradrenaline (NA) in the reserpine-pretreated rabbit
   heart. *Naunyn-Schmiedeberg's Arch. Pharmacol.* 297, R48.

Bönisch, H., Uhlig, W. & Trendelenburg, U. (1974). Analysis of
   the compartments involved in the extraneuronal storage and
   metabolism of isoprenaline in the perfused heart. *Naunyn-
   Schmiedeberg's Arch. Pharmacol.* 283, 223-244.

Bogdanski, D.F. & Brodie, B.B. (1969). The effects of inorganic
   ions on the storage and uptake of ^{3}H-norepinephrine by rat
   heart slices. *J. Pharmacol. Exp. Ther.* 165, 181-189.

Bogdanski, D.F., Tissari, A. & Brodie, B.B. (1968). Role of
   sodium, potassium, ouabain, and reserpine in uptake, storage
   and metabolism of biogenic amines in synaptosomes. *Life
   Sciences* 7, 419-428.

Bogdanski, D.T., Tissari, A.H. & Brodie, B.B. (1970). Mechanism
   of transport and storage of biogenic amines. III. Effects of
   sodium and potassium on kinetics of 5-hydroxytryptamine and
   norepinephrine transport by rabbit synaptosomes. *Biochim.
   Biophys. Acta* 219, 189-199.

Brodie, B.B., Costa, E., Groppetti, A. & Matsumoto, C. (1968).
   Interaction between desipramine, tyramine and amphetamine at
   adrenergic neurones. *Br. J. Pharmacol.* 34, 648-658.

Carlsson, H., Hillarp, N.A. & Waldeck, B. (1963). Analysis of
   the ATP-Mg^{++} dependent storage mechanism in the amine granules
   of the adrenal medulla. *Acta Physiol. Scand.* 59, Suppl. 215.

Eckert, E., Henseling, M., Gescher, A. & Trendelenburg, U.
   (1976a). Stereoselectivity of the distribution of labelled
   noradrenaline in rabbit aortic strips after inhibition of the
   noradrenaline-metabolizing enzymes. *Naunyn-Schmiedeberg's
   Arch. Pharmacol.* 292, 219-229.

Eckert, E., Henseling, M. & Trendelenburg, U. (1976b). The effect
   of inhibitors of extraneuronal uptake on the distribution of
   ^{3}H-(±)-noradrenaline in nerve-free rabbit aortic strips.
   Naunyn-Schmiedeberg's Arch Pharmacol. 293, 115-127.

Farnebo, L.-O. (1971).   Effect of reserpine on release of ^{3}H-noradrenaline, ^{3}H-dopamine and ^{3}H-metaraminol from field stimulated rat iris. *Biochem. Pharmacol.* 20, 2715-2726.

Giachetti, A. & Hollenbeck, R.A. (1976).   Extra-vesicular binding of noradrenaline and guanethidine in the adrenergic neurones of the rat heart; a proposed site of action of adrenergic neurone blocking agents. *Br. J. Pharmacol.* 58, 497-504.

Golko, D.S. & Paton, D.M. (1976).   Characteristics of accumulation of ephedrine in rabbit atria. *Can. J. Physiol. Pharmacol.* 54, 93-100.

Graefe, K.-H., Bönisch, H., Fiebig, R. & Trendelenburg, U. (1975). Extraneuronal uptake and metabolism of catecholamines in isolated perfused hearts. *Proc. Sixth Int. Cong. Pharmacol.* Helsinki, 2, 117-130.

Graefe, K.-H., Bönisch, H. & Keller, B. (1978).   Transient kinetics and saturation kinetics of the adrenergic neurone uptake system in the perfused rabbit heart. *Nauyn-Schmiedeberg's Arch. Pharmacol.*, in press.

Graefe, K.-H., Stefano, F.J.E. & Langer, S.Z. (1973).   The distribution of (±)-noradrenaline (NA) or (±)-metaraminol (MA) in the adrenergic nerve endings of the rat vas deferens.
• *Nauyn-Schmiedeberg's Arch. Pharmacol.* 277, R22.

Graefe, K.-H., Stefano, F.J.E. & Langer, S.Z. (1977).   Stereoselectivity in the metabolism of ^{3}H-noradrenaline during uptake into and efflux from the isolated rat vas deferens. *Nauyn-Schmiedeberg's Arch. Pharmacol.* 299, 225-238.

Haeusler, G., Haefely, W. & Huerlimann, H. (1969).   On the mechanism of the adrenergic nerve blocking action of bretylium. *Nauyn-Schmiedeberg's Arch. Pharmacol.* 265, 260-277.

Heinz, E. & Walsh, P.M. (1958).   Exchange diffusion, transport and intracellular level of amino acids in Ehrlich carcinoma cells. *J. Biol. Chem.* 233, 1488-1493.

Henseling, M., Eckert, E. & Trendelenburg, U. (1976a).   The distribution of ^{3}H-(±)-noradrenaline in rabbit aortic strips after inhibition of the noradrenaline-metabolizing enzymes. *Nauyn-Schmiedeberg's Arch. Pharmacol.* 292, 205-217.

Henseling, M., Eckert, E. & Trendelenburg, U. (1976b).   The effect of cocaine on the distribution of labelled noradrenaline in rabbit aortic strips and on efflux of radioactivity from the strips. *Nauyn-Schmiedeberg's Arch. Pharmacol.* 292, 231-241.

Henseling, M. & Trendelenburg, U. (1978).   Stereoselectivity of the accumulation and metabolism of noradrenaline in rabbit aortic strips. *Nauyn-Schmiedeberg's Arch. Pharmacol.* in press.

Iversen, L.L. (1967). The uptake and storage of noradrenaline
    in sympathetic nerves.   p. 253, Cambridge University Press,
    England.

Iversen, L.L. & Salt, P.J. (1970).   Inhibition of catecholamine
    uptake by steroids in the isolated rat heart. *Br. J. Pharmacol.*
    40, 528-530.

Iversen, L.L., Salt, P.J. & Wilson, H.A. (1972).   Inhibition of
    catecholamine uptake in the isolated rat heart by haloalkyl-
    amines related to phenoxybenzamine. *Br. J. Pharmacol.* 46,
    647-657.

Jacquot, C., Bralet, J., Cohen, Y. & Valette, G. (1972).   Fixa-
    tion de la dl-ephedrine-^{14}C par le cour isolé perfuse de rat.
    Biochem. Pharmacol. 18, 903-914.

Leitz, F.H. & Stefano, F.J.E. (1971).   The effect of tyramine,
    amphetamine and metaraminol on the metabolic disposition of
    ^{3}H-norepinephrine released from the adrenergic neuron. *J.
    Pharmacol. Exp. Ther.* 178, 464-473.

Lentzen, H. & Philippu, A. (1977).   Uptake of tyramine into
    synaptic vesicles of the caudate nucleus. *Naunyn-Schmiedeberg's
    Arch. Pharmacol.*, 300, 25-30.

Lindmar, R. & Löffelholz, K. (1972).   Differential effects of
    hypothermia on neuronal efflux, release and uptake of nor-
    adrenaline. *Naunyn-Schmiedeberg's Arch. Pharmacol.* 274, 410-
    414.

Lindmar, R. & Löffelholz, K. (1974).   Neuronal and extraneuronal
    uptake and efflux of catecholamines in the isolated rabbit
    heart. *Naunyn-Schmiedeberg's Arch. Pharmacol.* 284, 63-92.

Luchelli-Fortis, M.A. & Langer, S.Z. (1974).   Reserpine-induced
    depletion of the norepinephrine stores: Is it a reliable
    criterion for the classification of the mechanism of action of
    sympathomimetic amines? *J. Pharmacol. Exp. Ther.* 188, 640-
    653.

Lundborg, P. & Waldeck, B. (1966).   Two different mechanisms for
    incorporation of ^{3}H-metaraminol into the amine-storing
    granules. *J. Pharm. Pharmacol.* 18, 762-764.

Matthaei, H., Lentzen, H. & Philippu, A. (1976).   Competition of
    some biogenic amines for uptake into synaptic vesicles of the
    striatum. *Naunyn-Schmiedeberg's Arch. Pharmacol.* 293, 89-96.

Paton, D.M. (1973).   Mechanism of efflux of noradrenaline from
    adrenergic nerves in rabbit atria. *Br. J. Pharmacol.* 49,
    614-627.

Paton, D.M. (1976). Characteristics of efflux of noradrenaline
from adrenergic neurons. In: *The Mechanism of Neuronal and
Extraneuronal Transport of Catecholamines* (ed.) D.M. Paton,
pp. 155-174, Raven Press, New York.

Raiteri, M., del Carmine, R. & Bertolini, A. (1977). Effect of
desmethylimipramine on the release of (^{3}H)norepinephrine
induced by various agents in hypothalmic synaptosomes. *Mol.
Pharmacol.* 13, 746-758.

Raiteri, M., Levi, G. & Federico, R. (1974). d-Amphetamine and
the release of ^{3}H-norepinephrine from synaptosomes. *Eur. J.
Pharmacol.* 28, 237-240.

Rosenberg, T. & Wilbrandt, W. (1957). Uphill transport induced
by counterflow. *J. Gen. Physiol.* 41, 289-296.

Ross, S.B. & Gosztonyi, T. (1975). On the mechanism of the
accumulation of ^{3}H-bretylium in peripheral sympathetic nerves.
Naunyn-Schmiedeberg's Arch. Pharmacol. 288, 283-293.

Ross, S.B., Kelder , D. (1976). Active transport of ^{3}H-bretylium
in the rat vas deferens *in vitro*. *Acta Physiol. Scand.* 97,
209-221.

Ross, S.B. & Renyi, A.L. (1966a). Uptake of some tritiated
sympathomimetic amines by mouse brain cortex slices *in vitro*.
Acta Pharmacol. Toxicol. 24, 297-309.

Ross, S.B. & Renyi, A.L. (1966b). Uptake of tritiated tyramine
and (+)-amphetamine by mouse heart slices. *J. Pharm.
Pharmacol.* 18, 756-757.

Ross, S.B., Renyi, A.L. & Brunfelter, B. (1968). Cocaine-
sensitive uptake of sympathomimetic amines in nerve tissue.
J. Pharm. Pharmacol. 20, 283-288.

Stein, W.D. (1967). *The Movement of Molecules Across Cell
Membranes*. Academic Press, New York, London.

Thoenen, H., Hürlimann, A. & Haefely, W. (1968). Mechanism of
amphetamine accumulation in the isolated perfused heart of
the rat. *J. Pharm. Pharmacol.* 20, 1-11.

Trendelenburg, U. (1972). Classification of sympathomimetic
amines. In: *Handbook of Experimental Pharmacology* (eds.)
H. Blaschko & E. Muscholl, Vol. 33, pp. 336-362, Springer-
Verlag, Berlin.

Uhlig, W., Bönisch, H. & Trendelenburg, U. (1974). The O-methylation of extraneuronally stored isoprenaline in the perfused
heart. *Naunyn-Schmiedeberg's Arch. Pharmacol.* 283, 245-261.

White, T.D. (1976). Models for neuronal noradrenaline uptake.
In: *The Mechanism of Neuronal and Extraneuronal Transport of
Catecholamines* (ed.) D.M. Paton, pp. 175-194, Raven Press, N.Y.

Wilbrandt, W. & Rosenberg, T. (1961). The concept of carrier
     transport and its corollaries in pharmacology. *Pharmacol.
     Rev.* 13, 109-183.

BIOCHEMICAL ASSESSMENT OF PERIPHERAL ADRENERGIC ACTIVITY

I. J. Kopin

I   INTRODUCTION

Eighty years ago, adrenaline, the pressor substance found in the adrenal glands, was isolated and identified as N-methyl-3,4-di-hydroxyphenylethanolamine (Abel & Crawford, 1897). Langley (1901) noted the similarities between the actions of adrenaline and the effects of stimulating the sympathetic nerves. This led Elliot (1905), who was then a student of Langley, to propose that an ad-renaline-like substance was released from sympathetic nerve end-ings and was responsible for the effects of nerve stimulation. A generation later Loewi (1921) and Cannon & Uridil (1921) provided direct evidence that an active substance was indeed released when sympathetic nerves to the heart or liver were stimulated.   The definitive demonstration by Euler (1948) that noradrenaline was the active substance released from sympathetic nerves made possi-ble biochemical approaches to the study of the sympathetic ner-vous system.

Early bioassay methods were tedious, nonspecific and of limited sensitivity. The development by Lund (1950) of a fluorimetric method for determining adrenaline and noradrenaline in plasma led to several useful chemical procedures for assay of these catechol-amines. Although not particularly convenient because of technical difficulties and the large volumes of blood required, the fluori-metric methods developed could be used to measure levels of the catecholamines in blood. These methods are easily used, however, to assay catecholamines in urine. Euler, Franksson & Hellström (1954) showed that adrenaline excretion was markedly depressed after adrenalectomy, but that urinary noradrenaline was almost un-changed. Thus, adrenaline excretion provided an index of adrenal medullary secretion while noradrenaline excretion appeared to re-flect activity of the sympathetic nervous system.

Armstrong, McMillan & Shaw (1957) showed that 3-methoxy-4-hydroxy-mandelic acid (VMA) is a major urinary metabolite of adrenaline and noradrenaline (Fig. 1). It was known that the catecholamines were substrates for monamine oxidase (Blaschko, Richter & Shlossman, 1937) so that deamination appeared to be followed by O-methylation and excretion. Axelrod (1957) demonstrated that O-methylation of the catecholamines could precede deamination and that the metanephrines so formed were present in urine (Axelrod, Senoh & Witkop, 1958). Introduction of isotopic methods provided a simple means of assessing the disposition and metabolism of the catecholamines. With this information procedures for assay of metabolic products excreted in urine were soon developed (see below). The total of the urinary metabolites of the catechol-amines provides a direct measure of the amounts of these com-pounds formed and metabolized.

Plasma levels of catecholamines have been studied by using bio-assay procedures, by conversion to fluorimetrically measurable compounds, and by enzymatic formation of radio-actively labelled products (see below). These methods measure changes in levels of adrenaline and noradrenaline and are related to the amounts of the amines being released from the adrenal medulla or sympathetic nerve endings into the circulation.

When it was realized that the mechanism of release of catechol-amines involved a process in which the contents of the synaptic vesicles were extruded, release of proteins stored along with the catecholamines was sought. After the demonstration of release of dopamine-β-hydroxylase from sympathetic nerves (see references in Axelrod, 1972 and Kopin, Kaufman, Viveros, Jacobowitz, Lake, Ziegler, Lovenberg & Goodwin, 1976), Weinshilboum & Axelrod (1971) showed that the enzyme was present in human and animal plasma. Levels of this enzyme are easily measured and numerous attempts have been made to relate the amounts of dopamine-β-hydroxylase in plasma to sympathetic nerve activity.

Measurement of the rates of urinary excretion of the catechol-amines and their metabolites and of the plasma levels of adren-aline, noradrenaline and dopamine-β-hydroxylase have been used to assess the activity of the sympatho-adrenal medullary system in various physiologic states, in diseases, and after administration of drugs. It is the purpose of this chapter to review the valid-ity and limitations of these various procedures in assessing ad-renergic activity.

II   URINARY EXCRETION OF CATECHOLAMINES

Shortly after Euler (1948) demonstrated that noradrenaline is re-leased from sympathetic nerves, chemical methods were developed to measure each of the catecholamines in urine and plasma. Bio-assay of the separated catecholamines (see Gaddum, 1959) was the first method to be used, but with the development of more con-venient and specific chemical procedures, use of bioassay dimini-shed. Most of the chemical procedures involve adsorption of the catecholamines on alumina, elution with acid, and controlled oxi-dation of the catecholamines to form fluorescent trihydroxyindole derivatives using MnO_2 (Lund, 1952; Goldenberg, Serlin, Edwards & Rapport, 1954), iodine (Sourkes & Drujan, 1957), or potassium ferricyanide (Euler & Floding, 1955; Weil Malherbe & Bone, 1957).

Increases in catecholamine excretion have been elicited by the wide variety of stimuli which Cannon (1929) associated with en-hanced sympatho-adrenal medullary secretion. Euler & Luft (1952) demonstrated that striking increases in urinary catecholamine ex-cretion attend insulin-induced hypoglycemia. Physiological vari-

ables such as age, diurnal variation, and muscular work (Karki,
1956) were examined and found to influence catecholamine excretion. Euler & Lundberg (1954) showed that airplane flying raised
adrenaline excretion and attributed that response to the psychological stress rather than any hypoxia. There are many other
studies which demonstrate that a host of psychosocially stressful
situations induce increases in catecholamine excretion (see reviews in Levi, 1972). As predicted by Cannon (1929) a wide
variety of physical as well as mental, stresses such as physical
exertion, cold, hypoxia, and surgery produce increases in urinary
catecholamines.

Although there can be little disagreement that excretion of catecholamines in urine does provide an index of discharge of adrenaline from the adrenal medulla and of noradrenaline from sympathetic nerves, there are several disadvantages and possible pit-
falls in the use of urinary catecholamines as an index of sympathetic nerve activity. Only a small percentage of catecholamines infused intravenously is recovered in urine. Bygdeman,
Euler & Hökfelt (1960) found that, in rabbits, at infusion rates
below 14 μg/kg/min only about 2.5% of administered adrenaline
appeared in the urine, but at higher rates of infusion the per-
cent recovered increased. In similar studies in humans,
Elmadjian, Lamson, Freedman, Neri & Varjabedian (1956) found that
only 0.5 - 2.0% of infused adrenaline was recovered in the urine.
When radioactively-labelled catecholamines became available, the
fractions of the administered compound and its metabolites which
appeared in the urine were also determined. During the first 24
hrs after administration of $(\pm)-[^{14}C]$noradrenaline to normal
humans, the unchanged catecholamine in urine was only about 4% of
the administered dose (Kirshner, Goodall & Rosen, 1958). Other
studied using tritium-labelled catecholamines have reported that
7% of administered $(\pm)-[^{3}H]$adrenaline (LaBrosse, Axelrod, Kopin &
Kety, 1961) and 11% of $(\pm)-[^{3}H]$noradrenaline (Maas & Landis, 1971)
to be excreted unchanged. The higher proportion of administered
noradrenaline excreted unchanged may reflect the more specific
uptake of the physiologic levo-isomer. When racemic catecholamines are infused, the dextro-isomer may be excreted to a
greater extent than the endogenous levo-isomer. It is evident,
however, that only small, and perhaps variable, fractions of circulating catecholamines are excreted. Changes in blood flow to
the kidney and other tissues or alterations in metabolism could
alter significantly the rate of catecholamine excretion in the
absence of changes in the rate of catecholamine release. This
factor becomes important if the amounts of catecholamines excreted are to be used to quantitate the amounts of amine released
into the circulation. Empirically, however, it is clear that
large changes in urinary excretion of the amines do occur when
there is enhanced release of catecholamines.

The major limitation in use of urinary excretion of catecholamines
as an index of sympathetic activity is the time interval over
which the urine must be collected. Short-term changes in release
of catecholamines cannot be accurately assessed because they must
be distributed over the interval of the urine collection. A ten-

fold increase in noradrenaline release for a three-minute interval would appear as a 5% increase in excretion of the amine in
urine collected over a one-hour interval, assuming the fraction
of released noradrenaline which is excreted remains constant.
Urinary excretion rates of the catecholamines are, however, valid
indices of relatively prolonged (over one hour) changes in catecholamine release.

III   EXCRETION OF URINARY METABOLITES

After intravenous administration of radioisotope-labelled catecholamines, it is possible to account for over 95% of the excreted
radioactivity as unchanged amine or its metabolites (Kirshner *et
al.*, Goodall, Kirshner & Rosen, 1959; LaBrosse *et al.*, 1961; Maas
& Landis, 1971). Armstrong *et al.*, (1957) showed that VMA (Fig.
1) was a major metabolite of noradrenaline and the isotopic studies demonstrated that 30 - 40% of the urinary radioactivity is
present as VMA (Table 1). The O-methylated amines, metanephrine
or normetanephrine (free + conjugated) account for 20 - 40% of
the excreted radioactivity. Conjugates of the catecholamines and
3-methoxy-4-hydroxyphenylglycol (MOPEG) account for most of the
remainder of the isotope. The metabolism of exogenously administered noradrenaline is clearly different from the endogenously
formed catecholamine. From isotopic studies it has been calculated that about 90% of excreted VMA is derived from noradrenaline
(Kopin, 1963). Excretion of endogenous normetanephrine is less
than 1/10 that of VMA (Table 1) while isotopically-labelled VMA
represents only 1.5 - 3 times the amount of labelled normetanephrine derived from exogenously administered labelled noradrenaline. This suggests that a major fraction of noradrenaline is
metabolized before it ever reaches the circulation.

The total of the excretion rates of all of the metabolites of the
catecholamines provides an accurate measure of their rate of formation and metabolism. Since monoamine oxidase is present on the
mitochondria at sympathetic nerve terminals, a considerable fraction of the noradrenaline may be deaminated before it is released
(see Kopin, 1964). This occurs when reserpine interferes with
storage of noradrenaline in the synaptic vesicles. The catecholamine is released from the storage vesicles, destroyed by
monoamine oxidase and excreted as VMA and MOPEG. When noradrenaline is released into the circulation, however, O-methylation is
the major route of metabolism (Kopin & Gordon, 1962, 1963). These
results and those of Maas & Landis (1971) suggest that the excretion of noradrenaline, normetanephrine, and their conjugates may
be a more sensitive index of sympathetic nerve activity than the
total of all of the metabolites.

The first methods used for assay of the various endogenous O-methylated metabolites of the catecholamines were based on paper or
column chromatography and colorimetric assay (Armstrong *et al.*,
1957; Weise, McDonald & LaBrosse, 1961; Kakimoto & Armstrong,
1962). Subsequently more sensitive and convenient assays were
developed which are based on formation of fluorescent derivatives

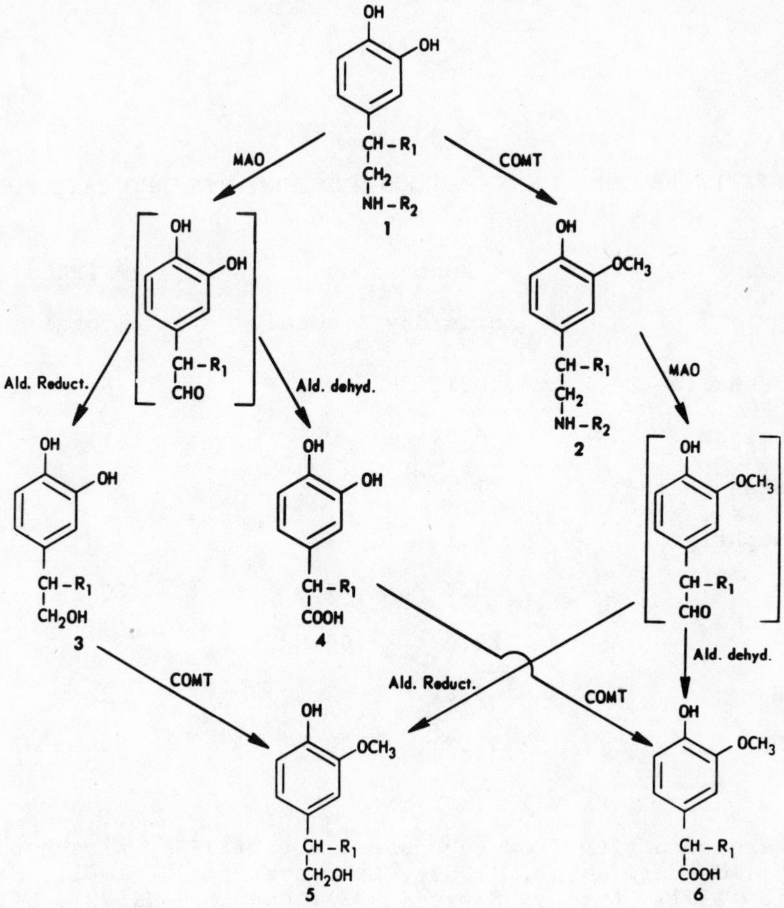

Fig. 1   Metabolism of noradrenaline and adrenaline (R_1=OH)
Compound 1. Adrenaline if R_2=CH$_3$, Noradrenaline if R_2=H
Compound 2. Metanephrine if R_2=CH$_3$, Normetanephrine if
        R_2=H
Compound 3. 3,4-Dihydroxyphenylglycol (DOPEG)
Compound 4. 3,4-Dihydroxymandelic acid (DOMA)
Compound 5. 3-Methoxy-4-hydroxyphenylglycol (MOPEG)
Compound 6. 3-Methoxy-4-hydroxymandelic acid (VMA)
COMT = Catechol-O-methyltransferase
Ald Reduct = Aldehyde Reductase
Ald dehyd = Aldehydedehydrogenase
MAO = Monamine oxidase

I. J. Kopin

TABLE 1

URINARY EXCRETION OF ENDOGENOUS AND ADMINISTERED CATECHOLAMINES

| | Endogenous | | $[^3H]NA$ | $[^3H]ADR$ |
	μmoles/day	% total	% total	% total
Noradrenaline	0.15	0.5	6	
Adrenaline	0.04	0.1		8
Normetanephrine	1.4	3.5	25	
Metanephrine	1.1	4.5		40
MOPEG	8.7	27.9	20	7
VMA	19.0	60.9	35	40
Other	0.8	2.6	3	2
Total	31.2	100	89	97

Data are composite from LaBrosse *et al.* (1958), Kirshner *et al.* (1958), Goodall *et al.* (1959), LaBrosse *et al.* (1961), Maas & Landis (1971), Anton & Sayre (1972), Engelman (1972), Wilk *et al.* (1972) and Pisano (1972).

of the O-methylated compounds (Anton & Sayre, 1972), radioenzymatic procedures for the catechols (Engelman, 1972) or gas
liquid chromatography (Wilk, Gitlow & Vertani, 1972). A particularly simple and useful technique is based on conversion by oxidation with periodate of O-methylated products of catecholamines
to vanillin (Pisano, 1972). Average excretion rates of the various metabolites of adrenaline and noradrenaline are shown in
Table 1.

Adrenaline is probably not metabolized to a significant extent in
the adrenal medulla. When adrenaline release is stimulated, its
rate of synthesis increases and the catecholamine levels are
rapidly restored (Bygdeman *et al.*, 1960). The catecholamine released into the circulation is metabolized in the same way as is
radioactively-labelled adrenaline injected intravenously. This
is reflected by the similar ratios (0.15) of excreted endogenous
adrenaline to metanephrine and radioactively-labelled adrenaline
to labelled metanephrine (Table 1).

As in the case of urinary excretion rates of the free catecholamines, the rates of excretion of their metabolites must be measured during relatively prolonged intervals and provide information of catecholamines. The deaminated compounds may also be
derived from brain, thus confounding any interpretation relating
only to peripheral sympatho-adrenal medullary activity.

IV   MEASUREMENT OF PLASMA LEVELS OF ADRENALINE AND
      NORADRENALINE

Plasma levels of the catecholamines are very low so that high
orders of sensitivity and specificity are required for their
accurate determination. Bioassay procedures can be used if sufficient care is taken to separate the amines or distinguish them
from each other and from other vasoactive substances present in
plasma. The blood pressure of a rat, particularly after treatment with a drug (such as cocaine) which inhibits uptake of injected catecholamines into sympathetic nerves (e.g., Gunne &
Reis, 1963), provides a sufficiently sensitive system. Vane
(1969) has described a cascade system of superfusing isolated
selected tissues (hen rectal caecum, rat stomach strip, etc.)
which can be used to detect various active substances, including
catecholamines, in blood.

The development of chemical methods for estimating catecholamine
levels in plasma depended upon their preliminary isolation by absorption on, and subsequent elution from, alumina or an ion exchange resin and conversion to a fluorescent derivative (see
above). The difficulties with the fluorimetric assays and their
usefulness when carefully performed have been reviewed by
Callingham (1968).

Recently, highly sensitive and specific radioenzymatic techniques
have been developed for assay of catecholamines in plasma and
cerebrospinal fluid. These are based on the enzyme-catalysed

transfer of the radioactively-labelled methyl group from S-adeno-sylmethionine to the catecholamines.

Initially a double-isotope procedure (Engelman & Portnoy, 1970) was used to determine the extent of conversion of the catechol-amines to their O-methylated products. A small, tracer amount of tritium-labelled adrenaline and/or noradrenaline is added to the plasma, the catecholamines are isolated by adsorption on an ion exchange resin and then enzymatically O-methylated using catechol-O-methyl-transferase and S-adenosylmethionine-methyl-[^{14}C] as methyl donor. The amine products are adsorbed on an ion exchange resin, eluted, and separated by thin layer chromatography. After elution, the separated O-methylated catecholamines are oxidized to vanillin which is extracted into toluene and assayed for ^{3}H and ^{14}C.

Subsequently, the efficiency of O-methylation has been improved and conversion of a constant, major portion of the catecholamines to the corresponding O-methylated derivatives achieved. Efficient O-methylation and use of high specific activity S-adenosylmethio-nine-methyl-C[^{3}H$_3$] has resulted in development of extremely sensi-tive enzymatic single isotopic assay methods which can measure accurately the catecholamine content of less than one ml blood or cerebrospinal fluid (Coyle & Henry, 1973; Passon & Peuler, 1973; Cryer, Santiago & Shah, 1974; DePrada & Zurcher, 1976; Weise & Kopin, 1976; Peuler & Johnson, 1977).

The more recently described of these techniques do not require preliminary isolation of the catecholamines. O-Methylation is carried out directly on plasma or immediately after precipitation of proteins. The products are extracted into an organic solvent and separated by rapid thin-layer chromatography so that the pro-cedure has been shortened considerably and several dozen samples may be conveniently assayed in one or two days.

Another radioenzymatic technique is based on conversion of nor-adrenaline to adrenaline-methyl-C[^{3}H$_3$] using phenylethanolamine-N-methyl transferase and S-adenosylmethionine-methyl-C[^{3}H$_3$] (Saelens, Schoen & Kovacsics, 1967; Henry, Starman, Johnson & Williams, 1975). This technique measures only noradrenaline, but has been adapted so that over 100 samples of plasma or CSF can be assayed (Lake, Ziegler & Kopin, 1976).

V   SIGNIFICANCE OF PLASMA CATECHOLAMINE LEVELS

The level of any substance in plasma is determined by the rate of its removal as well as the rate of its entry. The effects of intravenously administered catecholamines are extremely transient, consistent with the rapid disappearance from blood of exogenously administered catecholamines. Stable levels of adrenaline or nor-adrenaline in plasma must be maintained by continuous release or intravenous infusion of the catecholamines. Using a fluorimetric assay, Cohen, Holland & Goldenberg (1959) studied, in man, plasma concentrations of catecholamines during and after infusion of

adrenaline or noradrenaline. With infusion rates of about 0.4
µg/kg/min, after 10 min concentrations of about 3.5 µg/l noradrenaline or 2.5 µg/l adrenaline were found in the plasma. The
relationship between amine concentrations in plasma and rates of
infusion appear linear over a range of 0.02 - 0.5 µg/kg/min.
Because somewhat longer infusion times (up to 40 - 70 min) did
not appear to further increase the plasma catecholamine levels,
Cohen *et al.* (1959) assumed that a steady state had been attained.
From this data and an estimate of the resting plasma levels or
noradrenaline (0.35 µg/l) and adrenaline (0.06 µg/l), they calculated that about 0.04 µg/kg/min noradrenaline and 0.01 µg/kg/min
adrenaline reaches the circulation from endogenous sources. After
cessation of the infusions, the plasma catecholamine levels fell
rapidly and approached normal levels with a half-life of one to
two min. Vendsalu (1960) performed a similar study and found
only slightly slower rates of formation and turnover rate. Similar initial rates of decline have been obtained after infusion of
(±)-[^{3}H]adrenaline (LaBrosse, Mann & Kety, 1961) and (±)-[^{3}H]nor-
adrenaline (Gitlow, Mendelowitz, Smith, Gall, Wolf & Naftchi,
1961). In these studies, however, it was possible to follow the
decline in levels of the isotopically-labelled amine well beyond
the times possible when non-isotopic catecholamines are infused.
After the initial rapid decline (half-life of less than two min)
the rate of fall in concentration of the labelled amines was
markedly slowed. The multiphasic decline indicated that the
labelled catecholamines had been taken up in tissues and were
slowly being returned to the circulation. The slowest rates of
decline had half-lives of about 75 min for adrenaline (LaBrosse
et al., 1961) and 90 min for noradrenaline (Gitlow *et al.*, 1961)
and accounted for about one-third of the infused catecholamine.
These results suggest that in the studies of Cohen *et al.* (1959)
and Vendsalu (1960), a steady state had not been achieved and the
estimates of rates of endogenous secretion of the catecholamines
into the circulation were about 33% too high. The combined results of the isotopic and non-isotopic studies suggest that the
rates of catecholamine secretion from endogenous sources at rest
are 0.027 µg/kg/min for noradrenaline and 0.0067 µg/kg/min for
adrenaline. This is equivalent to 2.7 mg (14.8 µmole)/day noradrenaline and 0.67 (4.0 µmole)/day adrenaline for a 70 kg man.
These secretion rates appear to be excessively high. Only about
5% of intravenously administered isotopically-labelled catecholamines are excreted in the urine unchanged. Since the daily
urinary excretion of noradrenaline is less than 50 µg (0.3 µmoles)
per day, it would be expected that about 20 times this amount or
1 mg (6.0 µmoles) would be released into the circulation.

The total amount of catecholamine released into the circulation
can be considered to be a maximum of 10 - 20 µmoles/day. The
total urinary excretion products of the catecholamines, however,
is in excess of 30 µmoles/day (Table 1). Most of the adrenaline
formed is released into the blood; therefore, a considerable
fraction of the noradrenaline formed must be metabolized in the
tissues before it reaches the circulation. This is consistent
with observations on the fate of [^{3}H]noradrenaline released by
stimulation of sympathetic nerves to isolated tissues of several

species. In cat nictitating membrane (Langer, 1970) and spleen (Dubocovich & Langer, 1973), rat vas deferens (Langer, 1970), guinea pig atria and vas deferens (Tarlov & Langer, 1971) and rabbit aorta (Levin, 1974), 3,4-dihydroxyphenylglycol is the major substance which accounts for the increment in tritium when the nerves are stimulated, while noradrenaline makes up only one-third of the released radioactivity. Inhibition of neuronal up-take of the released amine by cocaine results in almost no change in the total tritium released from cat nictitation membrane, but increases the proportion of tritium released as noradrenaline at the expense of the deaminated metabolite (Langer & Enero, 1974). There was no change in the normetanephrine released. These ob-servations indicate that after being taken up into the nerve ending, the released noradrenaline is normally metabolized by deamination while the catecholamine which reaches the extra-neuronal tissues is O-methylated. The exact proportion of the released noradrenaline which reaches the circulation, is metabo-lized in the neuron after re-uptake, or O-methylated, cannot be determined since the proportion which is taken into the synaptic vesicles after uptake is not known. The results obtained with cocaine (Langer & Enero, 1974), however, suggest that the propor-tion of neuronally released amine which is reused is small.

The relative importance of re-uptake of noradrenaline in termin-ating the action of the released neurotransmitter depends on the density and pattern of innervation, and width of the synaptic cleft. The narrower the synaptic cleft, the greater the role of neuronal uptake in terminating the action of the released trans-mitter (Verity, 1971). Deamination appears to be the major route of metabolism in the neurone, and O-methylation in extraneuronal tissues. Escape into the blood of released noradrenaline there-fore varies between tissues and the plasma levels of the catechol-amines differ with the site from which blood is sampled. Since catecholamines are metabolized to some extent in the lungs, arterial levels are somewhat lower than in mixed venous blood. Peripheral venous blood contains less adrenaline than arterial blood because some of the catecholamine is taken up and metabo-lized. There are also significant differences in the noradren-aline content of venous plasma from different regions of the body (see Callingham, 1968) presumably because of different rates of uptake and release of the catecholamines and different rates of blood flow. Plasma levels of catecholamines in the venous blood from an antecubital vein, however, do seem to reflect adequately the state of sympathetic neuron and adrenal medullary activity.

Plasma catecholamine levels may fluctuate rapidly because of the rapid rate of metabolism and the numerous environmental, emotion-al, and endogenous stimuli which provoke a sympathetic response (Cannon, 1928). Exposure to cold, pain, anxiety, anger, exertion or anticipation of exercise, certain anesthetics, hypoglycemia, hypoxia, hypercapnia, hemorrhage, fluid loss with hypotension, etc., are among the numerous stimuli which are associated with clinical evidence of sympathetic responses, increased urinary ex-cretion of catecholamines and elevated plasma levels of adren-aline and noradrenaline.

VI   SERUM DOPAMINE-β-HYDROXYLASE

Dopamine-β-hydroxylase is the enzyme which converts dopamine to
noradrenaline. It is present in the storage vesicles of the
sympathetic nerve endings and is released along with the neurotransmitter (see Axelrod, 1972 and Kopin *et al.*, 1976). Because
the enzyme is present in blood and appears to be derived from
the sympathetic nerves, the levels of the enzyme in blood were
at first thought to reflect the level of function of the sympathetic nerves (Weinshilboum & Axelrod, 1971). There are, however, extremely wide variations between individuals in serum
dopamine-β-hydroxylase levels while the function of the sympathetic nervous system seems perfectly normal in individuals with
extremely low levels of enzyme activity in the plasma. Since
there is a good correlation between enzyme activity and immunoreactive dopamine-β-hydroxylase (Wooten & Ciaranello, 1974;
Dunnette & Weinshilboum, 1976) the variation in enzyme activity
cannot be attributed to the presence in plasma of an inhibitor
of the enzyme. Studies of members of the same family have established the importance of genetic factors in determining levels of
serum dopamine-β-hydroxylase (Weinshilboum, Raymond, Elveback &
Weidman, 1973; Ross, Wetterberg & Myrhed, 1973; Ogihara, Nugent,
Shen & Goldfein, 1975). In studies of families in which there
are individuals with extremely low levels of the enzyme in serum,
Weinshilboum, Schorott, Raymond, Weidman & Elveback (1975) found
that the occurrence of this characteristic was consistent with
the existance of an allele for low levels of the enzyme which was
inherited in an autosomal recessive fashion. Levels of dopamine-
β-hydroxylase also vary with age, but in older adults the levels
of enzyme activity remain remarkably constant over intervals of
up to seven years (Lamprecht, Andres & Kopin, 1975).

There have been many clinical studies which have shown that
dopamine-β-hydroxylase levels in plasma are increased when there
is stimulation of the sympathetic nervous system. However, the
magnitude of the changes in enzyme levels are small, there are
also changes in levels of other proteins in the plasma (suggesting that redistribution of protein, e.g., via lymphatics, may
play a role), and the changes in enzyme levels are not necessarily related to the increases in plasma levels of noradrenaline
(see references in Kopin *et al.*, 1976). These factors, and the
strong genetic determinants of the levels of serum dopamine-β-
hydroxylase make it unlikely that measurements of the activity of
this enzyme can be used to determine acute changes in the level
of sympathetic nerve activity.

Altered levels of dopamine-β-hydroxylase in association with
familial disorders such as dysautonomia or dystonia may be useful
genetic markers for these disorders even if they are not directly
involved in the pathogenesis of the disorder (see references in
Kopin *et al.*, 1976).

A prolonged increase in sympatho-adrenal medullary secretion is
attended by an increase in the rate of synthesis and tissue
levels of the enzymes concerned with catecholamine biosynthesis,

including dopamine-β-hydroxylase (Axelrod, 1972). The enzyme is synthesized in the perikaryon and transported in the synaptic vesicles to the nerve ending. At the nerve ending there is a proportional release of noradrenaline and the soluble dopamine-β-hydroxylase. Most of the dopamine-β-hydroxylase, however, is not soluble and remains bound to the synaptic vesicle. The fate of this major portion of the enzyme is unknown. If genetic factors determine the extent to which the vesicular-bound dopamine-β-hydroxylase is released, by a non-exocytotic mechanism, into the circulation or destroyed before it is released, the wide range of normal levels of the enzyme in plasma could be explained. In any individual, however, when there is intense stimulation of the sympathetic nerves, levels of the enzyme could be increased. If there is sufficiently prolonged increase in sympathetic neuronal activity, the rate of synthesis of the enzyme might be increased and more of the active enzyme appear in the plasma. Thus, in a single individual changes in levels of dopamine-β-hydroxylase might reflect changes in overall sympathetic nerve activity over a long interval. This hypothesis would adequately explain the apparent relationship between urinary catecholamine excretion and dopamine-β-hydroxylase in patients with labile hypertension (Schanberg & Kirshner, 1976), the increases in serum levels of the enzyme after myocardial infaction (Gutteberg, Borud & Stromme, 1976), and the decreases in enzyme levels when established hypertension develops (Lamprecht *et al.*, 1975). The occurrence of familial diseases associated with high or low levels of serum dopamine-β-hydroxylase, independent of the level of sympathetic nerve activity, is consistent with genetic determination of the fate of the enzyme independent of its role in the nerve endings (see references in Kopin *et al.*, 1976; Lake, Ziegler & Murphy, 1977).

VII   CONCLUSION

Urinary excretion of catecholamines provides a useful index of the level of sympatho-adrenal medullary activity over intervals sufficiently long to collect adequate urine specimens. Measurement of the amine metabolites as well as the catecholamines, particularly as a fraction of the total of the metabolites may provide a somewhat better index of sympathetic activity, but may not be worth the effort.

Plasma levels of adrenaline or noradrenaline are particularly useful in measurement of acute changes in levels of sympatho-adrenal medullary activity. The recent development of sensitive, specific and reasonably simple methods for such measurements should markedly increase the use of this index of sympatho-adrenal medullary activity.

Plasma levels of dopamine-β-hydroxylase may be useful as a genetic marker for some disorders and may reflect, in a single individual, prolonged changes in the level of sympathetic activity, but is of limited value in assessing acute changes in activity of the sympathetic nervous system.

VIII REFERENCES

Abel, J.J. & Crawford, A.C. (1897). On the blood pressure raising constituent of the suprarenal capsule. *Bull. Johns
Hopkins Hosp.* 8, 151-157.

Anton, A.H. & Sayre, D.F. (1972). Fluorimetric assay of catechol-
amines, serotonin and their metabolites. In: *Methods in
Investigative and Diagnostic Endocrinology*, Vol. I. *The
Thyroid and Biogenic Amines* (eds.) J.E. Rall & I.J. Kopin,
North-Holland Publishing Co., Amsterdam-London, pp. 398-436.

Armstrong, M.D., McMillan, A. & Shaw, K.N.F. (1957). 3-Methoxy-
4-hydroxy-D-mandelic acid, a urinary metabolite of norepinephrine. *Biochem. Biophys. Acta* 25, 422.

Axelrod, J. (1957). O-methylation of catechol amines *in vitro*
and *in vivo*. *Science* 126, 400-401.

Axelrod, J. (1972). Dopamine-β-hydroxylase: regulation of its
synthesis and release from nerve terminals. *Pharmacol. Rev.*
23, 233-244.

Axelrod, J., Senoh, S. & Witkop, B.B. (1958). O-methylation of
catechol amines *in vivo*. *J. Biol. Chem.* 233, 697-701.

Blaschko, H., Richter, D. & Schlossman, H.J. (1937). Inactivation
of adrenaline. *J. Physiol.* 90, 1-17.

Bygdeman, S., Euler, U.S. von & Hökfelt, B. (1960). Resynthesis
of adrenaline of rabbit's adrenal medulla during insulin-
induced hypoglycemia. *Acta Physiol. Scand.* 49, 21-28.

Callingham, B.A. (1968). In: *The Catecholamines. Adrenaline,
Noradrenaline, Hormones in Blood*, 2nd edition, Vol. 2,
Academic Press, N.Y.

Cannon, W.B. (1929). Organisation for physiological homeostasis.
Physiol. Rev. 9, 399-431.

Cannon, W.B. & Uridil, J.E. (1921). Studies on the conditions of
activity in endocrine glands. VIII. Some effects on the denervated heart of stimulating the nerves of the liver. *Am.
J. Physiol.* 58, 353-354.

Cohen, G., Holland, B. & Goldenberg, M. (1959). Disappearance
rates of infused epinephrine and norepinephrine from plasma.
A comparison of normal and schizophrenic subjects. *Arch.Gen.
Psychiatry* 1, 228.

Coyle, J.T. & Henry, D. (1973). Catecholamines in fetal and new-
born rat brain. *J. Neurochem.* 21, 61-67.

Cryer, P.E., Santiago, J.V. & Shah, S. (1974). Measurement of norepinephrine and epinephrine in small volumes of human plasma by a single-isotope derivative method: Response to the upright posture. *J. Clin. Endocrinol. Metab.* 39, 1025-1029.

DaPrada, M. & Zurcher, G. (1976). Simultaneous radio-enzymatic determination of plasma and tissue adrenaline, noradrenaline and dopamine within the femtomole range. *Life Sci.* 19, 1161-1174.

Dubocovich, M. & Langer, S.Z. (1973). Effects of flow-stop on the metabolism of noradrenaline released by nerve stimulation in the perfused spleen. *Naunyn-Schmiedeberg's Arch. Pharmacol.* 278, 179-194.

Dunnette, J. & Weinshilboum, R. (1976). Human serum dopamine-beta-hydroxylase: correlation of enzymatic activity with immunoreactive protein in genetically defined samples. *Am. J. Hum. Genet.* 28, 155-166.

Elliot, T.R. (1905). The action of adrenaline. *J. Physiol.* *(Lond)* 32, 401.

Elmadjian, F., Lamson, E.T., Freeman, H., Neri, R. & Varjabedian, L. (1956). Excretion of epinephrine and norepinephrine after administration of insulin and methacholine. *J. Clin. Endocrinol. Metab.* 16, 876-886.

Engelman, K. (1972). Isotopic methods of assay of catecholamines and their metabolites. In: *Methods in Investigative and Diagnostic Endocrinology,* Vol. I. *The Thyroid and Biogenic Amines* (eds.) J.E. Rall & I.J. Kopin, North-Holland Publishing Co., Amsterdam-London, pp. 437-451.

Engelman, K. & Portnoy, B. (1970). Sensitive double-isotope derivative assay for norepinephrine and epinephrine. *Circ. Res.* 26, 53-57.

Euler, U.S. von (1948). Identification of the sympathomimetic ergone in adrenergic nerves of cattle (Sympathin N) with laevo-noradrenaline. *Acta Physiol. Scand.* 16, 63-74.

Euler, U.S. von & Floding, I. (1955). Fluorimetric estimation of noradrenaline (NA) and adrenaline (A) in urine. *Acta Physiol. Scand.* 33, 57-62 [Suppl.]118].

Euler, U.S. von, Franksson, C. & Hellström, J. (1954). Adrenaline and noradrenaline output in urine after unilateral and bilateral adrenalectomy in man. *Acta Physiol. Scand.* 31, 1.

Euler, U.S. von & Luft, R. (1952). Effect of insulin on urinary excretion of adrenaline and noradrenaline. *Metabolism* 1, 528-532.

Euler, U.S. von & Lundberg, U. (1954). Effect of flying on the epinephrine excretion in air force personnel. *J. Appl. Physiol.* 6, 551-555.

Gaddum, J.H. (1959). Bioassay procedures. *Pharmacol. Rev.* 11, 241-249.

Gitlow, S.E., Mendelowitz, M., Smith, A., Gall, E., Wolf, R.L. & Naftchi, N.E. (1961). The dynamics of norepinephrine metabolism. In: *Hypertension: Recent Advances on Hypertensive Disease*, 2nd Hannemann Symposium, (eds.) A.N. Brest & Mo J.H. Moyer, Lea & Febiger, Phila., pp. 335-341.

Goldenberg, M., Serlin, I., Edwards, T. & Rapport, M.M. (1954). Chemical screening methods for the diagnosis of pheochromocytoma. I. Norepinephrine and epinephrine in human urine. *Am. J. Med.* 16, 310-327.

Goodall, McC., Kirshner, N. & Rosen, L. (1959). Metabolism of noradrenaline in human. *J. Clin. Invest.* 38, 707-714.

Gunne, L.-M. & Reis, D.J. (1963). Changes in brain catecholamines associated with electrical stimulation of amygdaloid nucleus. *Life Sci.* 2, 804-809.

Gutteberg, T., Borud, O. & Stromme, J.H. (1976). Dopamine-beta-hydroxylase activity in serum following acute myocardial infarction; an evaluation of this parameter for routine use as an index of sympathetic activity. *Clin. Chim. Acta* 69, 61-66.

Henry, D.P., Starman, B.J., Johnson, D.G. & Williams, R.H. (1975). A sensitive radioenzymatic assay for norepinephrine in tissue and plasma. *Life Sci.* 16, 375-384.

Kakimoto, Y. & Armstrong, M.D. (1962). The phenolic amines of human urine. *J. Biol. Chem.* 237, 208.

Karki, N.T. (1956). The urinary excretion of noradrenaline and adrenaline in different age groups, its diurnal variation and the effect of muscular work on it. *Acta Physiol. Scand.* 39, 1-96.

Kirshner, N., Goodall, McC. & Rosen, L. (1958). Metabolism of DL-adrenaline-2-C[14] in the human. *Proc. Soc. Exp. Biol. Med.* 98, 627-635.

Kopin, I.J. (1963). Estimation of relative magnitudes of alternative metabolic pathways. In: *Methods of Biochemical Analysis*, Vol. XI (ed.) D. Glick, John Wiley & Sons, N.Y., pp. 247-278.

Kopin, I.J. (1964). Storage and metabolism of catecholamines: The role of monoamine oxidase. *Pharmacol. Rev.* 16, 179-191.

Kopin, I.J. & Gordon, E.K. (1962). Metabolism of norepinephrine-H^3 released by tyramine and reserpine. *J. Pharmacol.* 138, 351-357.

Kopin, I.J. & Gordon, E.K. (1963). Metabolism of administered and drug-released norepinephrine-7-H^3 in the rat. *J. Pharmacol.* 140, 207-216.

Kopin, I.J., Kaufman, S., Viveros, H., Jacobowitz, D., Lake, C.R., Ziegler, M.G., Lovenberg, W. & Goodwin, F.K. (1976). Dopamine-β-hydroxylase - basic and clinical studies. *Ann. Int. Med.* 85, 211-223.

LaBrosse, E.H., Axelrod, J., Kopin, I.J. & Kety, S.S. (1961). Metabolism of 7-H^3-epinephrine-D-bitartrate in normal young men. *J. Clin. Invest.* 40, 253-260.

LaBrosse, E.H., Mann, J.D. & Kety, S.S. (1961). The physiological and psychological effects of intravenously administered epinephrine and its metabolism in normal and schizophrenic men. III. Metabolism of 7-^{3}H-epinephrine as determined in studies on blood and urine. *J. Psychiat. Res.* 1, 68-75.

Lake, C.R., Ziegler M.G. & Kopin, I.J. (1976). Use of plasma norepinephrine for evaluation of sympathetic neuronal function in man. *Life Sci.* 18, 1315-1325.

Lake, C.R. Ziegler, M.G. & Murphy, D.L. (1977). Increased norepinephrine levels and decreased dopamine-β-hydroxylase activity in primary autism. *Arch. Gen. Psychiatry* 34, 553-556.

Lamprecht, F., Andres, R. & Kopin, I.J. (1975). Serum dopamine-beta-hydroxylase: constancy of levels in normotensive adults and decreases with development of blood pressure elevation. *Life Sci.* 17, 749-754.

Langer, S.Z. (1970). The metabolism of [^{3}H]noradrenaline released by electrical stimulation from the isolated nictitating membrane of the cat and from the vas deferens of the rat. *J. Physiol. (Lond)* 208, 515-546.

Langer, S.Z. & Enero, M.A. (1974). The potentiation of responses to adrenergic nerve stimulation in the presence of cocaine: its relationship to the metabolic fate of released norepinephrine. *J. Pharmacol. Exp. Ther.* 191, 431-443.

Langley, J.N. (1901). The difference of behavior of central and peripheral pilomotor nerve cells. *J. Physiol. (Lond)* 27, 224-236.

Levi, L. (1972). Stress and distress in response to psychosocial stimuli. *Acta Medica Scand.* [Suppl. 528].

Levin, J.A. (1974). The uptake and metabolism of ^{3}H-l and ^{3}H-dl-norepinephrine by intact rabbit aorta and isolated aventation and media. *J. Pharmacol. Exp. Ther.* 190, 210-226.

Loewi, O. (1921). Ober humorale Ubertragberkeit der Herznerven-
    wirkung. *Pfluggers Arch. Ges. Physiol.* 189, 239-242.

Lund, A. (1952). Adrenaline and noradrenaline in blood and urine
    in cases of pheochromocytoma. *Scand. J. Clin. Lab. Invest.*
    4, 263-265.

Lund, A. (1950). Simultaneous fluorimetric determinations of
    adrenaline and noradrenaline in blood. *Acta Pharm. Tox. Kbh.*
    6, 137-146.

Maas, J.W. & Landis, D.H. (1971). The metabolism of circulating
    norepinephrine by human subjects. *J. Pharmacol. Exp. Ther.*
    177, 600.

Ogihara, T., Nugent, C.A., Shen, S.W. & Goldfein, S. (1975).
    Serum dopamine-beta-hydroxylase activity in parents and
    children. *J. Lab. Clin. Med.* 85, 566-573.

Passon, P.G. & Pauler, J.D. (1973). A simplified radiometric
    assay for plasma norepinephrine and epinephrine. *Anal.
    Biochem.* 51, 518-631.

Peuler, J.D. & Johnson, G.A. (1977). Simultaneous single isotope
    radioenzymatic assay of plasma norepinephrine, epinephrine
    and dopamine. *Life Sci.* 21, 625-636.

Pisano, J. (1972). Assay of catecholamine metabolites based on
    vanillin formation. In: *Methods in Investigative and Diagnos-
    tic Endocrinology*, Vol. I, *The Thyroid and Biogenic Amines*,
    (eds.) J.E. Rall & I.J. Kopin, North-Holland Publishing Co.,
    Amsterdam-London, pp. 474-488

Ross, S.B., Wetterberg, L. & Myrhed, M. (1973). Genetic control
    of plasma dopamine-β-hydroxylase. *Life Sci.* 12, 529-532.

Saelens, J.K., Schoen, M.S. & Kovacsics, G.B. (1967). An enzyme
    assay for norepinephrine in brain tissue. *Biochem. Pharmacol.*
    16, 1403-1409.

Schanberg, S.M. & Kirshner, N. (1976). Serum dopamine-beta-
    hydroxylase as an indicator of sympathetic activity and
    primary hypertension. *Biochem. Pharmacol.* 25, 617-621.

Sourkes, T.L. & Drujan, B.D. (1957). A routine procedure for the
    determination of catecholamines in urine and tissues. *Can.
    J. Biochem. Physiol.* 35, 711-719.

Tarlov, S.R. & Langer, S.Z. (1971). The fate of ^{3}H-norepineph-
    rine released from isolated atria and vas deferens: Effect
    of field stimulation. *J. Pharmacol. Exp. Ther.* 179, 186-197.

Vane, J.R. (1969). The release and fate of vaso-active hormones
    in the circulation. *Br. J. Pharmacol.* 35, 209-242.

Vendsalu, A. (1960). Studies on the adrenaline and noradrenaline in human plasma. *Acta Physiol. Scand.* [Suppl. 173] 1-123.

Verity, M.A. (1971). Morphologic studies of vascular neuro-effector apparatus. In: *Proceedings of the Symposium on Physiological and Pharmacological Vascular Neuroeffector Systems*, S. Karger, Basel, pp. 2-12.

Weil-Malherbe, H. & Bone, A.D. (1957). The estimation of catecholamines in urine by a chemical method. *J. Clin. Path.* 10, 138-147.

Weinshilboum, R.M. & Axelrod, J. (1971). Serum dopamine-beta-hydroxylase activity. *Circ. Res.* 28, 307-315.

Weinshilboum, R.M., Raymond, F.A., Elveback, L.R. & Weidman, W.H. (1973). Serum dopamine-β-hydroxylase activity: sibling-sibling correlation. *Science* 181, 943-945.

Weinshilboum, R.M., Schorott, H.G., Raymond, F.A., Weidman, W.H. & Elveback, L.R. (1975). Inheritance of very low serum dopamine-beta-hydroxylase activity. *Am. J. Hum. Genet* 27, 573-585.

Weise, V.K. & Kopin, I.J. (1976). Assay of catecholamines in human plasma: Studies of a single isotope radioenzymatic procedure. *Life Sci.* 19, 1673-1686.

Weise, V.K., McDonald, R.K. & LaBrosse, E.L. (1961). Determination of urinary 3-methoxy-4-hydroxymandelic acid in man. *Clin. Chim. Acta* 6, 79.

Wilk, S., Gitlow, S.E. & Bertani, L.M. (1972). Gas liquid chromatographic methods for assay of catecholamine metabolites. In: *Methods in Investigative and Diagnostic Endocrinology*, Vol. I, *The Thyroid and Biogenic Amines* (eds.) J.E. Rall & I.J. Kopin, North-Holland Publishing Co., Amsterdam-London, pp. 452-472.

Wooten, G.F. & Ciaranello, R.D. (1974). Proportionally between dopamine-beta-hydroxylase activity and immunoreactive protein concentration in human serum. *Pharmacology* 12, 272-282.

THE CLINICAL PHARMACOLOGY OF ADRENERGIC NEURON BLOCKING AGENTS

D. M. Paton

I   INTRODUCTION

The adrenergic neuron blocking agents were introduced into clinical practice in 1959 (Boura, Green, McConbrey, Lawrence, Moulton & Rosenheim, 1959) and represented an important advance in the management of hypertension. Since then hundreds of publications have appeared describing various aspects of the biochemistry, pharmacology and clinical pharmacology of these agents. Detailed reviews have appeared on their biochemistry and metabolism (Lukas, 1973), pharmacology (Boura & Green, 1967), hemodynamic effects (Sannerstedt & Conway, 1970), clinical application (Woosley & Nies, 1976) and their involvement in drug interactions (Koch-Weser, 1975; Stafford & Fann, 1977). In this section, only certain aspects of their pharmacology will be reviewed.

II   MECHANISM OF ACTION

This has been extensively discussed in the chapter by Hausler and Haefely, and will therefore only be summarized here. Adrenergic neuron blocking agents are transported into adrenergic neurons by the carrier mechanism utilised by noradrenaline and related amines. This transport or uptake results in the accumulation of these drugs against the concentration gradient within the neuron and is essential for the inhibition of release of noradrenaline that they produce.

III   HEMODYNAMIC EFFECTS

The hemodynamic effects of treatment with adrenergic neuron blocking agents have been reviewed by Sannerstedt and Conway (1970), Jandhyala, Clarke and Buckley (1974) and Woosley and Nies (1976). After short-term treatment with guanethidine, the main effect is on cardiac output which is reduced while the systemic resistance is only moderately lower. However, after long-term treatment there is mainly a reduction in the systemic vascular resistance with little change in cardiac output.

The hypotensive effect of adrenergic neuron blocking agents is markedly increased in the upright posture because the normal sympathetic reflexes are blocked resulting in a loss of the usual compensatory changes in resistance and capacitance vessels with changes in posture. Talbot and Smith (1975) studied the factors

373

predisposing to symptoms of postural hypotension in 448 patients
during treatment with guanethidine, bethanidine or debrisoquine.
Guanethidine typically caused postural hypotensive symptoms in
the early morning, whereas hypotensive symptoms caused by bethanidine and debrisoquine occurred at other times of the day and
particularly 1-2 hrs after taking the drug. Hypotensive symptoms
occurred in 29% of patients receiving guanethidine and in 17-19%
of patients receiving bethanidine or debrisoquine. Evidence of
vascular and renal disease were significantly more frequent in
patients who experienced hypotensive symptoms.

Goldberg and Raftery (1976) continuously recorded the intra-
arterial blood pressure in 11 patients on adrenergic neuron blocking agents. During the day time all patients had large and ab-
rupt variations in pressure which were not accompanied by changes
in heart rate. On sudden standing and after exercise, the systo-
lic pressures fell, on the average, by 97 and 54 mm Hg respectively. The authors concluded that postural hypotension is more common than generally reported in patients on such drugs. They also
pointed out that the alternating periods of high and low pressure
may predispose to cerebral or myocardial infarction.

Guanethidine caused an increase in the plasma volume and in total
body exchangeable sodium in hypertensive patients (Smith, 1965).
The mechanism for this was unclear but may possibly have involved
a decrease in the glomerular filtration rate. In normal subjects,
guanethidine increased the plasma volume by 24% after a week and
13% after three weeks (Weil & Chidsey, 1968). These changes occurred in the absence of sodium retention and were associated
with a reduction in venous sympathetic reflexes and an increase i
in venous compliance. It was therefore suggested that the blood
volume may be affected by changes in venous resistance. The most
important effect of the increase in plasma volume is that it can
result in the development of tolerance to the antihypertensive
effects of guanethidine. This can be avoided by reducing the
plasma volume with diuretics or a low sodium diet (Dustan, Tarazi
& Bravo, 1972).

                    IV   DRUG INTERACTIONS

The adrenergic neuron blockers have been implicated in a number
of clinically important drug interactions. These have been reviewed by Koch-Weser (1975) and Stafford and Fann (1977).

In addition to the adrenergic neuron blocking agents, a large
number of other drugs have an affinity for the transport mechanism present in the plasma membrane of adrenergic nerve terminals;
these include sympathomimetic drugs, the tricyclic antidepressants,
nomifensine, chlorpromazine, certain antihistaminics etc. The
antihypertensive action of the adrenergic neuron blockers is significantly impaired when patients also take such drugs. This
occurs because the neuronal transport of the adrenergic neuron
blockers is reduced thus reducing their intraneuronal concentration. This interaction has been described with the tricyclic
antidepressants (imipramine, desipramine, amitriptyline, nor-

triptyline), chlorpromazine and sympathomimetic agents (e.g., amphetamine, methamphetamine, ephedrine, pseudoephedrine, phenyl-ephrine, phenylpropanolamine and methylphenidate). The sympatho-mimetics may also antagonize the adrenergic neuron blockers by causing their displacement from the neuron.

The pharmacological effects of noradrenaline are terminated as a result of the transport of noradrenaline into adrenergic nerve terminals. Consequently the administration of an adrenergic neuron blocker will interfere with the transport of noradrenaline and hence potentiate and prolong the pharmacological effects of noradrenaline. For this reason the use of such agents is con-traindicated in patients who have a phaeochromocytoma.

V PHARMACOKINETICS

The metabolism and pharmacokinetics of adrenergic neuron blocking agents have been reviewed by Lukas (1973). Here only the metabo-olism and pharmacokinetics of guanethidine and bethanidine in man will be considered.

Guanethidine

Guanethidine appeared to be absorbed continuously over a period of at least 12 hr after oral administration (McMartin, Rondel, Vinter, Allan, Humberstone, Leishman, Sandler & Thirkettle, 1970). However, absorption was incomplete and varied from patient to patient (McMartin & Simpson, 1971). Following its absorption, guanethidine is metabolised to guanethidine N-oxide and 2-(6-carboxyhexylamino)ethylguanidine (McMartin & Simpson, 1971). These metabolites have less than one-tenth of the pharmacological activity of guanethidine. The metabolism of guanethidine was much more extensive after oral than after intramuscular adminis-tration suggesting that an appreciable fraction of absorbed drug was metabolised during its first pass through the liver (McMartin et al., 1970). The fraction of guanethidine that was metabolised varies from patient to patient and from day to day (McMartin & Simpson, 1971).

The plasma levels of guanethidine declined rapidly after intra-venous (Rahn, 1971) or intramuscular administration (McMartin et al., 1970). However, the drug was only slowly eliminated from the body due to extensive tissue binding in adrenergic nerve terminals. Guanethidine and its metabolites are almost entirely eliminated from the body by urinary excretion. The renal clear-ance of guanethidine was considerably greater than the glomerular filtration rate indicating that there was active tubular secretion of guanethidine and its metabolites (McMartin et al., 1970). Patients with impaired renal function excreted guanethidine and its metabolites more slowly (Rahn, 1971). After the first 2 to 3 days the amount of guanethidine and metabolites left in the body declined with a half-life of 9-10 days (McMartin et al., 1970).

Bethanidine

The absorption of bethanidine after oral administration appeared
to be quite rapid with peak excretion in the urine after 6 hr
(Shen, Gibaldi, Throne, Bellward, Cunningham, Israili, Dayton &
McNay, 1975).   Bethanidine is excreted unchanged in the urine.
The renal excretion of bethanidine was subject to substantial
fluctuations possibly as a result of changes in renal plasma flow
(Shen *et al.*, 1975).   There was a highly significant correlation
between creatinine clearance and urinary excretion of bethanidine
(Doyle & Morley, 1965).   The time-course of urinary excretion of
bethanidine could be resolved into 3 exponential phases and a 3-
compartment open model has been suggested.   The apparent half-
life of the terminal urinary excretion phase was 7-11 hr and was
reduced by imipramine (Shen *et al.*, 1975).   After an intravenous
dose, the half-life of bethanidine was 2-2.5 hr and was increased
to 8-10 hr in a subject with impaired renal function (Doyle &
Morley, 1965).

Implications

The pharmacokinetics of guanethidine and bethanidine have important implications for therapy.   Guanethidine has a long half-life
and this results in a long duration of action, whereas bethanidine
has a much shorter half-life and a much shorter duration of action.
When therapy with such agents was stopped suddenly, the effects
observed were different (Goldberg, Raftery & Wilkinson, 1977).
In two patients on bethanidine, there was a relatively rapid increase in arterial pressure and episodes of ventricular and supra-
ventricular tachycardia; by contrast, in a patient on guanethidine
there was little change in arterial pressure or in heart rate.
Similarly the addition of the tricyclic antidepressant, desipramine, caused more rapid antagonism of the antihypertensive
action of bethanidine and debrisoquin than of guanethidine
(Mitchell, Cavanaugh, Arias & Oates, 1970).

The long half-life of guanethidine means that if a constant dose
is given each day a steady-state will only be reached after many
days.   In order to avoid this delay, Shand, Nies, McAllister and
Oates (1975) have described a loading scheme for guanethidine to
achieve control of severe hypertension within a few days.   According to this scheme, loading is begun with an initial dose of
80 mg.   Subsequent doses are calculated to increase the body
stores by about 30%, and are given every 6 hr, the night-time dose
being omitted.   The maintenance dose is calculated as one-seventh
of the amount of drug in the body pool since it is estimated that
about one-seventh of the body stores would be lost daily.   No evidence of a sympathomimetic effect was observed with the first dose
(Walter & Nies, 1977).

VI   RELATIONSHIP OF PLASMA CONCENTRATION
TO ADRENERGIC NEURON BLOCKADE

The relationship between the dose of guanethidine and the hypotensive response in patients with hypertension is not predictable.

One possible explanation is that there are individual differences
in the sensitivity of adrenergic nerve terminals to such blockade. To determine whether this is so, Walter, Khandelwal,
Falkner and Nies (1975) examined the relationship of plasma
levels to adrenergic blockade in patients on guanethidine. All
the subjects received diuretics or were maintained in 10 mEq
sodium balance. The degree of adrenergic blockade was measured
by determining the venous reflex response to the Valsalva manoeuvre or to a deep breath. A high degree of adrenergic blockade
(i.e., venous reflex response of 2.5 mm Hg or less) was observed,
in all patients, at plasma levels of 8 ng/ml. Above 17 ng/ml no
patient had any detectable venous response while 5-8 ng/ml represented a border zone. These results show that plasma levels
can be used to predict the degree of adrenergic blockade and also
suggest that there is unlikely to be a great deal of variation in
the sensitivity of adrenergic neurons to blockade by guanethidine.
On the average, a daily maintenance dose of guanethidine of 15 mg
resulted in a plasma level of 5.5 ng/ml, 25 mg resulted in 9.3
ng/ml and 50 mg resulted in 18 ng/ml (Walter *et al.*, 1975). However, there was a 6-fold variation in the individual plasma
levels resulting from a given dose. Walter *et al.* (1975) also
demonstrated that the hypotensive effect of guanethidine depended
not only on the degree of adrenergic blockade produced but apparently also on the plasma volume since in some patients the blood
pressure decreased further with adequate diuresis and restriction
of dietary·sodium.

The plasma concentration of such agents will be misleading in
patients who are also taking drugs such as the tricyclic antidepressants. In such patients adrenergic blockade will not occur
at plasma concentrations that are usually associated with this
effect.

VII RESISTANCE TO TREATMENT WITH
ADRENERGIC NEURON BLOCKING AGENTS

Woosley and Nies (1976) have reviewed the causes of resistance to
therapy with guanethidine. They have pointed out that it is important to determine in such patients whether sympathetic reflexes
are present or not, and have reviewed the methods for assessing
this. The easiest test is to observe the pulse rate when the
patient stands. If the pulse rate increases, it is unlikely that
sympathetic reflexes have been blocked. If sympathetic reflexes
are present, then the drug is not producing its pharmacological
effect. This could result from inadequate dosage, non-compliance
or drug interaction (e.g., from tricyclic antidepressants, sympathomimetics etc.). If sympathetic reflexes are absent, then
the absence of an adequate antihypertensive response probably results from an expanded plasma volume; this can usually be managed
by adequate diuresis.

VIII   CONCLUSIONS

The introduction of the adrenergic neuron blocking agents represented a major advance in the treatment of hypertension, and provided valuable pharmacological aids in the studies of drug action.   The side effects of these agents are generally attributable to the sympathetic blockade they produce and to unopposed
parasympathetic activity.   As indicated previously, a major dis-
advantage is the occurrence of orthostatic hypotension.   Other
side effects are diarrhoea, fluid retention and failure of ejacu-
lation.   Because of this, many would now relegate the use of
adrenergic neuron blocking agents to patients with severe hypertension who have not responded adequately to previous combination
therapy with adequate doses of other agents (see for example
Koch-Weser, 1974).

IX   REFERENCES

Boura, A.L.A., Green, A.F., McCoubrey, A., Laurence, D.R.,
    Moulton, R. & Rosenheim, M.L. (1959). Darenthin: hypertensive
    agent of new type. *Lancet* 2, 17-21.

Doyle, A.E. & Morley, A. (1965).   Studies on the absorption and
    excretion of [^{14}C]-bethanidine in man. *Br. J. Pharmacol.* 24,
    701-704.

Dustan, H.P., Tarazi, R.C. & Bravo, E.L. (1972).   Dependence of
    arterial pressure on intravascular volume in treated hyper-
    tensive patients. *New Eng. J. Med.* 286, 861-866.

Goldberg, A.D. & Raftery, E.B. (1976).   Patterns of blood pres-
    sure during chronic administration of postganglionic sympath-
    etic blocking drugs for hypertension.   2, 1052-1054.

Goldberg, A.D., Raftery, E.B. & Wilkinson, P. (1977). Blood pres-
    sure and heart rate and withdrawal of antihypertensive drugs.
    Br. Med. J. 1, 1243-1246.

Jandhydala, B.S., Clarke, D.E. & Buckley, J.P. (1974).   Effects
    of prolonged administration of certain antihypertensive
    agents. *J. Pharm. Sci.* 63, 1497-1513.

Koch-Weser, J. (1974).   Vasodilator drugs in the treatment of
    hypertension. *Arch. Intern. Med.* 133, 1017-1027.

Koch-Weser, J. (1975).   Drug interactions in cardiovascular
    therapy. *Am. Heart J.* 90, 93-116.

Lukas, G. (1973).   Metabolism and biochemical pharmacology of
    guanethidine and related compounds. *Drug Metabolism Rev.*
    2, 101-116.

McMartin, C., Rondel, R.K., Vinter, J., Allan, B.R., Humberstone, P.M., Leishman, A.W.D., Sandler, G. & Thirkettle, J.L. (1970). The fate of guanethidine in two hypertensive patients. *Clin. Pharmacol. Ther.* 11, 423-431.

McMartin, C. & Simpson, P. (1971). The absorption and metabolism of guanethidine in hypertensive patients requiring different doses of the drug. *Clin. Pharmacol. Ther.* 12, 73-77.

Mitchell, J.R., Cavanaugh, J.H., Arias, L. & Oates, J.A. (1970). Guanethidine and related agents. III. Antagonism by drugs which inhibit the norepinephrine pump in man. *J. Clin. Invest.* 49, 1596-1604.

Rahn, Von K.H. (1971). Plasmaspiegel und renale Ausscheidung von guanethidin bei hypertonikern. *Arzneim-Forsch (Drug Res.)* 21, 1487-1489.

Sannerstedt, R. & Conway, J. (1970). Hemodynamic and vascular responses to antihypertensive treatment with adrenergic blocking agents: A review. *Am. Heart J.* 79, 122-127.

Shand, D.G., Nies, A.S., McAllister, R.G. & Oates, J.A. (1975). A loading-maintenance regimen for more rapid initiation of the effect of guanethidine. *Clin. Pharmacol. Ther.* 18, 139-144.

Shen, D., Gibaldi, M., Throne, M., Bellward, G., Cunningham, R., Israili, Z., Dayton, P. & McNay, J. (1975). Pharmacokinetics of bethanidine in hypertensive patients. *Clin. Pharmacol. Ther.* 17, 363-373.

Smith, A.J. (1965). Fluid retention produced by guanethidine. *Circulation* 31, 490-496.

Stafford, J.R. & Fann, W.E. (1977). Drug interactions with guanidinium antihypertensives. *Drugs* 13, 57-64.

Talbot, S. & Smith, A.J. (1975). Factors predisposing to postural hypotensive symptoms in the treatment of high blood pressure. *Br. Heart J.* 37, 1059-1063.

Walter, I.E., Khandelwal, J., Falkner, F. & Nies, A.S. (1975). The relationship of plasma guanethidine levels to adrenergic blockade. *Clin. Pharmacol. Ther.* 18, 571-580.

Walter, I.E. & Nies, A.S. (1977). Safety of single large oral doses of guanethidine. *Clin. Pharmacol. Ther.* 21, 706-708.

Weil, J.V. & Chidsey, C.A. (1968). Plasma volume expansion resulting from interference with adrenergic function in normal man. *Circulation* 37, 54-61.

Woosley, R.L. & Nies, A.S. (1976). Guanethidine. *New Eng. J. Med.* 295, 1053-1057.

INDEX